Magnetic Resonance Imaging in Movement Disorders

A Guide for Clinicians and Scientists

Magnetic Resonance Imaging in Movement Disorders

A Guide for Clinicians and Scientists

Paul Tuite
Director of Movement Disorders and Associate Professor in the Department of Neurology at the
University of Minnesota, Minneapolis, MN, USA

Alain Dagher
Associate Professor, Montreal Neurological Institute, McGill University, Montreal, QC, Canada

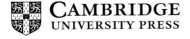

CAMBRIDGE
UNIVERSITY PRESS

University Printing House, Cambridge CB2 8BS, United Kingdom

Published in the United States of America by Cambridge University Press, New York

Cambridge University Press is part of the University of Cambridge.

It furthers the University's mission by disseminating knowledge in the pursuit of education, learning and research at the highest international levels of excellence.

www.cambridge.org
Information on this title: www.cambridge.org/9781107026360

© Cambridge University Press 2013

First published 2013

Printed in Spain by Grafos AS, Arte sobre papel

A catalog record for this publication is available from the British Library

Library of Congress Cataloging in Publication data

Magnetic resonance imaging in movement disorders : a guide for clinicians and scientists / [edited by] Paul Tuite, Alain Dagher.
    p. ; cm.
Includes bibliographical references.
ISBN 978-1-107-02636-0 (Hardback)
I. Tuite, Paul   II. Dagher, Alain.
[DNLM: 1. Movement Disorders.   2. Magnetic Resonance Imaging–methods. WL 390]
RC376.5
616.8'307548–dc23   2013014373
ISBN 978-1-107-02636-0 Hardback

DAMAGED

....

Every effort has been made in preparing this book to provide accurate and up-to-date information which is in accord with accepted standards and practice at the time of publication. Although case histories are drawn from actual cases, every effort has been made to disguise the identities of the individuals involved. Nevertheless, the authors, editors, and publishers can make no warranties that the information contained herein is totally free from error, not least because clinical standards are constantly changing through research and regulation. The authors, editors, and publishers therefore disclaim all liability for direct or consequential damages resulting from the use of material contained in this book. Readers are strongly advised to pay careful attention to information provided by the manufacturer of any drugs or equipment that they plan to use.

Contents

v

Contributors

Aviva Abosch, MD, PhD
Department of Neurosurgery, University
of Minnesota Medical School, Minneapolis,
MN, USA

Nazanin Baradaran, MD
Pacific Parkinson's Research Centre, University of
British Columbia, Vancouver, BC, Canada

Ferdinand Binkofski
Division for Clinical and Cognitive Neuroscience,
Department of Neurology, RWTH Aachen
University, Aachen, Germany

Richard Camicioli, MD
Department of Medicine (Neurology), University of
Alberta, Edmonton, AB, Canada

Alain Dagher, MD
Montreal Neurological Institute, McGill University,
Montreal, QC, Canada

Janet Dubinsky, PhD
Department of Neuroscience, University of
Minnesota, Minneapolis, MN, USA

Uzay E. Emir, PhD
Center for Magnetic Resonance Research (CMRR),
Department of Radiology, Medical School,
University of Minnesota, Minneapolis, MN, USA

Cecile Gallea, PhD
ICM – Institut du Cerveau et de la Moelle épinière,
CENIR – Centre de NeuroImagerie de Recherche,
Groupe Hospitalier Pitie-Salpetriere; Université
Pierre et Marie Curie-Paris 6, Centre de Recherche
de l'Institut du Cerveau et de la Moelle épinière;
Inserm and CNRS, Paris, France

Noam Harel, PhD
Center for Magnetic Resonance Research,
Department of Radiology and Department of

Neurosurgery, University of Minnesota Medical
School, Minneapolis, MN, USA

Andreas Hartmann
Département de Neurologie, Pôle des Maladies du
Système Nerveux, and Centre de Recherche de
l'Institut du Cerveau et de la Moelle épinière,
UPMC/INSERM, Paris, France

Bernhard Haslinger
Neurologische Klinik und Poliklinik, Klinikum rechts
der Isar, Technische Universität München, München,
Germany

Isabelle Iltis, PhD
Center for Magnetic Resonance Research (CMRR),
University of Minnesota, Minneapolis, MN, USA

Jozef Jarosz
Department of Neuroradiology, King's College Hospital,
King's Health Partners, Denmark Hill, London, UK

Keith A. Josephs, MD, MST, MSc
Department of Neurology, Mayo Clinic, Rochester,
MN, USA

Stephane Lehericy, MD, PhD
ICM – Institut du Cerveau et de la Moelle épinière,
CENIR – Centre de NeuroImagerie de Recherche,
Groupe Hospitalier Pitie-Salpetriere;
Université Pierre et Marie Curie-Paris 6,
Centre de Recherche de l'Institut du Cerveau
et de la Moelle épinière; Inserm and CNRS,
Paris, France

Elan D. Louis, MD, MS
Department of Neurology; the Taub Institute for
Research on Alzheimer's Disease and the Aging
Brain; the GH Sergievsky Center, College of
Physicians and Surgeons; and Department of
Epidemiology, Mailman School of Public Health,
Columbia University, New York, NY, USA

Silvia Mangia, PhD
Center for Magnetic Resonance Research (CMRR),
Department of Radiology, University of Minnesota,
Minneapolis, MN, USA

W. R. Wayne Martin, MD, FRCPC
Department of Medicine (Neurology), University of
Alberta, Edmonton, AB, Canada

Martin J. McKeown, BEng, MD, FRCP(C)
Pacific Parkinson's Research Centre; Departments of
Neuroscience, Electrical and Computer Engineering,
and Medicine (Neurology), University of British
Columbia, Vancouver, BC, Canada

Shalom Michaeli, PhD
Center for Magnetic Resonance Research (CMRR),
Department of Radiology, University of Minnesota,
Minneapolis, MN, USA

Christoph Mueller, MD
Department of Neurology, Innsbruck Medical
University, Innsbruck, Austria

Gülin Öz, PhD
Center for Magnetic Resonance Research (CMRR),
Department of Radiology, Medical School, University
of Minnesota, Minneapolis, MN, USA

Cyril Poupon, PhD
CEA, NeuroSpin, Gif-Sur-Yvette, France

Kathrin Reetz
JARA – Translational Brain Medicine, Department
of Neurology, RWTH Aachen University, Aachen,
Germany

Michael Samuel
Department of Neurology, King's College Hospital,
King's Health Partners, Denmark Hill, London, UK

Michael Schocke, MD
Department of Radiology, Innsbruck Medical
University, Innsbruck, Austria

Norbert Schuff, PhD
Center for Imaging of Neurodegenerative Diseases,
Veterans Affairs Medical Center, and
Department of Radiology and Biomedical Imaging,
University of California at San Francisco,
San Francisco, CA, USA

Klaus Seppi, MD
Department of Neurology, Innsbruck Medical
University, Innsbruck, Austria

Hiral Shah, MD
Department of Neurology, College of Physicians
and Surgeons, Columbia University,
New York, NY, USA

Alison Simioni
Montreal Neurological Institute, McGill University,
Montreal, QC, Canada

Paul Tuite, MD
Department of Neurology,
University of Minnesota, Minneapolis, MN, USA

Tobias Wächter, MD
German Centre of Neurodegenerative
Diseases (DZNE), and Department of
Neurodegenerative Diseases at the Centre of
Neurology and Hertie Institute for Clinical
Brain Research, University of Tübingen,
Tübingen, Germany

Gregor K. Wenning, MD, PhD, MSc
Department of Neurology, Innsbruck Medical
University, Innsbruck, Austria

Jennifer L. Whitwell, PhD
Department of Radiology, Mayo Clinic, Rochester,
MN, USA

Yulia Worbe, PhD
Behavioural and Clinical Neuroscience Institute,
Cambridge University, Cambridge, UK

Preface

The field of magnetic resonance imaging (MRI) has recently undergone dramatic changes with a proliferation of methodologies. These techniques have been applied to Parkinson's disease and other movement disorders and provide insights not previously foreseen with MRI. This book represents the first comprehensive published collections of clinical and research MRI findings related to movement disorders. The chapters of this book focus on Parkinson's disease, progressive supranuclear palsy, corticobasal degeneration/syndrome, multiple system atrophy, Huntington's disease, essential tremor, dystonia, and others and provides a focus on imaging methods and their clinical applications. Most of the space is devoted to Parkinson's disease, the most common degenerative movement disorder. Chapters focus on the motor versus cognitive aspects of the disease and on the application of different imaging methods to Parkinson's disease, notably functional MRI, which is poised to take on a clinical role in movement disorders. Another section covers imaging for deep brain stimulation (DBS) surgery and there is a chapter on MRI as a potential clinical outcome measure in clinical trials. As we expect the field to continue to grow, this book represents a starting point to future brain mapping of movement disorders. Hopefully, this provides a background on imaging methods and their research and clinical applications. This handbook should be of interest to MRI physicists, research scientists, physicians (neurologists, neurosurgeons, and radiologists), neuropsychologists, and other individuals in the field. We have attempted to cover all the current fundamental aspects of movement disorders' imaging and show where the field is heading.

Presently there is no single atlas of brain imaging for movement disorders; thus we have provided a chapter (17) with numerous examples of MRI findings in different movement disorders. Another goal is to enhance awareness of novel imaging methods for movement disorders neurologists and radiologists as many have had little training or exposure to this field.

In some sense movement disorders has lagged behind other neurological specialties such as multiple sclerosis or vascular disease, in which MRI is a crucial diagnostic tool. We also foresee MRI methods as having a useful role in monitoring disease progression and the effect of therapy.

While positron emission tomography (PET) and single-photon emission computed tomography (SPECT) scanning provide a measure of dopamine signaling in the nigrostriatal pathway, there are still limitations to nuclear imaging and its promise is unfulfilled to a degree. MRI provides information that is unavailable with nuclear imaging. MRI as a research tool may improve understanding of disease mechanisms as well as uncovering endophenotypes for genetic studies (or other at-risk populations, for example idiopathic rapid eye movement (REM) behavior disorder). Ultimately it is hoped that MRI may prove useful as a diagnostic tool and a potential means for monitoring disease progression and response to symptomatic and disease-modifying therapies.

We would like to acknowledge funding from the Minnesota Medical Foundation which helped make this project a reality as well as the support from Cambridge University Press who had faith in the importance of this project. We would also like to thank the numerous authors who provided their time to craft chapters with little reward for their efforts. PT would like to thank physicians who have helped him along the way with training and collaborations: John Stewart, Tony Lang, Alain Dagher, Ted Fon, Liam Durcan, Vera Brill, Joe Bruni, Edward Neuwelt, James Ashe, Nestor Galvez-Jimenez, Antonio Strafella, Bob and Karen Pascuzzi, David Anderson, David Knopman, Gareth Parry, Brent Clark, and Jerry Vitek. Additionally he acknowledges his family John and Camille Tuite and siblings Kathy, Frances, Brian, Ann, and Clare, wife Marilee, and children John and Audrey who have kept him grounded. AD thanks his parents and his wife Celesti for their immense support.

Abbreviations

AC	anterior commissure		ED	embouchure dystonia
ACC	anterior cingulate cortex		EEG	electroencephalogram
AD	Alzheimer's disease		EPI	echo-planar imaging
ADC	apparent diffusion coefficient		ET	essential tremor
ADHD	attention-deficit hyperactivity disorder		FA	fractional anisotropy
ADNI	Alzheimer's Disease Neuroimaging Initiative		FAHN	fatty acid hydroxylase-associated neurodegeneration
AFP	α-fetoprotein		FC	functional connectivity
AFP	adiabatic full passage		fcMAP	functional connectivity map
ALFF	amplitude of low frequency fluctuations		FDG-PET	^{18}F-fluorodeoxyglucose positron emission tomography
AM	amplitude modulation			
AOA1/2	autosomal recessive ataxia with oculomotor apraxia type 1 and 2		FDR	false discovery rate
			FLAIR	fluid-attenuated inversion recovery
APD	atypical parkinsonian disorder		FM	frequency modulation
ASL	arterial spin labeling		fMRI	functional magnetic resonance imaging
A-T	ataxia telangiectasia		FOV	field of view
AUC	area under the curve		FPN	frontoparietal network
AUN	auditory network		FRDA	Friedreich's ataxia
AVED	ataxia with isolated vitamin E deficit		FSE	fast spin echo
BOLD	blood oxygen level-dependent		FTD	frontotemporal dementia
BTX	botulinum toxin		FTLD	frontotemporal lobar degeneration
bvFTD	behavioral variant of FTD		GABA	γ-aminobutyric acid
CBD	corticobasal degeneration		GCI	glial cytoplasmic inclusion
CBF	cerebral blood flow		GDNF	glial cell-derived neurotrophic factors
CBS	corticobasal syndrome		Gln	glutamine
CD	cervical dystonia		Glu	glutamate
CDR	Clinical Dementia Rating		GM	gray matter
Cho	choline		GPe	globus pallidus externa
CMR$_{ATP}$	cerebral metabolic rate of ATP		GPi	globus pallidus internus
cMRI	conventional magnetic resonance imaging		GRE	gradient echo
CMRO$_2$	cerebral metabolic rate of oxygen		GTS	Gilles de la Tourette syndrome
CNS	central nervous system		H & Y	Hoehn and Yahr Scale
Cr	creatine		^{1}H MRS	proton magnetic resonance spectroscopy
CRW	Cosman–Roberts–Wells		HC	healthy controls
CSF	cerebrospinal fluid		HD	Huntington's disease
CT	computed tomography		HS	hyperbolic secant
CW	continuous wave		IBZM-	$[^{123}$I]-iodobenzamide single-photon emission
DA	dopamine		SPECT	computed tomography
DAT	dementia of Alzheimer's type		ICA	independent component analysis
DAT	dopamine transporter		ICD	impulse control disorder
DBM	deformation-based morphometry		ICP	inferior cerebellar peduncle
DBN	dynamic Bayesian network		IDCA-P	idiopathic cerebellar ataxia and parkinsonism
DBS	deep brain stimulation		IGF-1	insulin growth factor 1
DLB	dementia with Lewy bodies		iRBD	idiopathic rapid eye movement sleep behavior disorder
DLPFC	dorsolateral prefrontal cortex			
DMN	default mode network		LC	locus coeruleus
DTI	diffusion tensor imaging		LD	laryngeal dystonia
DWI	diffusion-weighted imaging		MAOA	monoamine oxidase subtype A
ECN	executive control network			

MAPT	microtubule-associated protein tau	PPAOS	primary progressive apraxia of speech
MCI	mild cognitive impairment	PPMI	Parkinson's Disease Progression Marker Initiative
MCP	middle cerebellar peduncle		
MD	mean diffusivity	PPN	pedunculopontine nucleus
MIBG	[^{123}I]-meta-iodobenzylguanidine	PRESTO	principles of echo shifting with a train of observations
MMSE	Mini-Mental State Examination		
MPAN	mitochondrial protein-associated neurodegeneration	PRIME	partially refocused interleaved multiple-echo
		PSP	progressive supranuclear palsy
m/p-ratio	midbrain-to-pontine ratio	QSM	quantitative susceptibility mapping
MRI	magnetic resonance imaging	R_1	T_1 relaxation rate
MRPI	magnetic resonance parkinsonism index	R_2	T_2 relaxation rate
MRS	magnetic resonance spectroscopy	RAFF	relaxations along a fictitious field
MRSI	magnetic resonance spectroscopic imaging	RBD	rapid eye movement sleep behavior disorder
MRV	magnetic resonance volumetry	REM	rapid eye movement
MSA	multiple system atrophy	RF	radiofrequency
MSA-C	cerebellar variant of multiple system atrophy	RM	Riechert–Mundinger
MSA-P	parkinsonian variant of multiple system atrophy	ROC	receiver operating characteristic
		ROI	region of interest
MSC	mesenchymal stem cell	RPE	reward prediction error
M_{ss}	steady-state magnetization	rs-fMRI	resting-state functional MRI
MT	magnetization transfer	RSN	resting-state network
MTI	magnetization transfer imaging	SAR	specific absorption rate
MTR	magnetization transfer ratio	SARA	Scale for the Assessment and Rating of Ataxia
myo-Ins	myo-inositol		
n	number	SCA	spinocerebellar ataxia
NAA	N-acetylaspartate	SCP	superior cerebellar peduncle
NAA/Cho	N-acetylaspartate to choline ratio	SMA	supplementary motor area
NAA/Cr	N-acetylaspartate to creatine ratio	SMN	sensorimotor network
NAAG	N-acetylaspartyl glutamate	SN	substantia nigra
NBIA	neuronal brain iron accumulation	SNc	substantia nigra pars compacta
OCD	obsessive–compulsive disorder	SND	striatonigral degeneration
OPCA	olivopontocerebellar atrophy	SNR	signal-to-noise ratio
PAPT	progressive ataxia with palatal tremor	SNr	substantia nigra pars reticulata
PC	posterior commissure	SPECT	single-photon emission tomography
PCA	posterior cortical atrophy	SS	steady state
PCC	posterior cingulate cortex	SSPE	subacute sclerosing panencephalitis
PCr	phosphocreatine	STEAM	stimulated echo acquisition mode
PD	Parkinson's disease	STN	subthalamic nucleus
PD-CN	Parkinson's disease cognitively normal	SWI	susceptibility-weighted imaging
PDD	Parkinson's disease with dementia	T	Tesla
PD-MCI	Parkinson's disease with mild cognitive impairment	TE	echo time
		UHDRS	Unified Huntington Disease Rating Scale
PEP	postencephalitic parkinsonism	UMSARS	Unified Multiple System Atrophy Rating Scale
PET	positron emission tomography		
PFC	prefrontal cortex	UPDRS	Unified Parkinson's Disease Rating Scale
P_i	inorganic phosphate	VBM	voxel-based morphometry
PiD	Pick's disease	VBR	voxel-based relaxometry
PKAN	pantothenate kinase-associated neurodegeneration	Vc	ventral caudalis
		VIM	ventral intermediate nucleus
PLAN	phospholipase A2-associated neurodegeneration	VIN	visual network
		Vop	ventro-oralis posterior
PLS	primary lateral sclerosis	WC	writer's cramp
PMC	primary motor cortex	WM	white matter

Key words

Brain
Cerebellum
Default mode network
Diffusion imaging
Essential tremor
Magnetic resonance imaging (MRI)
Magnetization transfer
Neurodegeneration

Neuroimaging
Parkinson's disease
Positron emission tomography
Relaxometry
Resting-state functional magnetic resonance imaging (fMRI)
Substantia nigra

Chapter 1

Magnetic resonance imaging (MRI) methods in Parkinson's disease

Silvia Mangia, Shalom Michaeli, and Paul Tuite

Introduction

The revolution created by magnetic resonance imaging (MRI) is a result of its ability to utilize the intrinsic differences in the magnetic properties of tissues to provide information about function, structure, and chemistry. This book provides background on a variety of MRI methods and focuses on their application to neurological conditions that manifest with movement disorders. These disorders include neurodegenerative conditions such as Parkinson's disease (PD), Huntington's disease, and ataxia which are characterized by progressive neuronal loss with accompanying neuropathological changes. Meanwhile other movement disorders are not clearly degenerative and tend to have more subtle structural, functional, and neurochemical changes.

The focus of many chapters herein will be on PD, which constitutes the second most common neurodegenerative disease after Alzheimer's disease (AD), and is the principle focus of many clinicians and researchers in the movement disorders field. It is stated that approximately 1% of those over 65 years of age have PD [1]. As a result there is substantial focus on PD research, and the discoveries made in basic neuroscience that relate to pathogenic mechanisms of PD (or AD for that matter) are often relevant for lesser known neurodegenerative parkinsonian conditions such as multiple system atrophy (MSA) or progressive supranuclear palsy (PSP). Along with the progress made in basic science research, MRI developments have been applied to PD and have begun to show promise as a surrogate biomarker in research studies. As well these techniques may be more useful clinically in looking at other parkinsonian conditions such as MSA and PSP. While MRI is presently not able directly to image dopaminergic neuronal loss that underlies degenenerative parkinsonian conditions, it can provide complementary data to those obtained with nuclear tracer imaging. First, this chapter will provide an overview of MRI methods which will be discussed in much greater depth in subsequent chapters, and we will cover nascent techniques that we are employing at the University of Minnesota that may ultimately help provide an imaging biomarker of disease.

Iron imaging in PD

Initial MRI work in PD began in the mid 1980s as several groups focused on the paramagnetic effects of iron, which is present in increasing quantities in the basal ganglia in PD [2]. This was followed by the frequently referenced work by Gorell *et al.* in 1995 who utilized T_2 and T_2^* imaging of the substantia nigra (SN) and showed a separation between those with PD and control participants; the change in relaxation time constants was attributed to increased iron in patients with PD [3]. T_2^* imaging is especially sensitive to local magnetic field inhomogeneities induced for example by iron. The focus on iron in PD imaging has remained an important topic and researchers have often utilized T_2^*, or its reciprocal R_2^*, in nigral imaging protocols. Visually obvious changes have been observed at 7 tesla (T) in patients with PD as compared to controls (Figure 1.1) [4]. When the term "iron" is employed in PD imaging manuscripts, this typically refers to non-heme iron as opposed to heme iron, and also relates to bound iron that may be present in ferritin or neuromelanin [5]. However, a small pool of free labile iron may actually be a pathogenic culprit as opposed to iron that is safely bound and tucked away. Nonetheless the overall increase in bound iron seen in PD – which is more

Magnetic Resonance Imaging in Movement Disorders, ed. Paul Tuite and Alain Dagher. Published by Cambridge University Press. © Cambridge University Press 2013.

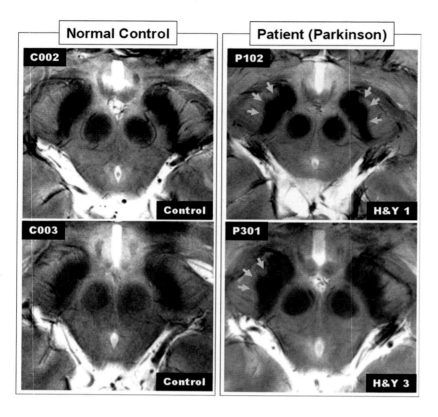

Normal Control | **Patient (Parkinson)**

C002 — Control | P102 — H&Y 1
C003 — Control | P301 — H&Y 3

Figure 1.1 Three-dimensional T_2^*-weighted gradient echo MRI at 7T of the midbrain. These two PD cases (H&Y 1 and 3 = Hoehn & Yahr stage 1 and 3, respectively) show substantially serrated substantia nigra (SN) in their lateral boundaries compared with normal controls that may represent increased iron accumulation. (Cho *et al.*, 2011 [4].)

than occurs with "normal aging" – may represent a marker of disease and possibly a source for increased free and presumably pathogenic iron [5]. Other important issues to consider about brain iron are the higher concentrations seen in men, as well as the potential for effects from dietary and environmental toxins. Serum ceruloplasmin levels may help address potential confounds in imaging studies [6]. Another factor is the location of iron; whether it is present in neurons or glia such as astrocytes or oligodendrocytes [7]. It is currently not possible to determine whether the imaging abnormalities in PD reflect changes in neuromelanin in dopaminergic neurons or ferritin in glia or neurons. Additionally, while iron changes have been noted in PD, it remains to be determined if iron-sensitive MRI methods will serve as a surrogate of disease – to monitor progression or characterize the severity of disease. This topic will be covered more completely in Chapter 2 by Wayne Martin.

Meanwhile other iron-sensitive methods have been recently developed. These include adiabatic $T_{2\rho}$ [8, 9], magnetization transfer (MT) imaging [10–15], and susceptibility-weighted imaging (SWI) [16–20].

Susceptibility-weighted imaging (SWI)

SWI is a technique that is available on clinical MRI platforms which exploits the differences in magnetic susceptibility between tissues. SWI is based on gradient echo (GRE) pulse sequences with long echo time (TE), and it achieves enhanced image contrast for detecting susceptibility variations from combining magnitude and phase data of the GRE acquisitions. Since iron induces magnetic susceptibility differences, SWI is inherently sensitive to the presence of iron, and is able to demonstrate anatomical structure as well as potentially providing measures of iron content [21]. Much of the recent excitement in movement disorders has arisen from studies conducted at 7T – including work in enhanced visualization of brain surgical targets [16–20], as discussed in Chapter 8.

Magnetization transfer imaging (MTI)

MTI utilizes the transfer of magnetization between bulk (free) water protons and protons associated with macromolecules [22] and is generally accepted as a correlate of tissue integrity. The detection of the magnetization transfer (MT) effect in clinical practice is usually limited to the measurement of MT ratios (MTRs), that is, ratios of signal intensity measured with and without the saturation pulse [22]. However, MTRs have appeared to be more useful in atypical parkinsonian conditions than in PD except for one group which showed the potential utility of MTR in PD [10, 12–15]. In contrast to MTR, we have developed an easy-to-implement *quantitative* MT method to estimate MT parameters, which relies on an inversion-prepared MT protocol [11]. By progressively incrementing the duration of the off-resonance continuous wave (CW) pulse, the T_1 of water in the presence of saturation (T_{1sat}) and the steady-state (SS) magnetization (M_{ss}) can be estimated. In addition, the forward exchange rate from the solid to the free pool, k_f, can be calculated as $(1 - M_{ss}/M_0)/T_{1sat}$. The basic source of instability in the fitting procedure of T_{1sat} and M_{ss} originates from the impossibility of using MT pulses that are long enough to achieve the steady state, due to safety limitations imposed by the specific absorption rate (SAR) of radiofrequency (RF) power deposition. To circumvent this limitation, we developed a protocol where two consecutive sets of measurements are acquired with the magnetization initially along the −z or +z-axis, that is with or without an on-resonance inversion prior to the off-resonance irradiation. Whereas the usage of inversion recovery approaches has been suggested to measure MT effects [23, 24], the implementation of an on-resonance inversion pulse prior to the off-resonance irradiation has not been exploited so far. We have used the inversion-prepared MT protocol together with adiabatic $T_{1\rho}$ in a study which aimed at assessing the integrity of the brainstem structures of PD [25]. Results from this study will be discussed in the next section.

Adiabatic rotating frame relaxation methods

Conventionally, MRI contrast is generated by the tissue variation of free-precession longitudinal (time constant, T_1) and/or transverse (time constant, T_2) relaxation of the ^1H_2O MR signal. These time constants are measured in the laboratory frame, in which the direction of the main magnetic field defines the longitudinal or z-axis. The free precession relaxation rate constant (R_1) is particularly sensitive to magnetic fluctuations that occur as a result of molecular motion at frequencies near the Larmor precession frequency (ω_0), which falls in the MHz range. However, there is reason also to probe lower frequencies in tissue (i.e., in the kHz range) in order to evaluate for pathology. Rotating frame relaxation rate constants, $R_{1\rho}$ and $R_{2\rho}$, characterize relaxation during radiofrequency (RF) irradiation when the magnetization vector is aligned along or perpendicular to the direction of the effective magnetic field (ω_{eff}), respectively, where the effective magnetic field depends on the applied RF (ω_1) and the frequency offset ($\Delta\omega$). $R_{1\rho}$ and $R_{2\rho}$ reflect the features of the spin dynamic processes and depend on the properties of the RF irradiation [26, 27]. Importantly, $R_{1\rho}$ and $R_{2\rho}$ are driven principally by dipolar fluctuations at frequencies near the effective precession frequency. Since ω_{eff} can be "tuned" by adjustment of the RF amplitude and the frequency offset, $R_{1\rho}$ and $R_{2\rho}$ can provide experimental access to the relevant lower frequencies in the range of kHz.

Rotating frame relaxation constants can be measured during the application of adiabatic pulses [28]. In this case, the adiabatic $R_{1\rho}(t)$ and $R_{2\rho}(t)$ are time-dependent longitudinal and transverse relaxation rate constants, which characterize decay of magnetization during application of RF pulses operating in the adiabatic regime, that is, when the adiabatic condition (i.e., $|\gamma^{-1}d\alpha/dt| << B_{eff}$), is well satisfied. Here α is the angle between B_{eff} and the first rotating frame z'-axis. The pulses used for the measurements are adiabatic full passage (AFP) of the hyperbolic secant family (HSn) (where n = 1, 2, 4, 8,...). Detailed descriptions of HSn adiabatic pulse modulation functions are given in Michaeli *et al.* [26, 27]. Briefly, HSn pulses are stretched versions of the hyperbolic secant (HS) pulse [29] and n denotes the stretching factor. According to this description, the original hyperbolic secant pulse is referred to as the HS1 pulse. As n becomes larger, the HSn pulse amplitude modulation (AM) function becomes flatter. Thus, the time evolution of magnetization during an HSn pulse can change significantly with a change of n. During adiabatic pulses the $R_{1\rho}(t)$ is time dependent as a result of modulating the pulse functions, $\omega_1(t)$ and $\omega_{RF}(t)$. Here, $\omega_1(t)$ and $\omega_{RF}(t)$ each have units of radian/s. We have shown that the instantaneous relaxation rate constants during AFP pulse resemble pulse modulation functions and their magnitude depends on the effective frequency $\omega_{eff}(t)$. If the magnetization M is initially not perturbed and the train of the AFP pulses

3

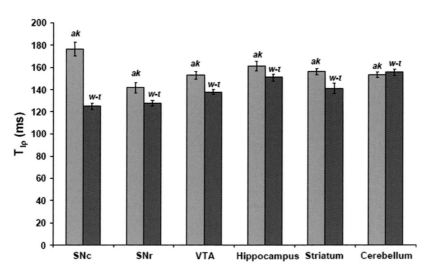

Figure 1.2 $T_{1\rho}$ time constants measured in different areas of *aphakia* (**ak**) and wild-type (**w-t**) mice using HS1 AFP pulses. SNc = substantia nigra pars compacta; SNr = substantia nigra reticulate; VTA = ventral tegmental area. (Michaeli *et al.*, 2009 [31].) These findings show that in **ak** mice with absence of SNc neurons there is an increase in $T_{1\rho}$ as compared to the **w-t** mice in this region.

is applied, the relaxation is governed solely by $R_{1\rho}$ mechanisms. If magnetization M is initially excited to 90° and is located in the *xy* plane of the laboratory frame and the train of AFP pulses is applied, relaxation is solely $R_{2\rho}$. Overall, adiabatic $R_{1\rho}$ ($= 1/T_{1\rho}$) and $R_{2\rho}$ ($= 1/T_{2\rho}$) provide novel tissue MRI contrast [26, 27, 30], and allow for determination of fundamental MR parameters, which are rotational correlation times at specific sites, τ_c, apparent populations, and exchange relaxation rate constants [31]. The $R_{1\rho}$ and $R_{2\rho}$ measured during adiabatic pulses were demonstrated to be sensitive to neural integrity and iron accumulation, respectively [8, 9, 31, 32]. In a validation study of an *aphakia* mouse model, $T_{1\rho}$ was indeed able to separate *aphakia* versus wild-type mice in the substantia nigra pars compacta (SNc), where there is a congenital absence of dopaminergic neurons (Figure 1.2) [31]. In human studies of PD patients and healthy controls, we have shown the ability of adiabatic methods to detect midbrain changes in PD (Figure 1.3) [8, 9]. Table 1.1 shows the separation of group data using these techniques [8]. Additional recent work has shown that adiabatic methods were able to demonstrate midbrain and medullary changes in PD as compared to controls, as demonstrated in Figure 1.4 [25]. In this figure, the representative $R_{1\rho}$ and R_{1sat} maps from control (top) and PD (bottom) subjects are shown. All PD patients were Hoehn and Yahr stage 2, average motor Unified Parkinson Disease Rating Scale (part III) scores were 33.8 (off medication), and average disease duration

was 6 years. Analyses were performed with ten age-matched control subjects. The regions of interest (ROIs) are indicated on the T_2-weighted images. The differences between the $R_{1\rho}$ values measured from a rostral region used as internal control per subject (here identified by ROI-1) minus the $R_{1\rho}$ values measured from medullary nuclei (i.e., ROI-5 and ROI-1 versus ROI-6) were altered in patients relative to control subjects (p = 0.004 and p = 0.033, respectively). Differences in $R_{1\rho}$ values were six and eight times larger in patients than in controls when comparing ROI-1 versus ROI-5 and ROI-1 versus ROI-6, respectively. Since $R_{1\rho}$ values in ROI-1 were not different between patients and controls (p = 0.25), these findings represent a change in imaging parameters from areas that contain medullary nuclei that are known to be affected in PD. Interestingly, no statistical differences were observed between patients and controls when considering R_{1sat}. This could be attributed to differential sensitivity to the exchange regime between $T_{1\rho}$ and T_{1sat} [11]. Together, the findings of this study might indicate functional changes that occur prior to neuronal death within the medullary nuclei.

Relaxations along a fictitious field (RAFF)

A potential limitation to the widespread exploitation of rotating frame relaxation in PD is the required RF power delivered to the sample (i.e., specific absorption rate – SAR), which can result in tissue heating. However, RF power can sometimes be reduced by using off-resonance irradiation to create the locking field, B_{eff} [33, 34]. Recently we have developed a novel rotating frame relaxation

Table 1.1. Averaged calculated $T_{2\rho}$, $T_{1\rho}$, and T_2 time constants in PD patients and controls

Time constants (ms)	$T_{2\rho}$ [a]	T_2 [b]	$T_{1\rho}$ [c]
Controls	72.3 ± 3.4	59.4 ± 4.3	156 ± 6.7
PD	64.6 ± 3.4	57.1 ± 4.2	178 ± 11.6

[a] Significant difference between PD and controls ($p < 0.01$, two-tailed).
[b] No difference between PD and controls ($p = 0.32$, two-tailed).
[c] Significant difference between PD and controls ($p = 0.036$, two-tailed).

experiment called Relaxation Along a Fictitious Field (RAFF). RAFF does not require an initial rotation of the magnetization to a specific locking angle. As compared to CW $T_{1\rho}$ and adiabatic $T_{1\rho}$ and $T_{2\rho}$ methods, RAFF experiments can be performed with reduced RF power because the spin-locking field (i.e., the so-called fictitious field **E**) is produced by taking advantage of both amplitude and frequency modulation functions (AM *sine* and FM *cosine*, respectively) operating in a sub-adiabatic condition [34]. RAFF comprises $T_{1\rho}$ and $T_{2\rho}$ mechanisms by exploiting relaxation in a second rotating frame. RAFF was able to provide a greater contrast in tissues of the SN as compared to $T_{1\rho}$ and $T_{2\rho}$, and specifically it was better than all other methods in separating the SN into its various subregions, that is, the pars compacta from pars reticulata [35]. Additional studies are warranted to sort out its utility.

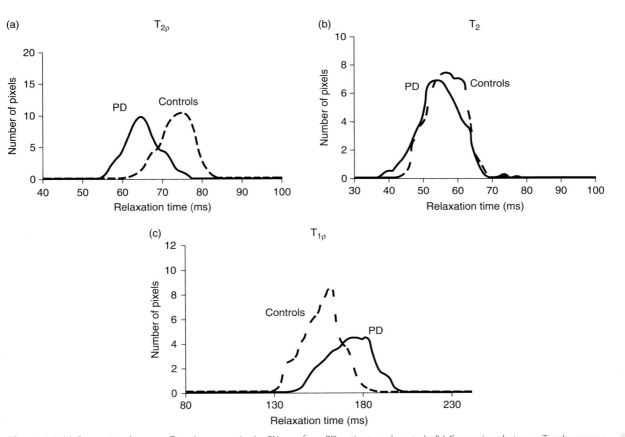

Figure 1.3 (a) Comparison between $T_{2\rho}$ relaxograms in the SN area from PD patients and controls. (b) Comparison between T_2 relaxograms in the SN area from PD patients and controls. (c) Comparison between $T_{1\rho}$ relaxograms in the SN between PD patients and controls. ROI obtained from 8 healthy controls and 8 patients with PD. (Michaeli *et al.*, 2007 [8].) ROI, region of interest.

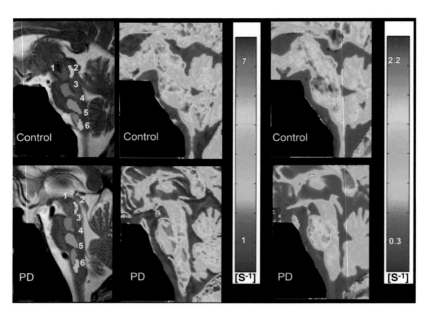

Figure 1.4 Rotating frame $R_{1\rho}$ maps (middle column), MT rate maps (R_{1sat}) (right column), with relative T_2-weighted (T_2w) images (left column) from representative control subject (top row) and PD patient (bottom row). Regions of interest (ROIs) – as depicted on T_2w images – were obtained in maps from six areas: (1) medial raphe nucleus; (2) dorsal raphe nucleus; (3) nucleus raphe pontis; (4) nucleus raphe magnus; (5) nucleus raphe pallidus; (6) nucleus raphe obscuris. (Tuite et al., 2012 [25].) See text for details.

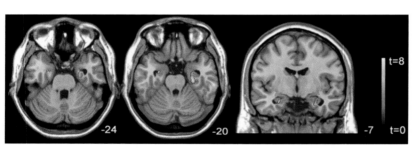

Figure 1.5 Statistical parametric mapping (t-statistic) axial intensity projection maps rendered onto a stereotactically normalized magnetic resonance imaging (MRI) scan, showing areas of significant increases (colour code, yellow to orange) of gray matter density values in a cohort of patients with idiopathic rapid eye movement sleep behaviour disorder versus healthy control subjects. The number at the bottom right corner of each MRI scan corresponds to the z coordinate in Talairach space. (Scherfler et al., 2011 [39].)

Volumetric measurements and diffusion tensor imaging (DTI)

Meanwhile researchers have pursued other imaging methods to confirm the known loss of neurons and shrinkage of the SN in PD, with measurements of area or volumes beginning in the early 1990s [36]. These attempts utilized a preselected ROI and subsequently compared affected to unaffected individuals. However, there has been greater refinement with the utilization of methods that do not employ a-priori ROIs. One such method is voxel-based morphometry (VBM), in which there is standardization of data and then voxel-by-voxel comparison between group data to determine if there are differences in signal intensity. VBM discussions will be covered in an assortment of chapters as they relate

to different movement disorders. These methods utilize 1.5 or 3T T_1 anatomical data, which may not be sufficiently sensitive to detect structural changes in PD until there is substantial disease progression and the presence of accompanying dementia [37, 38]. Conditions such as Huntington's disease, MSA, PSP, along with AD and atypical dementias may lend themselves to greater utilization of these methods because atrophy is more prominent and therefore detected earlier. One example of the potential utility of VBM is from a rapid eye movement sleep behavior disorder (RBD) study that showed changes in a population of individuals with RBD as opposed to controls – RBD may represent a precursor to PD in some situations (Figure 1.5) [39]. Meanwhile, researchers are utilizing higher field strengths along with potentially

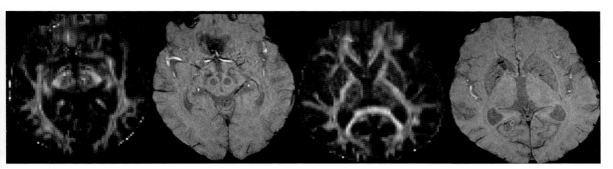

Figure 1.6 Representative fractional anisotropy (FA) maps from different slices with the corresponding susceptibility weighted imaging (SWI) images in a PD subject demonstrating feasibility of methods on clinical 3T platforms. (Images provided courtesy of P Tuite, K. Lim, and B. Mueller, University of Minnesota, unpublished data.)

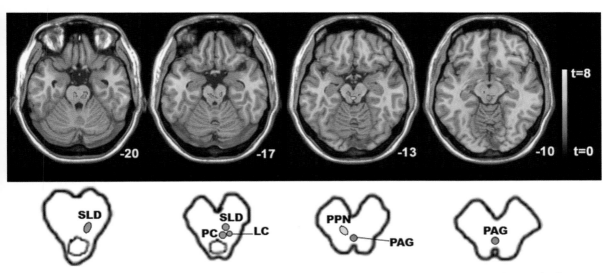

Figure 1.7 Statistical parametric mapping (t-statistic) axial intensity projection maps rendered onto a stereotactically normalized magnetic resonance imaging (MRI) scan, showing areas of significant increases of mean diffusivity values (colour code, yellow to orange) in a cohort of patients with idiopathic rapid eye movement (REM) sleep behaviour disorder versus healthy control subjects. The number at the bottom right corner of each MRI scan corresponds to the z coordinate in Talairach space. Schematic drawings below correspond to the MRI and visualize proposed nuclei involved in REM sleep control. The REM-off region is represented by the periaqueductal gray matter (PAG) in red, and the REM-on region is represented by the precoeruleus (PC) and sublaterodorsal nucleus (SLD) in green. Nuclei in yellow and blue are known to influence REM and non-REM sleep circuits. LC = locus coeruleus; PPN = pedunculopontine nucleus. (Scherfler *et al.*, 2011 [39].)

more sensitive methods such as $T_{1\rho}$ or others to generate raw structural data that may provide renewed interest in VBM for PD.

Diffusion tensor imaging (DTI)

DTI provides structural data based on the directionally restrained diffusion of water within fiber tracts. The movement of water, and hence protons, in white matter tends to be constrained to the long axis of fiber tracts, leading to anisotropy, that is, greater random motion in certain directions. Pathological processes disturb this natural state of anisotropy and this can be exploited with imaging. Specifically, the loss of restriction of water movement within damaged fiber bundles results in reduced anisotropy, which can be characterized as a reduction in fractional anisotropy or FA. Figure 1.6 (P. Tuite, K. Lim, and B. Mueller, unpublished data) demonstrates FA and SWI imaging of the SN and striatum in PD. Figure 1.7 shows changes in mean diffusivity in a cohort of individuals with RBD, a possible precursor to PD [39]. DTI has its limitations in determining directional and spatial anisotropy; hence some individuals have resorted to methods such as tractography, which include probabilistic and streamline tractography. Several groups have funded but unpublished studies that are evaluating these methods as a means for tracking disease and differentiating parkinsonian conditions from one another as well as appreciating the structural substrates that underlie clinical features. A large-scale effort called the human connectome project (www.humanconnectomeproject.org) is under way to advance DTI methods by generating normative imaging along with neurobehavioral and genomic data. This project applies established and novel methods to evaluate structure and function in the brain. The hope is that these data will allow a reference for disease states such as movement disorders.

Resting-state MRI

The focus of resting-state MRI is on brain activity that occurs in the absence of externally triggered activity. Even in a "resting state" there are physiological variations in brain activity and accompanying blood flow alterations that manifest as fluctuations in the MRI blood oxygen level-dependent (BOLD) signal. Spontaneous correlations in BOLD signal can be utilized to determine the "functional connectivity" between different regions. There have been a fair number of studies in PD [40–45]. Measurement of this fluctuation can be done using a variety of methods, including the amplitude of low frequency fluctuations or ALFF to assess for an index of resting-state brain activity based on the blood flow variability [44]. Resting-state methods allow the determination of spontaneously occurring brain networks, which may distinguish PD from controls; however, in one study 1/3 of those with PD and 1/5 of controls had unusable data due to motion artifact, which may be partially due to the need to assess subjects when they had been off medications for at least 12 hours [44]. Hence while resting-state functional MRI (fMRI) methods are able to provide a rapid and whole brain view of PD their practicality remains to be determined due to possible need for medication withdrawal for imaging.

In vivo magnetic resonance spectroscopy (MRS)

MRS has failed to demonstrate great utility in movement disorders until recently. This has been due to the low sensitivity of methods and the low concentrations of metabolites of interest. High-field MRS with its greater sensitivity has overcome some limitations and will be discussed in several chapters, including one by Emir and Öz (Chapter 15) who have demonstrated the ability to measure absolute concentrations of various neurochemicals within the SN and other brainstem regions.

Meanwhile, MRS imaging (MRSI) has begun to measure cerebral metabolic rates of oxygen ($CMRO_2$) and ATP (CMR_{ATP}) and to correlate neuroenergetics with specific brain functions. $CMRO_2$ measurements are achieved using inhaled $^{17}O_2$ gas which is ultimately incorporated into labeled water ($H_2^{17}O$) in brain tissue, which is detectable by in vivo ^{17}O MRS [46, 47]. This method allows the determination of the role of oxygen metabolism in normal brain function and disease to complement functional MRI studies that utilize the BOLD contrast and are sensitive to cerebral blood flow.

Another important development includes in vivo ^{31}P MRSI which generates measurements of intracellular pH and metabolites of ATP, ADP, and phosphocreatine (PCr), among others [47]. The combination of MRSI and magnetization transfer imaging allows for the measurement of CMR_{ATP}, and hence oxidative phosphorylation, a measure of cerebral mitochondrial function. This may prove useful in PD and Huntington's disease, in which mitochondrial dysfunction is thought to play a key role.

Clinical applications

MRI methods are seemingly making their way into the clinic; most rapidly by aiding the neurosurgeon in planning targeting for deep brain stimulation (DBS) surgery (Figure 1.8) [48], also discussed in more detail in Chapter 8. Combining information from different modalities may increase sensitivity to disease states, as shown for example in the combination of structural and iron-sensitive imaging (Figures 1.9, 1.10, and 1.11) [49, 50]. It is hoped that cross-sectional and longitudinal studies that are funded through the M. J. Fox Foundation and the

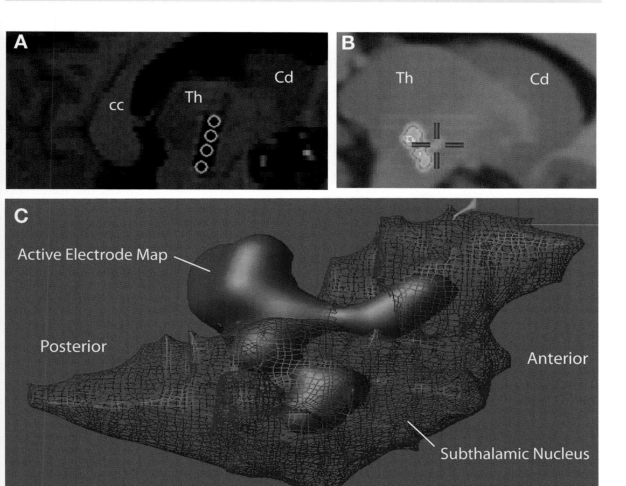

Figure 1.8 (A) Postoperative sagittal T_1-weighted MRI scan of a patient who underwent insertion of subthalamic stimulators for Parkinson's disease. The hypointense signal artifact shows the electrode tip (Medtronic 3387) with four contacts indicated by circles that traverse the subthalamic nucleus. The electrode contacts are within, and dorsal to, the subthalamic nucleus. Abbreviations: cc, corpus callosum; Cd, caudate; Th, thalamus. (B) The automatic non-linear image matching and automatic labeling (ANIMAL) algorithm was used to integrate each patient's MRI scan with the canonical high-resolution MRI (Colin27), resulting in a common space for evaluation of electrode positions from different patients. A probabilistic average map of active contacts of subthalamic stimulators associated with the best outcome for motor symptoms of the contralateral side is shown. (C) The voxel-labeled 3D atlas was integrated with the probabilistic volume map of the most effective active electrode contacts in patients with Parkinson's disease with subthalamic stimulator implants. The subthalamic nucleus is represented as a net. A 90% probability map of most effective electrode positions shows they are localized in the dorsolateral subthalamic nucleus, and areas dorsal and posterior to the subthalamic nucleus, including the zona incerta, Forel's fields, and ventral thalamus. (Sadikot *et al.*, 2011 [48].)

National Institutes of Health will provide additional insights for determining the ability of such methods to provide a correlate to disease severity and progression. With a recent dramatic increase in sales of 7T clinical MRI platforms, there has been great haste to use higher-field magnets over the 3T but whether this proves useful as well as feasible for clinical research studies as well as care of patients will remain to be seen. At our institution 7T preoperative images already have altered surgical planning; however, whether 7T can improve outcomes has not been proven yet, and researchers will need to be creative to find funding to address this question.

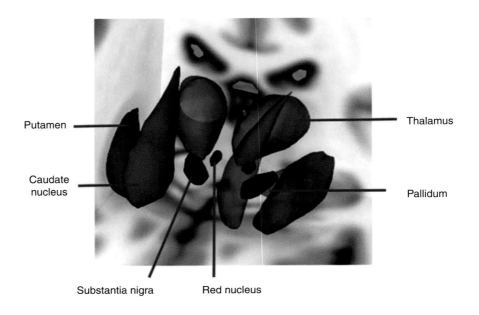

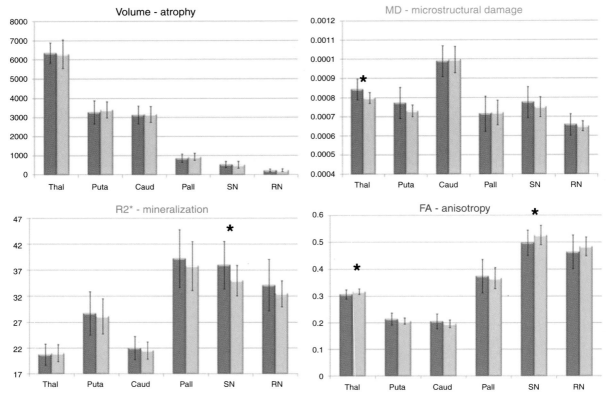

Figure 1.9 3D reconstruction of subcortical regions considered in this work (top). Volume (mm^3), R_2^* (s^{-1}), mean diffusivity (mm^2 s^{-1}), and fractional anisotropy mean values from whole subcortical structures (bottom). Light bars = controls, darker bars = Parkinson's disease. *Significant difference. (Peran *et al.*, 2010 [49].)

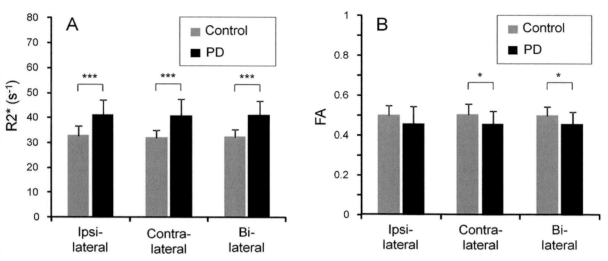

Figure 1.10 Comparison of R_2^* and FA values in PD and controls. Comparison of R_2^* (A) and FA (B) values between PD and control subjects in ipsilateral, contralateral, and bilateral SN (gray bars, control subjects; black bars, PD subjects). Significant differences between PD and control subjects are represented as: *p <0.05; ***p <0.001. (Du et al., 2011 [50].)

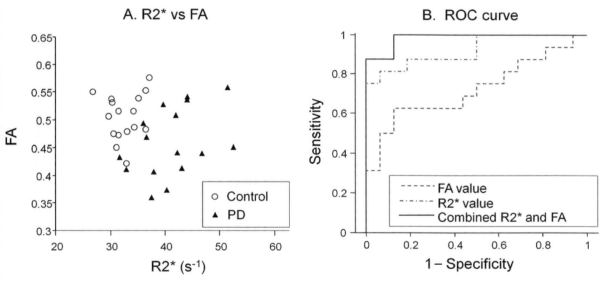

Figure 1.11 Correlation of R_2^* and FA, along with receiver operating characteristic (ROC) curves. (A) Scatter plot of bilateral R_2^* and FA. (B) ROC curves for discriminating between PD and control subjects generated by using FA (dashed line), R_2^* (dashed dotted line), or their combination (solid line). (Du et al., 2011 [50].)

Acknowledgements

NIH grant R01NS061866 (DR. Michaeli), R21N5059813 (Dr. Michaeli), NIH grant KL2 RR033182 to the University of Minnesota Clinical and Translational Science Institute (Dr. Mangia). Additional CMRR Funding is From P41 RR008079, P41 EB015894, P30 N5057091, S10 RR023730, and S10 RR027290, and from Minnesota Medical Foundation (Dr. Tuite).

References

1. Tanner CM, Goldman SM. Epidemiology of Parkinson's disease. *Neurol Clin.* 1996; **14**(2):317–35.

2. Rutledge JN, Hilal SK, Silver AJ, Defendini R, Fahn S. Study of movement disorders and brain iron by MR. *AJR Am J Roentgenol.* 1987;**149**(2):365–79.

3. Gorell JM, Ordidge RJ, Brown GG, *et al.* Increased iron-related MRI contrast in the substantia nigra in Parkinson's disease. *Neurology.* 1995;**45**(6):1138–43.

4. Cho ZH, Oh SH, Kim JM, *et al.* Direct visualization of Parkinson's disease by in vivo human brain imaging using 7.0T magnetic resonance imaging. *Mov Disord.* 2011;**26**(4):713–18.

5. Zecca L, Youdim MB, Riederer P, Connor JR, Crichton RR. Iron, brain ageing and neurodegenerative disorders. *Nat Rev Neurosci.* 2004;**5**(11):863–73.

6. Jin L, Wang J, Zhao L, *et al.* Decreased serum ceruloplasmin levels characteristically aggravate nigral iron deposition in Parkinson's disease. *Brain.* 2011;**134**(Pt 1):50–8.

7. Zecca L, Wilms H, Geick S, *et al.* Human neuromelanin induces neuroinflammation and neurodegeneration in the rat substantia nigra: implications for Parkinson's disease. *Acta Neuropathol.* 2008;**116**(1):47–55.

8. Michaeli S, Oz G, Sorce DJ, *et al.* Assessment of brain iron and neuronal integrity in patients with Parkinson's disease using novel MRI contrasts. *Mov Disord.* 2007;**22**(3):334–40.

9. Nestrasil I, Michaeli S, Liimatainen T, *et al.* T1rho and T2rho MRI in the evaluation of Parkinson's disease. *J Neurol.* 2010;**257**(6):964–8.

10. Tambasco N, Belcastro V, Sarchielli P, *et al.* A magnetization transfer study of mild and advanced Parkinson's disease. *Eur J Neurol.* 2011;**18**(3):471–7.

11. Mangia S, De Martino F, Liimatainen T, Garwood M, Michaeli S. Magnetization transfer using inversion recovery during off-resonance irradiation. *Magn Reson Imaging.* 2011;**29**(10):1346–50.

12. Anik Y, Iseri P, Demirci A, Komsuoglu S, Inan N. Magnetization transfer ratio in early period of Parkinson disease. *Acad Radiol.* 2007;**14**(2):189–92.

13. Eckert T, Sailer M, Kaufmann J, *et al.* Differentiation of idiopathic Parkinson's disease, multiple system atrophy, progressive supranuclear palsy, and healthy controls using magnetization transfer imaging. *Neuroimage.* 2004;**21**(1):229–35.

14. Morgen K, Sammer G, Weber L, *et al.* Structural brain abnormalities in patients with Parkinson disease: a comparative voxel-based analysis using T1-weighted MR imaging and magnetization transfer imaging. *AJNR Am J Neuroradiol.* 2011;**32**(11):2080–6.

15. Tambasco N, Pelliccioli GP, Chiarini P, *et al.* Magnetization transfer changes of gray and white matter in Parkinson's disease. *Neuroradiology.* 2003;**45**(4):224–30.

16. Wang Y, Butros SR, Shuai X, *et al.* Different iron-deposition patterns of multiple system atrophy with predominant parkinsonism and idiopathetic Parkinson diseases demonstrated by phase-corrected susceptibility-weighted imaging. *AJNR Am J Neuroradiol.* 2012; **33**(2):266–73.

17. Manova ES, Habib CA, Boikov AS, *et al.* Characterizing the mesencephalon using susceptibility-weighted imaging. *AJNR Am J Neuroradiol.* 2009; **30**(3):569–74.

18. Gupta D, Saini J, Kesavadas C, Sarma PS, Kishore A. Utility of susceptibility-weighted MRI in differentiating Parkinson's disease and atypical parkinsonism. *Neuroradiology.* 2010;**52**(12): 1087–94.

19. Lenglet C, Abosch A, Yacoub E, *et al.* Comprehensive in vivo mapping of the human basal ganglia and thalamic connectome in individuals using 7T MRI. *PLoS One.* 2012;**7**(1):e29153.

20. Abosch A, Yacoub E, Ugurbil K, Harel N. An assessment of current brain targets for deep brain stimulation surgery with susceptibility-weighted imaging at 7 tesla. *Neurosurgery.* 2010; **67**(6):1745–56; discussion 56.

21. Haacke EM, Mittal S, Wu Z, Neelavalli J, Cheng YC. Susceptibility-weighted imaging: technical aspects and clinical applications, part 1. *AJNR Am J Neuroradiol.* 2009;**30**(1): 19–30.

22. Balaban RS, Ceckler TL. Magnetization transfer contrast in magnetic resonance imaging. *Magn Reson Q.* 1992;**8**(2):116–37.

23. Gochberg DF, Gore JC. Quantitative imaging of magnetization transfer using an inversion recovery sequence. *Magn Reson Med.* 2003; **49**(3):501–5.

24. Gochberg DF, Gore JC. Quantitative magnetization transfer imaging via selective inversion recovery with short repetition times. *Magn Reson Med.* 2007;**57**(2):437–41.

25. Tuite PJ, Mangia S, Tyan AE, *et al.* Magnetization transfer and adiabatic R(1r) MRI in the brainstem of Parkinson's disease. *Parkinsonism Relat Disord.* 2012;**18**(5):623–5.

26. Michaeli S, Sorce DJ, Idiyatullin D, Ugurbil K, Garwood M. Transverse relaxation in the rotating frame induced by chemical exchange. *J Magn Reson.* 2004;**169**(2):293–9.

27. Michaeli S, Sorce DJ, Springer CS, Jr., Ugurbil K, Garwood M. T1rho MRI contrast in the human brain: modulation of the longitudinal rotating frame relaxation shutter-speed during an adiabatic RF pulse. *J Magn Reson*. 2006; **181**(1):135–47.

28. Michaeli S, Sorce D, Garwood M. T2rho and T1rho adiabatic relaxations and contrasts. *Curr Anal Chem*. 2008;**4**:8–25.

29. Silver MS, Joseph RI, Chen CN, Sank VJ, Hoult DI. Selective population inversion in NMR. *Nature*. 1984;**310**(5979):681–3.

30. Mangia S, Liimatainen T, Garwood M, Michaeli S. Rotating frame relaxation during adiabatic pulses vs. conventional spin lock: simulations and experimental results at 4 T. *Magn Reson Imaging*. 2009;**27**(8):1074–87.

31. Michaeli S, Burns TC, Kudishevich E, *et al*. Detection of neuronal loss using T1rho MRI assessment of ^1H_2O spin dynamics in the aphakia mouse. *J Neurosci Methods*. 2009; **177**(1):160–7.

32. Mitsumori F, Watanabe H, Takaya N. Estimation of brain iron concentration in vivo using a linear relationship between regional iron and apparent transverse relaxation rate of the tissue water at 4.7 T. *Magn Reson Med*. 2009;**62**(5):1326–30.

33. Bendall MR, Garwood M, Uğurbil K, Pegg DT. Adiabatic refocusing pulse which compensates for variable rf power and off-resonance effects. *Magn Reson Med*. 1987;**4**(5):493–9.

34. Bendall MR, Pegg DT. Uniform sample excitation with surface coils for in vivo spectroscopy by adiabatic rapid half passage. *J Magn Reson*. 1986;**67**(2):376–81.

35. Mangia S, Traaseth NJ, Veglia G, Garwood M, Michaeli S. Probing slow protein dynamics by adiabatic R(1rho) and R(2rho) NMR experiments. *J Am Chem Soc*. 2010;**132**(29): 9979–81.

36. Pujol J, Junqué C, Vendrell P, Grau JM, Capdevila A. Reduction of the substantia nigra width and motor decline in aging and Parkinson's disease. *Arch Neurol*. 1992;**49**(11):1119–22.

37. Price S, Paviour D, Scahill R, *et al*. Voxel-based morphometry detects patterns of atrophy that help differentiate progressive supranuclear palsy and Parkinson's disease. *Neuroimage*. 2004;**23**(2):663–9.

38. Focke NK, Helms G, Scheewe S, *et al*. Individual voxel-based subtype prediction can differentiate progressive supranuclear palsy from idiopathic parkinson syndrome and healthy controls. *Hum Brain Mapp*. 2011;**32**(11):1905–15.

39. Scherfler C, Frauscher B, Schocke M, *et al*. White and gray matter abnormalities in idiopathic rapid eye movement sleep behavior disorder: a diffusion-tensor imaging and voxel-based morphometry study. *Ann Neurol*. 2011;**69**(2):400–7.

40. Wu T, Wang L, Hallett M, *et al*. Effective connectivity of brain networks during self-initiated movement in Parkinson's disease. *Neuroimage*. 2011;**55**(1):204–15.

41. Wu T, Long X, Zang Y, *et al*. Regional homogeneity changes in patients with Parkinson's disease. *Hum Brain Mapp*. 2009;**30**(5): 1502–10.

42. Kwak Y, Peltier S, Bohnen NI, *et al*. Altered resting state cortico-striatal connectivity in mild to moderate stage Parkinson's

43. Baudrexel S, Witte T, Seifried C, *et al*. Resting state fMRI reveals increased subthalamic nucleus-motor cortex connectivity in Parkinson's disease. *Neuroimage*. 2011;**55**(4):1728–38.

44. Skidmore FM, Yang M, Baxter L, *et al*. Reliability analysis of the resting state can sensitively and specifically identify the presence of Parkinson disease. *Neuroimage*. 2013;**75**:249–61.

45. Krajcovicova L, Mikl M, Marecek R, Rektorova I. The default mode network integrity in patients with Parkinson's disease is levodopa equivalent dose-dependent. *J Neural Transm*. 2012;**119**(4): 443–54.

46. Zhu X, Chen W. In vivo oxygen-17 NMR for imaging brain oxygen metabolism at high field. *Prog Nucl Magn Reson Spectrosc*. 2011;**59**(4):319–35.

47. Zhu XH, Du F, Zhang N, *et al*. Advanced in vivo heteronuclear MRS approaches for studying brain bioenergetics driven by mitochondria. *Methods Mol Biol*. 2009;**489**:317–57.

48. Sadikot AF, Chakravarty MM, Bertrand G, *et al*. Creation of computerized 3D MRI-integrated atlases of the human basal ganglia and thalamus. *Front Syst Neurosci*. 2011;**5**:71.

49. Peran P, Cherubini A, Assogna F, *et al*. Magnetic resonance imaging markers of Parkinson's disease nigrostriatal signature. *Brain*. 2010;**133**(11):3423–33.

50. Du G, Lewis MM, Styner M, *et al*. Combined R2* and diffusion tensor imaging changes in the substantia nigra in Parkinson's disease. *Mov Disord*. 2011; **26**(9):1627–32.

disease. *Front Syst Neurosci*. 2010;**4**:143.

Imaging iron in Parkinson's disease

W. R. Wayne Martin

Introduction

In the early days of clinical magnetic resonance imaging (MRI), the exquisite anatomical detail evident in images of the midbrain led investigators to evaluate this new imaging modality in patients with Parkinson's disease (PD). It soon became apparent that the prominent low-signal regions evident in the brainstem and basal ganglia correlated with sites of ferric iron accumulation as determined in vitro by Perls' Prussian blue stain [1]. Since those early days of clinical MRI, new insights into the role of iron in the brain, combined with substantial advances in MRI technology, have had a significant impact on the role of iron imaging in the investigation of patients with PD and related disorders.

Iron in the brain

The adult brain has very high iron content, particularly in certain substructures of the basal ganglia. Direct postmortem measurements indicate that non-heme iron content is very low throughout the brain at birth and that it gradually increases during the first two decades of life [2]. Regional iron concentration in the adult brain is maximal in the globus pallidus, substantia nigra (SN), red nucleus, caudate, and putamen. Iron accumulation is primarily in the form of ferritin and seems to occur particularly in oligodendrocytes, although it is also present in neurons and microglia. Significant amounts of iron are sequestered in neuromelanin granules in dopaminergic neurons of the substantia nigra pars compacta (SNc) and in noradrenergic neurons of the locus coeruleus [3]. In normal subjects, about 20% of nigral iron is bound in its ferric form to neuromelanin [4],

with the remainder stored as soluble ferritin and its insoluble degradation product hemosiderin [5, 6].

Elevated iron levels are evident in selected brain areas not only with aging but also in neurodegenerative disorders, including PD where postmortem studies suggest an increase in regional iron content in the SN [7, 8]. Laser microprobe studies have confirmed not only that iron normally accumulates within neuromelanin granules of nigral neurons but also that iron levels within these granules are significantly increased in PD [9]. Although iron content within individual granules may be increased, however, there is a general decrease in neuromelanin granules in PD as a consequence of the loss of functional nigral neurons. There is evidence that, in patients with PD, iron is sequestered in Lewy bodies in SNc neurons, but, interestingly, not in cortical Lewy bodies [10]. Extended X-ray absorption fine structure experiments indicate that ferritin is the only storage protein that can be detected in both control and parkinsonian brain, and that there is increased loading of ferritin with iron in PD [11].

Iron is a critical component of the central nervous system, being involved in several important functions, including DNA synthesis, gene expression, myelination, neurotransmission, and mitochondrial electron transport. Iron is an essential cofactor for many of the proteins involved in normal neuronal function, including the enzyme tyrosine hydroxylase, which forms a critical part of the pathway involved in dopamine synthesis. Brain iron is relatively independent from total body iron content since it is excluded, for the most part, by the blood–brain barrier. While iron is transported in the periphery by transferrin and into the brain by interactions between transferrin and transferrin receptors on endothelial cells and on

Magnetic Resonance Imaging in Movement Disorders, ed. Paul Tuite and Alain Dagher. Published by Cambridge University Press. © Cambridge University Press 2013.

neurons, non-transferrin-bound iron is the main source of iron for oligodendrocytes and astrocytes. The sequestration of iron by the storage protein ferritin in the cytosol reduces levels of potentially toxic free iron. Neuromelanin–iron complexes in the SN and the locus coeruleus are responsible for sequestering large amounts of iron and may help protect against iron-mediated oxidative damage in these cells [12]. The role of iron in the brain and in neurodegenerative disease has recently been reviewed by Benarroch and others [13, 14].

It has been suggested that the copper transport protein ceruloplasmin may have an impact on iron accumulation in the brain, perhaps through a role in oxidizing ferrous iron to the ferric form, thereby minimizing the intracellular level of reactive ferrous iron. Jin et al. have suggested that nigral iron content correlates inversely with the level of serum ceruloplasmin and that decreased levels of serum ceruloplasmin may exacerbate nigral iron deposition in PD [15].

Quantitation of brain iron with MRI

The microstructural and physiological organization of tissue plays an important role in determining the local magnetic field behavior of a given region in the brain. Different regions demonstrate a specific behavior that is based on the intrinsic tissue properties. Several distinct MRI methods have been applied in the attempt to quantify regional brain iron content in the living human brain, including measurements of the relaxation rates R_2 and R_2^*, and their difference, R_2'. In addition, field-dependent relaxation rate increase and phase measurements have been used to characterize brain iron content. (In this review, the terms R_2, R_2^*, and R_2' are used interchangeably with the terms T_2, T_2^*, and T_2'. Mathematically, one set of terms is the reciprocal of the other, so that the expression $R_2^* = R_2 + R_2'$ is equivalent to the expression $1/T_2^* = 1/T_2 + 1/T_2'$.)

In proton MRI of the brain, the MR signal arises from mobile water protons within tissue. Image contrast develops primarily as a result of regional variations in proton density and in longitudinal (T_1) and transverse (T_2) relaxation of the protons. It is well established that paramagnetic ions, such as iron at concentrations seen in the human brain, will increase proton transverse relaxation (R_2), thereby shortening T_2 ($T_2 = 1/R_2$). The ability of ions to affect proton relaxation is dependent on several factors but, in

general, magnetic ions can be expected to affect contrast if they are present in sufficient concentrations (≥ 0.1 mM) [16]. Although paramagnetic ions such as copper and manganese can potentially affect contrast if present in sufficient quantities, their concentrations in the brain are normally too low to produce significant MR changes [16]. In normal basal ganglia, iron concentration is about 1.7–3.8 mM [2, 16], sufficient to increase transverse relaxation of protons, thereby shortening T_2 relaxation times. Langkammer et al. have recently reported a strong linear correlation ($r^2 = 0.67$) between transverse relaxation times and direct postmortem measurement of iron concentration in a series of prespecified gray and white matter regions obtained from seven subjects [17].

In aqueous solution, ferritin has a strong effect on transverse relaxation due to a loss of the MR signal resulting from the dephasing of proton spins related to the induction of microscopic magnetic fields surrounding the iron. In tissue, however, the associated T_2 changes are much less prominent. While shortened T_2 values have been reported in the SN and striatum in patients with PD, the changes have been small with substantial overlap between patients and controls [18, 19]. A more complex association between brain iron and PD has been suggested, with decreased nigral T_2 unrelated to disease duration, and increased T_2 in the putamen and pallidum in patients with longer disease duration [20]. Others have reported a poor correlation between T_2 times and direct measures of iron and ferritin, suggesting that factors other than iron, such as tissue water content, may have an overriding role in determining transverse relaxation parameters in tissue [21].

Alternate MR methods have been developed in an attempt to provide a more direct in vivo estimate of regional brain iron content. Ferritin affects transverse relaxation more in a high magnetic field than it does in a low field, a property that has been used to derive a regional index of ferritin content [22]. By measuring transverse relaxation in the same patient with instruments having two different field strengths, a specific measure of the tissue ferritin iron pool can be obtained. Field-dependent T_2 changes support the concept of an age-related increase in striatal iron [23]. In addition, this method has been used to provide evidence that patients with the onset of PD symptoms before 60 years of age have increased ferritin in the SNc, substantia nigra pars reticulata (SNr),

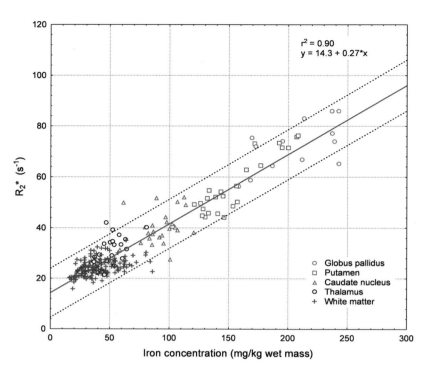

Figure 2.1 Graph shows the relationship between iron concentration and R_2^* as determined with linear regression analysis from a series of prespecified gray and white matter regions obtained post mortem from 7 subjects. The solid line is the regression line, and the dotted lines represent the 95% confidence limits. (Reprinted from *Radiology*. 2010;**257**:455–62, Langkammer C, *et al.* Quantitative MR imaging of brain iron: a postmortem validation study, with permission from the Radiological Society of North America [17].)

putamen, and globus pallidus, whereas later-onset patients may have decreased ferritin in the SNr [24].

Other methods have exploited the principle that paramagnetic substances such as iron create local magnetic field inhomogeneities, thereby altering transverse relaxation [25, 26]. T_2^* represents a combination of transverse relaxation and magnetic field inhomogeneity, with tissue iron being a major determinant of the latter. Gradient echo imaging sequences are particularly sensitive to the T_2^*-reducing effects of iron-induced local field inhomogeneities because, unlike spin echo sequences, they do not utilize a refocusing pulse. Recently, Langkammer *et al.* have shown that R_2^* values correlate very closely ($r^2 = 0.90$) with postmortem iron concentrations in human brain (Figure 2.1) [17]. These authors observed that R_2^* was more sensitive than R_2 to variations in brain iron concentration, suggesting that it is therefore the preferred parameter for the assessment of iron concentration in vivo. Gorell and colleagues used a T_2^*-based method to show a correlation between increased iron-related MR contrast in PD and simple reaction time, used as an indicator of disease severity [27].

Transverse relaxation measurements, both R_2 and R_2^*, are affected not only by iron but also by water

content; R_2' (the difference between R_2 and R_2^*) has been proposed as a parameter that is more specific for the field inhomogeneities due to iron by minimizing confounding effects of changes in water binding. Graham *et al.* used a partially refocused interleaved multiple-echo (PRIME) pulse sequence that yielded T_2^* and T_2 data from a single scan, thereby allowing for the calculation of T_2' [28]. This method suggested increased nigral but decreased putaminal iron in PD. A subsequent report used the PRIME sequence in a larger patient population and at a higher field strength (3T) to confirm the presence of increased nigral iron content and showed a correlation with the motor features of PD [29]. In contrast to the previous study, the 3T study indicated increased putaminal iron relative to healthy controls. The investigators suggested that their original study may have been biased by noisy data.

Another method for estimation of regional iron content, based on the effects of paramagnetic centers that are sequestered within cell membranes, has been developed [26]. This method exploits the interecho time dependence of the decay of transverse magnetization that is caused by the local field inhomogeneities resulting from intracellular paramagnetic ions.

Because the concentration of iron in the brain is much greater than that of other paramagnetic ions, this method enables the estimation of indices of brain iron content on a regional basis. We utilized this technique to show a correlation between increasing age and striatal iron content and suggested that this age-dependent increase may represent a risk factor for the development of nigrostriatal neuronal damage by increased oxidant stress [30]. An important caveat to this concept, however, is that ferritin-bound iron may be relatively non-reactive and therefore less likely to induce tissue damage than is free iron. We have also reported a significant increase in iron content in the putamen and pallidum in PD correlating with the severity of clinical symptomatology [31].

More recently, we have employed a modification of this method on a high-field imaging system (3T) to determine whether the observed SNc changes correspond anatomically to the neuropathological changes in the nigra that have been reported previously by Fearnley and Lees [32]. Our multiple gradient echo method was designed to minimize the magnetic field inhomogeneities that arise from tissue–tissue and air–tissue interfaces, thereby improving the specificity of transverse relaxation measurements for changes in regional iron content [33]. With this method, we acquired imaging data from the midbrain in 22 untreated patients with PD and 11 normal control subjects [34]. We observed a significant difference in measured $R_2{}^*$ values between patients and controls in the lateral (but not medial) SNc. Linear regression indicated a correlation between lateral SNc $R_2{}^*$ values and motor features of PD on the contralateral side. Our observation of lateral SNc changes that are consistent with increased iron content and correspond to the known distribution of neuronal loss occurring in early PD provides strong support for the notion that quantitation of regional iron with MRI may provide a marker for disease severity and progression in PD. Longitudinal studies are currently underway to address this hypothesis.

A related measurement, the rotating frame transverse relaxation $T_{2\rho}$, has been evaluated in studies of PD and controls performed at 4T [35, 36]. This parameter is said to be more sensitive to diffusion and exchange of water protons in environments with different local magnetic susceptibilities as compared to conventional T_2 measurements. The method was able to distinguish patients with PD from normal controls but there was no correlation with disease duration or severity. Direct comparisons between the $T_{2\rho}$ methodology and $T_2{}^*$ quantitation have not been published.

Multimodal approaches

Recent work has extended previous observations by using a multimodal approach that combines MRI techniques for imaging iron content with other MRI sequences. Péran and colleagues combined $T_2{}^*$ relaxation rate measurements with volumetric measurements and with diffusion tensor imaging (DTI), using a 3T imaging system [37]. Calculation of fractional anisotropy and mean diffusivity from DTI acquisitions provides information regarding microstructural integrity of tissue. Compared with control subjects, patients with PD displayed significantly higher $R_2{}^*$ values in the SN, lower fractional anisotropy values in the SN and thalamus, and higher mean diffusivity values in the thalamus. These authors also employed a voxel-based analysis to evaluate these parameters. This analysis confirmed the region-based results and, in addition, showed a significant difference in the mean diffusivity in the striatum (Figure 2.2). Logistic regression showed that combinations of three different markers were sufficient to obtain greater than 95% discrimination between patients with PD and controls. The three markers that provided this degree of discrimination were $R_2{}^*$ in the SN, fractional anisotropy in the SN, and mean diffusivity in the putamen or caudate nucleus. These findings demonstrate the utility of multimodal imaging of subcortical gray matter structures in the evaluation of PD.

Similar observations have been made by Du *et al.* in their report of transverse relaxation and fractional anisotropy measurements made at 3T in PD [38]. Compared with controls, PD subjects demonstrated a significantly increased transverse relaxation rate accompanied by reduced fractional anisotropy in the SN. There was no significant correlation between transverse relaxation rate and fractional anisotropy, indicating that these measurements reflect different aspects of parkinsonian pathophysiology. Although neither measurement correlated with clinical scores, the authors suggest that this type of multimodal MRI methodology may ultimately provide a practical tool for monitoring the progression of PD.

Another approach to multimodal imaging has been taken by Baudrexel *et al.* who utilized combined quantitative T_1-mapping (as a potential marker for

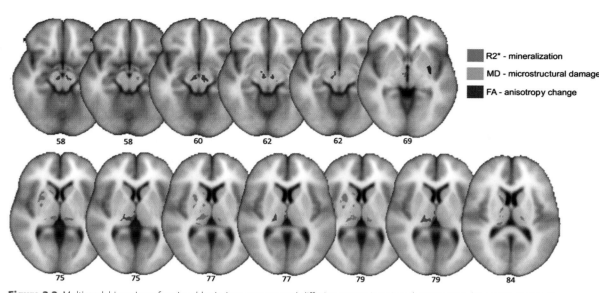

R2* - mineralization

MD - microstructural damage

FA - anisotropy change

Figure 2.2 Multimodal imaging of regional brain iron content and diffusion tensor imaging showing iron deposition (R_2^*) in the substantia nigra, microstructural damage (increased mean diffusivity (MD), and reduced fractional anisotropy (FA)) in the striatum, thalamus, and midbrain in patients with Parkinson's disease. Numbers under each image represent z-position on the template. (Reprinted from *Brain*. 2010;**133**:3423–33, Péran P, *et al.* Magnetic resonance imaging markers of Parkinson's disease nigrostriatal signature, with permission from Oxford University Press [37].)

gray matter loss) and T_2^*-mapping (as a marker of iron accumulation) at 3T to evaluate changes in local relaxation times in the midbrain and lower brainstem in patients with early PD [39]. These authors reported a large area of reduced T_1 in the midbrain and pons contralateral to the clinically most affected body side and interpreted this reduction as being indicative of neuronal loss from this region. In contrast, T_2^* reductions indicating increased tissue iron content were restricted primarily to the SN and showed a bilateral pattern. T_2^* did not correlate with disease duration and the correlation with disease severity was small, suggesting that nigral iron content remains relatively stable during the course of PD. Based on these data, the authors suggest that increased nigral iron may reflect a marker for disease susceptibility or vulnerability rather than for disease progression, a concept that was proposed previously by Berg *et al.* on the basis of their observations with transcranial sonography [40]. Baudrexel and colleagues point out that brainstem areas outside the SN affected by a decrease in T_1 did not show significant reductions in T_2^*, suggesting that increased iron deposition in extranigral regions is not a prerequisite for PD-related neuronal loss. They also highlight the fact that the pattern of nigral T_2^* decrease was different from that

associated with T_1-mapping. Within the nigra, the T_1 decrease matched the pattern of dopamine cell loss that has been shown in various postmortem studies, suggesting that T_1 is a marker for PD-related neuronal loss, whereas T_2^*-mapping revealed a bilateral increase in tissue iron content. Clearly, these relaxation parameters reflect different pathophysiological processes; the process that results in neuronal loss in PD may differ from the mechanisms that are associated with increased iron accumulation.

Susceptibility-based imaging

Most of the methods described above are indirectly dependent on the effects on magnetic susceptibility changes from tissue iron accumulation with a complex dependence on its microscopic distribution. MR-based measurements that are more directly related to magnetic susceptibility changes should be more closely related to iron content and less dependent on its microscopic spatial distribution. Local changes in the amount of tissue iron will lead to changes in magnetic susceptibility. A measurement of the phase difference between tissues is a potentially useful marker of susceptibility change. Images of the phase of the MR signal (phase maps), generated using gradient echo sequences at high magnetic field strength, show excellent contrast that has been attributed to perturbations in the local magnetic field that is produced by susceptibility differences between tissues [41]. Zhang *et al.* have reported a close relationship between measured phase shift values at 3T and direct measurement of tissue iron content [42]. While images determined by transverse relaxation rate (T_2 or T_2^*) are sensitive to changes in iron content, phase imaging should be more sensitive to iron because it depends on subtle phase shifts rather than the significant dephasing required to generate changes in transverse relaxation. In addition, unlike relaxation measurements, phase is not significantly affected by water content, which could be a confounder in cases of neurodegeneration [43]. Phase maps themselves, however, provide an imperfect indication of regional iron content due to a spatial mismatch between the contrast in a phase map and the underlying microscopic susceptibility distribution in tissue, particularly in large deep gray matter structures [44–46].

Susceptibility-weighted imaging (SWI) is a technique that uses magnetic susceptibility differences between different regions to generate image contrast. Unlike methods that generate images based on signal magnitude information alone or on the phase mapping described above, SWI utilizes both magnitude and phase information to generate images that are very sensitive to the changes in magnetic susceptibility that are caused by the presence of paramagnetic substances such as iron [6, 47].

The implementation of SWI on the very high-field imaging systems (e.g., 7T) that are currently in vogue has the potential for producing high-resolution images that allow for improved quantitation of regional iron content. Although putative quantitative iron measures have been reported with phase imaging, as noted above, the reliability of this method for iron measurement is inconsistent because phase can be confounded by several independent physical factors, including the three-dimensional geometry of the structure of interest in the brain and its relationship to the stationary magnetic field of the imaging system, neuronal fiber orientation, tissue myelin content, tissue calcium and phospholipid content, and the presence of neighboring susceptibility sources [48]. SWI is a useful alternative to simple phase imaging. While phase imaging itself is quantitative, there can be problematic artifacts. On the other hand, truly quantitative SWI is challenging and many of the concepts relating to these measurements remain to be validated in animal models [47].

In contrast to phase mapping, susceptibility mapping has been suggested as a tool that may provide a more direct measure of iron content and distribution and as an indirect marker of the spatial pattern of neuronal loss in the SN [49]. This is a method for retrieving the susceptibility distribution from the phase data, designed to overcome the spatial mismatch inherent in these data. These investigators have reported, in a small number of patients with PD, that magnetic susceptibility of the SNc is increased in patients as compared to controls. Their data indicated that, in control subjects, iron was higher in more caudal sections of the midbrain than in more rostral sections and that this effect was greater in some PD patients, suggesting a relative increase in iron in the caudal part of the SNc in this patient group (Figure 2.3). This is consistent with a previous study using DTI in which a loss in cell density in the caudal nigra was suggested [50].

Deep brain stimulation

Deep brain stimulation (DBS) plays an important role in the treatment of PD. Because of the critical importance of accurate anatomical localization of the structure of interest, typically either the subthalamic nucleus (STN) or the internal segment of the globus pallidus (GPi), there is a strong clinical interest in the use of MRI techniques for localization of these landmarks for the stereotactic implantation of stimulation electrodes. In general, T_2- or T_2^*-weighted sequences are employed for this purpose since the resulting images provide good anatomical contrast in iron-rich structures like the STN or GPi. A common procedure is to fuse T_2- or T_2^*-weighted images with datasets from other modalities that provide higher spatial resolution or improved contrast of other structures that are important to surgical planning. Dormont *et al.* showed that the decreased signal intensity located lateral to the red nucleus and dorsolateral to the SN on T_2-weighted images corresponds anatomically to the STN [51]. They emphasized, however, that although decreased signal was always present in the anterior part of the STN, the posterior part was not visible in most cases. In general, iron-related contrast in these structures is improved with increasing field strength [52].

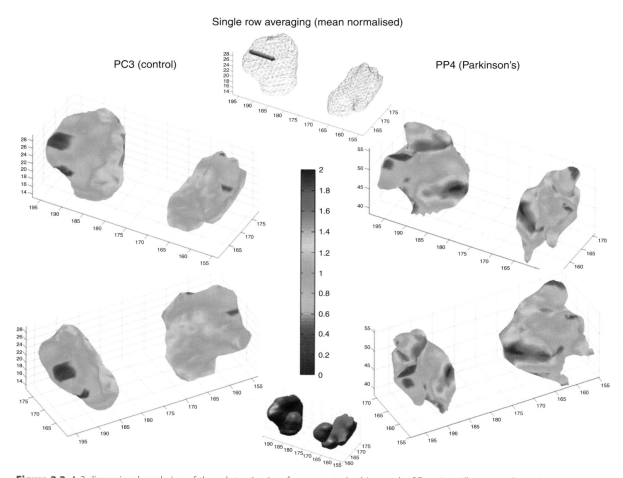

Figure 2.3 A 3-dimensional rendering of the substantia nigra from a control subject and a PD patient, illustrating the variation in susceptibility across the substantia nigra. This variation is greater in the patient than in the control. The color indicates the average susceptibility along a row through the nigra as indicated in the inset mesh image (top). The inset red, green and pink image (bottom) indicates the nigra and red nucleus mask for orientation. (Reprinted from *J Magn Reson Imaging*. 2012;**35**:48–55, Lotfipour AK, *et al.* High resolution magnetic susceptibility mapping of the substantia nigra in Parkinson's disease, with permission from John Wiley and Sons [49].)

One potentially valuable application of the SWI technique is in the identification of the STN for planning DBS surgery [53, 54]. The improved contrast and spatial resolution of SWI as compared to standard imaging methods allows for improved delineation of the iron-rich STN from the immediately adjacent SN, particularly at the very high magnetic field strength of 7T [55]. Enhanced STN visualization provides the potential for the development of a direct targeting approach for implantation of DBS electrodes, thereby leading to a simplified surgical procedure without the need for microelectrode recording [53].

A more complex method for stereotactic localization of the STN, again based on its high iron content but involving the use of five co-registered image contrasts (T_1-weighted navigation image, R_2^* map, SWI [phase, magnitude, and fusion image]), has been proposed more recently [56]. T_1-weighted images and R_2^* maps are illustrated in Figure 2.4.

Differential diagnosis

The regional distribution of brain iron may provide information that is useful for the differential diagnosis of parkinsonian syndromes. Boelmans *et al.* have suggested that a toxic interaction between tau and α-synuclein may lead to a toxic loss of neuronal function by affecting axonal transport, thereby resulting in

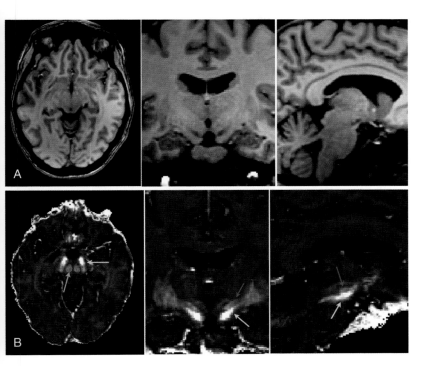

Figure 2.4 T_1-weighted images (Row A) and R_2* map (Row B) from a normal subject. The subthalamic nucleus is immediately adjacent to the rostral substantia nigra. Each contrast is demonstrated with three orthogonal sections: axial (left), coronal (middle) and sagittal (right). The midbrain nuclei appear in the images: red arrows – subthalamic nucleus, STN, green arrow – red nucleus, yellow arrows – substantia nigra. (Reprinted from *Magn Reson Imaging.* 2012;**30**:627–40, Xiao Y, *et al.* Multicontrast multiecho FLASH MRI for targeting the subthalamic nucleus, with permission from Elsevier [56].)

iron accumulation though impairment of iron secretion [57]. Based on this, they suggest that imaging markers of regional iron content may be used as an indirect marker of the accumulation and distribution of tau protein, potentially allowing for the discrimination of progressive supranuclear palsy (PSP) from PD. They obtained quantitative T_2 and T_2* maps at 1.5T from 30 patients with PD, 12 with PSP, and 24 age-matched healthy controls, and used these data to calculate regional T2'. This is essentially equivalent to a T_2* measurement that has been corrected for spin–spin relaxation according to the relationship $1/T_2' = 1/T_2^* - 1/T_2$. A significant shortening of T_2', consistent with iron accumulation, was observed in the caudate nucleus, globus pallidus, and putamen in PSP patients compared both to PD patients and to healthy controls. With further validation, this type of measurement could prove to be of diagnostic value in differentiating PSP from PD.

In a recent report, SWI was used to evaluate the pattern of iron accumulation in patients with the parkinsonian variant of multiple system atrophy (MSA-P) in comparison to PD [58]. SWI phase images suggested increased iron content in the putamen. These findings extend the previous reports in

MSA both of shortened T_2 in the putamen [19] and of decreased signal intensity in the putamen observed with T_2*-weighted sequences [59, 60]. The report from Wang *et al.* makes the interesting additional observation in MSA-P of increased iron accumulation in the pulvinar thalamus, a feature that may provide added information supporting a diagnosis of MSA-P [58].

Is the accumulation of iron in the SN specific for PD? This question has been addressed by Brar *et al.* who studied a series of patients with Alzheimer's disease who developed parkinsonism during the course of the disease [61]. Using T_2 shortening as an estimate of nigral iron content at 3T, they observed that individuals who developed parkinsonism superimposed on their pre-existing dementia had significantly more iron in the SN than did patients with dementia alone. The authors speculate that nigral iron accumulation in Alzheimer's disease may be a predictor of parkinsonism and more rapid disease progression.

Potential problems

Although most of the studies cited herein suggest the presence of increased iron in patients with PD, particularly in the SNc, a number of issues contribute to the variability in results amongst these reports. There are several challenges associated with the utilization of MRI to evaluate the structural integrity of the SN in a reproducible fashion. One issue is that the MRI methodology itself can vary from study to study. As described above, several different methods have been used to derive an index that corresponds to regional brain iron content. Little has been published in terms of a direct comparison between these methods although work is currently underway in this regard. Slice orientation, thickness, and spacing can differ significantly amongst studies.

Another major source of variability relates to accurate localization of the nigra itself on images of the midbrain. While one would anticipate that SNc changes would correlate best with the neuropathological changes associated with PD, many reports have not considered the nigral subdivisions of SNc and SNr. The low-signal area that is readily visualized on T_2- and T_2^*-weighted images of the ventrolateral midbrain probably corresponds most closely with the SNr, which has a significantly higher iron content than does the SNc [62]. The low-signal area in this part of the upper midbrain tends to extend beyond the border of the SNr and into the medial portion of the crus cerebri. While some authors state that the SNc corresponds best to the high-signal area that is interposed between the low signal of the SNr and the red nucleus, the parabrachial pigmented nucleus [63] as well as white matter of the nigrostriatal tracts may also separate the SNc from the red nucleus [27, 64]. Adachi and colleagues have suggested that the boundaries of the SN may be more accurately determined using DWI to depict the surrounding white matter but do not address the separation of the SNc from the SNr [64].

SN size and shape vary widely from subject to subject. Much of the nigra lies immediately below the red nucleus [62]. At its rostral border, there is an unclear boundary between the nigra and the STN [38]. This is particularly problematic in the dorsal region of the nigra. Studies of the three-dimensional structure of the SNc indicate a complex organization with clusters of tyrosine hydroxylase-positive neurons extending into the SNr [65, 66]. This fine structure is well beyond the resolving capability of most current clinical imaging systems. Whether it can be resolved with newer very high field systems is an important area for future study.

Future developments

MRI technology continues to evolve. In the early days of clinical MRI, 1.5T was considered to be a high-field imaging system. In many clinical centers, 3T is now the standard and we are seeing increasing deployment of progressively higher field strengths such as 7T and greater. Modern 7T scanners with 32-channel array detectors allow a 10- to 100-fold improvement in sensitivity over early low-field systems with single-channel detectors [67]. With the implementation of very high-field systems, new opportunities are becoming available to elucidate midbrain anatomy and the relationship between iron accumulation and parkinsonian symptomatology. Kwon *et al.* have recently reported T_2^*-weighted images obtained at 7T based on manual tracings of the SN and suggest that the boundaries between the SN and the crus cerebri have a different configuration in PD subjects compared to normal individuals [68].

Quantitative susceptibility mapping (QSM) is a post-processing technique that has the potential to estimate robustly the magnetic susceptibility of tissues from gradient echo phase measurments, although there are mathematical challenges associated with these measurements [46]. Optimized methods of dealing with these issues are currently being developed [69]. Langkammer *et al.* have recently reported a very close relationship between magnetic susceptibility measured with QSM and direct measurements of iron concentration in postmortem brain [70]. An example of a QSM map from Langkammer is illustrated in Figure 2.5. Currently, QSM allows only for the determination of susceptibility differences between tissues rather than absolute susceptibility values, requiring normalization of the susceptibility maps to a reference region such as occipital white matter [70]. A further limitation is the need for accurate removal of background field effects from air–tissue susceptibility differences.

Iron content is but one of the physiological variables that can be estimated with MRI in the basal ganglia of patients with PD. Iron imaging is best not considered in isolation. The value of multimodality imaging has already been illustrated by studies such as those of Péran *et al.* [37], Du *et al.* [38], and Baudrexel *et al.* [39]. We can anticipate additional insights into the relationship between brain iron content and PD as these multimodality techniques become more widely implemented on very high-field imaging systems.

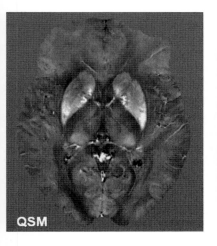 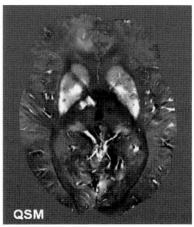

Figure 2.5 Quantitative susceptibility maps from a living 58-year-old subject (left) and a deceased 57-year-old subject (right). There is increased susceptibility in the posterior striatum and in the medial pallidum. More vessels are visible in the postmortem map because the blood is fully deoxygenated. (Reprinted from *Neuroimage.* 2012;**62**:1593–9, Langkammer C, *et al.* Quantitative susceptibility mapping (QSM) as a means to measure brain iron? A post mortem validation study, with permission from Elsevier [70].)

References

1. Rutledge JN, Hilal SK, Schallert T, *et al.* Magnetic resonance imaging of Parkinsonisms. In: Fahn S, Marsden CD, Calne D, Godstein M, editors. *Recent Development in Parkinson's Disease.* Florham Park, NH: Macmillan; 1987. 123–34.

2. Hallgren B, Sourander P. The effect of age on the nonhaemin iron in the human brain. *J Neurochem.* 1958;**3**:41–51.

3. Zecca L, Shima T, Stroppolo A, *et al.* Interaction of neuromelanin and iron in substantia nigra and other areas of human brain. *Neuroscience.* 1996;**73**:407–15.

4. Gerlach M, Double KL, Ben-Shachar D, *et al.* Neuromelanin and its interaction with iron as a potential risk factor for dopaminergic neurodegeneration underlying Parkinson's disease. *Neurotox Res.* 2003;**5**:35–43.

5. Schenck JF, Zimmerman EA. High-field magnetic resonance imaging of brain iron: birth of a biomarker? *NMR Biomed.* 2004;**17**:433–45.

6. Haacke EM, Cheng NY, House MJ, *et al.* Imaging iron stores in the brain using magnetic resonance imaging. *Magn Reson Imaging.* 2005;**23**:1–25.

7. Dexter DT, Wells FR, Lees AJ, *et al.* Increased nigral iron content and alterations in other metal ions occurring in brain in Parkinson's disease. *J Neurochem.* 1989;**52**: 1830–6.

8. Sofic E, Riederer P, Heinsen H, *et al.* Increased iron (III) and total iron content in post mortem substantia nigra of parkinsonian brain. *J Neural Transm.* 1988;**74**:199–205.

9. Good PF, Olanow CW, Perl DP. Neuromelanin-containing neurons of the substantia nigra accumulate iron and aluminum in Parkinson's disease: a LAMMA study. *Brain Res.* 1992; **593**:343–64.

10. Castellani RJ, Siedlak SL, Perry G, Smith MA. Sequestration of iron by Lewy bodies in Parkinson's disease. *Acta Neuropathol.* 2000;**100**:111–14.

11. Griffiths PD, Dobson BR, Jones GR, Clarke DT. Iron in the basal ganglia in Parkinson's disease: an in vitro study using extended X-ray absorption fine structure and cryo-electron microscopy. *Brain.* 1999;**122**:667–73.

12. Zecca L, Casella L, Albertini A, *et al.* Neuromelanin can protect against iron-mediated oxidative damage in system modeling iron overload of brain aging and Parkinson's disease. *J Neurochem.* 2008;**106**:1866–75.

13. Benarroch EE. Brain iron homeostasis and neurodegenerative disease. *Neurology.* 2009;**72**:1436–40.

14. Zecca L, Youdim MB, Riederer P, Connor JR, Crichton RR. Iron, brain ageing and neurodegenerative disorders. *Nat Rev Neurosci.* 2004;**5**:863–73.

15. Jin L, Wang J, Zhao L, *et al.* Decreased serum ceruloplasmin levels characteristically aggravate nigral iron deposition in Parkinson's disease. *Brain.* 2011;**134**:50–8.

16. Schenck JF. Magnetic resonance imaging of brain iron. *J Neurol Sci.* 2003;**207**:99–102.

17. Langkammer C, Krebs N, Goessler W, *et al.* Quantitative MR imaging of brain iron: a postmortem validation study. *Radiology.* 2010;**257**:455–62.

18. Antonini A, Leenders KL, Meier D, *et al.* T2 relaxation time in patients with Parkinson's disease. *Neurology.* 1993;**43**:697–700.

19. Vymazal J, Righini A, Brooks RA, *et al.* T1 and T2 in the brain of healthy subjects, patients with Parkinson disease, and patients with multiple system atrophy: relation to iron content. *Radiology.* 1999;**211**:489–95.

20. Ryvlin P, Broussolle E, Piollet H, *et al.* Magnetic resonance imaging evidence of decreased putamenal iron content in idiopathic Parkinson's disease. *Arch Neurol.* 1995;**52**:583–8.

21. Chen JC, Hardy PA, Kucharczyk W, *et al.* MR of human postmortem brain tissue: correlative study between T2 and assays of iron and ferritin in Parkinson and Huntington disease. *AJNR Am J Neuroradiol.* 1993;**14**:275–81.

22. Bartzokis G, Aravagiri M, Oldendorf WH, Mintz J, Marder SR. Field dependent transverse relaxation rate increase may be a specific measure of tissue iron stores. *Magn Reson Med.* 1993;**29**:459–64.

23. Bartzokis G, Mintz J, Sultzer D, *et al.* In vivo MR evaluation of age-related increases in brain iron. *AJNR Am J Neuroradiol.* 1994;**15**:1129–38.

24. Bartzokis G, Cummings JL, Markham CH, *et al.* MRI evaluation of brain iron in earlier- and later-onset Parkinson's disease and normal subjects. *Magn Reson Imaging.* 1999;**17**:213–22.

25. Ordidge RJ, Gorell JM, Deniau JC, Knight RA, Helpern JA. Assessment of relative brain iron concentrations using T2-weighted and T2*-weighted MRI at 3 Tesla. *Magn Reson Med.* 1994;**32**:335–41.

26. Ye FQ, Martin WRW, Allen PS. Estimation of the brain iron in vivo by means of the interecho time dependence of image contrast. *Magn Reson Med.* 1996;**36**:153–8.

27. Gorell JM, Ordidge RJ, Brown GG, *et al.* Increased iron-related MRI contrast in the substantia nigra in Parkinson's disease. *Neurology.* 1995;**45**:1138–43.

28. Graham JM, Paley MNJ, Grunewald RA, Hoggard N, Griffiths PD. Brain iron deposition in Parkinson's disease imaged using the PRIME magnetic resonance sequence. *Brain.* 2000;**123**:2423–31.

29. Wallis LI, Paley MN, Graham JM, *et al.* MRI assessment of basal ganglia iron deposition in Parkinson's disease. *J Magn Reson Imaging.* 2008;**28**:1061–7.

30. Martin WRW, Ye FQ, Allen PS. Increasing striatal iron content associated with normal aging. *Mov Disord.* 1998;**13**:281–6.

31. Ye FQ, Allen PS, Martin WRW. Basal ganglia iron content in Parkinson's disease measured with magnetic resonance. *Mov Disord.* 1996;**11**:243–9.

32. Fearnley JM, Lees AJ. Ageing and Parkinson's disease: substantia nigra regional selectivity. *Brain.* 1991;**114**:2283–301.

33. Wild JM, Martin WRW, Allen PS. A multiple gradient echo sequence optimized for rapid, single scan mapping of R2* at high B0. *Magn Reson Med.* 2002;**48**:867–76.

34. Martin WRW, Wieler M, Gee M. Midbrain iron content in early Parkinson disease: a potential biomarker of disease status. *Neurology.* 2008;**70**;1411–17.

35. Michaeli S, Oz G, Sorce DJ, *et al.* Assessment of brain iron and neuronal integrity in patients with Parkinson's disease using novel MRI contrasts. *Mov Disord.* 2007;**22**:334–40.

36. Nestrasil I, Michaeli S, Liimatainen T, *et al.* T1rho and T2rho MRI in the evaluation of Parkinson's disease. *J Neurol.* 2010;**257**:964–8.

37. Péran P, Cherubini A, Assogna F, *et al.* Magnetic resonance imaging markers of Parkinson's disease nigrostriatal signature. *Brain.* 2010;**133**:3423–33.

38. Du G, Lewis MM, Styner M, *et al.* Combined R2* and diffusion tensor imaging changes in the substantia nigra in Parkinson's disease. *Mov Disord.* 2011; **26**:1627–32.

39. Baudrexel S, Nürnberger L, Rüb U, *et al.* Quantitative mapping of T1 and T2* discloses nigral and brainstem pathology in early Parkinson's disease. *Neuroimage.* 2010;**51**:512–20.

40. Berg D, Roggendorf W, Schroder U, *et al.* Echogenicity of the substantia nigra: association with increased iron content and marker for susceptibility to nigrostriatal injury. *Arch Neurol.* 2002;**59**:999–1005.

41. Duyn JH, van Gelderen P, Li TQ, *et al.* High-field MRI of brain cortical substructure based on signal phase. *Proc Natl Acad Sci U S A.* 2007;**104**:11796–801.

42. Zhang J, Zhang Y, Wang J, *et al.* Characterizing iron deposition in Parkinson's disease using susceptibility-weighted imaging: an in vivo MR study. *Brain Res.* 2010;**1330**:124–30.

43. Mitsumori F, Watanabe H, Takaya N. Estimation of brain iron concentration in vivo using a linear relationship between regional iron and apparent transverse relaxation rate of the tissue water at 4.7 T. *Magn Reson Med.* 2009;**62**:1326–30.

44. Schafer A, Wharton S, Gowland P, Bowtell R. Using magnetic field simulation to study susceptibility-related phase contrast in gradient echo MRI. *Neuroimage.* 2009;**48**:126–37.

45. Wharton S, Bowtell R. Whole-brain susceptibility mapping at high field: a comparison of

multiple- and single-orientation methods. *Neuroimage*. 2010;**53**:515–25.

46. Schweser F, Deistung A, Lehr BW, Reichenbach JR. Quantitative imaging of intrinsic magnetic tissue properties using MRI signal phase: an approach to in vivo brain iron metabolism? *Neuroimage*. 2011;**54**:2789–807.

47. Haacke EM, Mittal S, Wu Z, Neelavalli J, Cheng Y-CN. Susceptibility-weighted imaging: technical aspects and clinical applications, Part 1. *AJNR Am J Neuroradiol*. 2009;**30**:19–30.

48. Walsh AJ, Wilman AH. Susceptibility phase imaging with comparison to R2* mapping of iron-rich deep grey matter. *Neuroimage*. 2011;**57**:452–61.

49. Lotfipour AK, Wharton S, Schwarz ST, *et al*. High resolution magnetic susceptibility mapping of the substantia nigra in Parkinson's disease. *J Magn Reson Imaging*. 2012;**35**:48–55.

50. Vaillancourt DE, Spraker MB, Prodoehl J, *et al*. High-resolution diffusion tensor imaging in the substantia nigra of de novo Parkinson disease. *Neurology*. 2009;**72**:1378–84.

51. Dormont D, Ricciardi KG, Tande D, *et al*. Is the subthalamic nucleus hypointense on T2-weighted images? A correlation study using MR imaging and stereotactic atlas data. *AJNR Am J Neuroradiol*. 2004;**25**:1516–23.

52. Slavin KV, Thulborn KR, Wess C, Nersesyan H. Direct visualization of the human subthalamic nucleus with 3 T MR imaging. *AJNR Am J Neuroradiol*. 2006;**27**:80–4.

53. Vertinsky AT, Coenen VA, Lang DJ, *et al*. Localization of the subthalamic nucleus: optimization with susceptibility-weighted phase MR imaging. *AJNR Am J Neuroradiol*. 2009;**30**:1717–24.

54. O'Gorman RL, Shmueli K, Ashkan K, *et al*. Optimal MRI methods for direct stereotactic targeting of the subthalamic nucleus and globus pallidus. *Eur Radiol*. 2011;**21**:130–6.

55. Schäfer A, Forstmann BU, Neumann J, *et al*. Direct visualization of the subthalamic nucleus and its iron distribution using high-resolution susceptibility mapping. *Hum Brain Mapp*. 2012;**33**:2831–42.

56. Xiao Y, Beriault S, Pike GB, Collins DL. Multicontrast multiecho FLASH MRI for targeting the subthalamic nucleus. *Magn Reson Imaging*. 2012;**30**:627–40.

57. Boelmans K, Holst B, Hackius M, *et al*. Brain iron deposition fingerprints in Parkinson's disease and progressive supranuclear palsy. *Mov Disord*. 2012;**27**:421–7.

58. Wang Y, Butros SR, Shuai X, *et al*. Different iron-deposition patterns of multiple system atrophy with predominant parkinsonism and idiopathic Parkinson diseases demonstrated by phase-corrected susceptibility-weighted imaging. *AJNR Am J Neuroradiol*. 2012;**33**:266–73.

59. Kraft E, Trenkwalder C, Auer DP. T2*-weighted MRI differentiates multiple system atrophy from Parkinson's disease. *Neurology*. 2002;**59**:1265–7.

60. von Lewinski F, Werner C, Jorn T, *et al*. T2*-weighted MRI in diagnosis of multiple system atrophy: a practical approach for clinicians. *J Neurol*. 2007;**254**:1184–8.

61. Brar S, Henderson D, Schenck J, Zimmerman EA. Iron accumulation in the substantia nigra of patients with Alzheimer disease and parkinsonism. *Arch Neurol*. 2009;**66**:371–4.

62. Oikawa H, Sasaki M, Tamakawa Y, Ehara S, Tohyama K. The substantia nigra in Parkinson disease: proton density-weighted spin-echo and fast short inversion time inversion-recovery MR findings. *AJNR Am J Neuroradiol*. 2002;**23**:1747–56.

63. Halliday G, Reyes S, Double K. Substantia nigra, ventral tegmental area and retrorubral fields. In: Mai JK, Paxinos G, editors. *The Human Nervous System*, 3rd edition. London: Elsevier; 2012. 439–55.

64. Adachi M, Hosoya T, Haku T, Yamaguchi K, Kawanami T. Evaluation of the substantia nigra in patients with Parkinsonian syndrome accomplished using multishot diffusion weighted MR imaging. *AJNR Am J Neuroradiol*. 1999;**20**:1500–6.

65. Damier P, Hirsch EC, Agid Y, Graybiel AM. The substantia nigra of the human brain. I. Nigrosomes and the nigral matrix, a compartmental organization based on calbindin D28K immunohistochemistry. *Brain*. 1999;**122**:1421–36.

66. Morel A, Loup F, Magnin M, Jeanmonod D. Neurochemical organization of the human basal ganglia: anatomofunctional territories defined by the distributions of calcium-binding proteins and SMI-32. *J Comp Neurol*. 2002;**443**:86–103.

67. Duyn JH, Koretsky AP. Novel frontiers in ultra-structural and molecular MRI of the brain. *Curr Opin Neurol*. 2011;**24**:386–93.

68. Kwon DH, Kim JM, Oh SH, *et al*. Seven-tesla magnetic resonance images of the substantia nigra in Parkinson disease. *Ann Neurol*. 2012;**71**:267–77.

69. Bilgic B, Pfefferbaum A, Rohlfing T, Sullivan EV, Adalsteinsson E. MRI estimates of brain iron concentration in normal aging using quantitative susceptibility mapping. *Neuroimage*. 2012;**59**:2625–35.

70. Langkammer C, Schweser F, Krebs N, *et al*. Quantitative susceptibility mapping (QSM) as a means to measure brain iron? A post mortem validation study. *Neuroimage*. 2012;**62**:1593–9.

25

Motor Parkinson's disease and structure

Stephane Lehericy, Cyril Poupon, and Cecile Gallea

Abstract

Magnetic resonance imaging (MRI) has long been unable to demonstrate changes in people with Parkinson's disease (PD). Recently, progress in MR sequences has provided improved contrast and enabled better visualization of deep brain nuclei, in particular the substantia nigra (SN) and the locus coeruleus (LC). Other developments in quantitative imaging, including relaxometry, magnetization transfer, and diffusion imaging, have provided useful insights into the neurodegeneration of PD that can aid in monitoring disease progression and improving understanding of the pathophysiology of parkinsonian syndromes. These advances in structural imaging are complemented by findings from functional connectivity studies that have used resting-state functional MRI (fMRI). This chapter presents an overview of new structural, quantitative, and resting-state fMRI techniques in parkinsonian syndromes.

Introduction

Idiopathic Parkinson's disease (PD) is the most common neurodegenerative cause of parkinsonism. Severe loss of the dopaminergic projection neurons of the substantia nigra (SN) is considered to be a hallmark of PD [1–3]. This degeneration results in further loss of dopaminergic innervation in the striatum, and is also often accompanied by extensive extranigral pathology [3].

Conventional magnetic resonance (MR) imaging (MRI) techniques typically have failed to show changes in PD or only demonstrated non-specific findings [4]. However, advanced MR techniques have provided useful information in PD. These techniques include new MR contrasts and image analysis techniques, and quantitative imaging, including relaxometry, diffusion imaging, and magnetization transfer (Table 3.1). Tractography and resting-state fMRI (rs-fMRI) have also been used to investigate anatomical and functional connectivity respectively in the brains of PD patients. It is now clear that MRI of the SN has the potential to quantify pathology and follow disease progression of PD.

This chapter reviews MR techniques from conventional structural MRI to advanced MRI (volumetry, magnetization transfer [MT], neuromelanin imaging, diffusion imaging, and rs-fMRI) and outlines the ways in which these techniques may be used to detect changes in the brain of PD patients and their relationships with parkinsonian symptoms.

Imaging methods
Structural imaging

Structural imaging refers to techniques that allow visualization of the anatomy of the brain. Structural imaging is used to assess various parameters such as volume, thickness, surface, or shape of brain regions. These parameters can be obtained manually or using automated tissue classification and segmentation methods.

Acquisition techniques

MR sequences that are commonly used for imaging brain structure include T_1-weighted three-dimensional datasets with high gray/white matter contrast. Such sequences allow accurate segmentation of the cortex as well as some subcortical structures such as the striatum (putamen, caudate nucleus), the globus pallidus, and the thalamus, although the inner boundary of the globus pallidus and the outer boundary of

Magnetic Resonance Imaging in Movement Disorders, ed. Paul Tuite and Alain Dagher. Published by Cambridge University Press. © Cambridge University Press 2013.

Table 3.1. Magnetic resonance imaging techniques

Method	Techniques	Measures	Information
Imaging techniques			
Structural	T_1w, T_2w, IR, MT	Volume, shape, surface, thickness	Morphometry
	Neuromelanin-sensitive	Signal intensity	Presence of melanin-containing cells
Functional	Resting-state fMRI	BOLD signal fluctuations	Functional connectivity within brain networks
Quantitative techniques			
Magnetization transfer	Images with (M_T) and without (M_0) MT pulse	MT ratio (MTR = $M_0 - M_T/M_0$)	Degree of myelination, axonal density
Relaxometry	T_1: T_2/T_2^*: multi-echo sequence	T_1, T_2, T_2^* $R_1 = 1/T_1$, $R_2 = 1/T_2$ $R_2^* = 1/T_2^*$	Microscopic architecture of brain tissue. Brain iron (T_2/T_2^*)
Susceptibility-weighted imaging	Phase images	Susceptibility	Brain iron
Diffusion imaging	DWI, DTI, HARDI Tractography	FA, GFA, MD, eigenvalues (lambdas) Number of tracks, probability of connection	Diffusion of water in biological tissues. Fiber tract-specific reconstruction

BOLD, blood oxygen level-dependent contrast; DTI, diffusion tensor imaging; DWI, diffusion-weighted imaging; FA, fractional anisotropy; GFA, generalized fractional anisotropy; HARDI, high angular resolution diffusion imaging; IR, inversion recovery; MD, mean diffusivity; MT, magnetization transfer; MTR, magnetization transfer ratio; T_1, T_1 relaxation time; T_2, T_2 relaxation time; T_2^*, gradient echo T_2 relaxation time; T_1w, T_1-weighted; T_2w, T_2-weighted; R_1, T_1 relaxation rate; R_2, T_2 relaxation rate; R_2^*, T_2^* relaxation rate.

the thalamus are less visible. Several basal structures (SN and subthalamic nucleus [STN], globus pallidus) and other midbrain nuclei (red nucleus) contain high iron levels [4], a property which shortens T_1 and reduces visibility on T_1-weighted sequences. On the other hand, increased iron content shortens T_2 and T_2^*, which reduces signal and provides good contrast on T_2- and T_2^*-weighted sequences. Increasing the static field of MRI systems is therefore indicated to reinforce the contrast between deep structures characterized by a high level of iron concentration and the rest of the brain. Better delineation of the SN and STN is thus obtained using 7T MRI, which also provides increased spatial resolution [5–8]. In addition, improved visualization of the SN and STN is also obtained using MT contrast [9], neuromelanin-sensitive sequences, MT (see below), or various inversion recovery sequences (Figure 3.1) [10, 11]. Neuromelanin-sensitive techniques use the paramagnetic T_1-shortening effects of neuromelanin when combined with metals such as iron and copper [12]. Neuromelanin is a pigment produced in noradrenergic neurons. Neuromelanin is present in

neurons of the pars compacta of the substantia nigra (SNc) and the locus coeruleus (LC) [13, 14]. The LC and SNc appear as areas of high neuromelanin-sensitive images (Figure 3.1) [15–17].

Data analysis

Region of interest

Regions of interest (ROI) can be segmented manually or using automated software. Structures such as the striatum, globus pallidus, and thalamus can be segmented automatically [18, 19]. Smaller structures such as the STN and SN are segmented manually. Tractography-based diffusion techniques are further used to segment the striatum, SN, and thalamus in sensorimotor, associative, and limbic territories based on connectivity profiles with the cortex [20–22]. Limitations of manual segmentation include inaccuracy in the definition of structural boundaries and require prior anatomical knowledge and training of the examiner. Manual segmentation is subject to inter- and intra-rater variability.

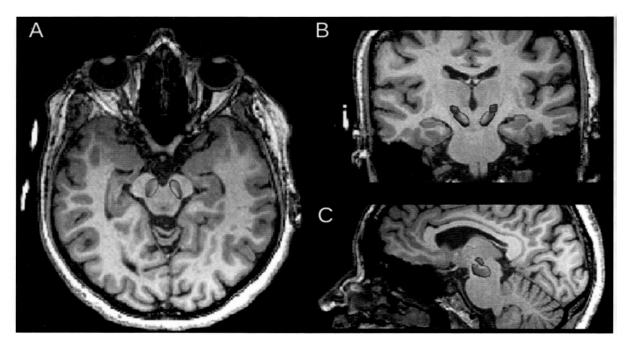

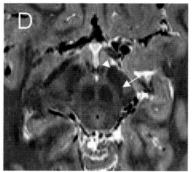 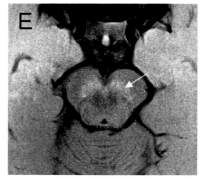 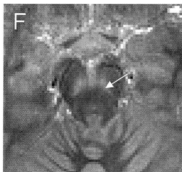

Figure 3.1 Anatomy of the substantia nigra. Three-dimensional reconstruction of the SN (yellow) and the sensorimotor territory of the STN (red) obtained using a postmortem atlas [141] superimposed on (A) axial, (B) coronal, and (C) sagittal T_1-weighted MR images of a control brain. (D) Axial T_2-weighted, (E) neuromelanin-sensitive, and (F) magnetization transfer images showing the SN (arrow). Contours of the SN differ depending on the type of contrast: in T_2-weighted images (D), the ventral limit of the area of reduced signal intensity extends into the cerebral peduncle (arrow) whereas in the neuromelanin-sensitive image (E), the area of high signal intensity is smaller and more posterior, probably restricted to the SNc.

Automated methods

One of the most popular methods to study the anatomical differences between groups of subjects is voxel-based morphometry (VBM). VBM is sensitive to structural differences in gray matter, white matter or cerebrospinal fluid between groups of subjects. The first step of VBM is spatial normalization, which removes positional and global volume differences.

Local changes in gray or white matter density are then detected by comparing voxel-by-voxel differences in the intensity of tissue maps after smoothing [23]. VBM is a whole brain statistical analysis, automated by software, and not dependent on rater abilities. Another widely used method relies on measurements of *cortical thickness* [19, 24, 25]. Following cortical segmentation of the cerebral cortex, topographic

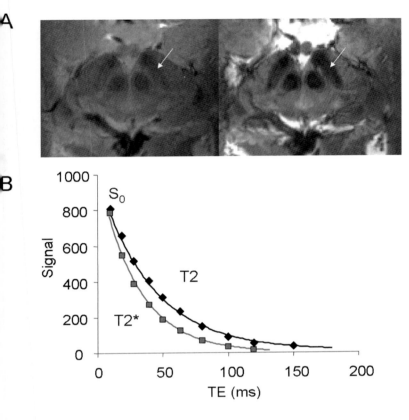

Figure 3.2 Relaxometry of the substantia nigra. (A) T_2^*-weighted MR images of the SN at short (left) and long (right) echo times. At longer echo times, signal will drop variably depending on local tissue properties. As the SN contains iron, signal decrease is greater than in the surrounding tissue (arrow). (B) Signal decrease with echo time presents an exponential decay. The T_2 (black diamonds) and T_2^* (gray squares) relaxation times correspond to the time taken to return to two-thirds of the baseline value (in milliseconds) and can be calculated using the formula $S = S0^*e^{-TE/T2}$. The R_2 and R_2^* relaxation rates correspond to $1/T_2$ and $1/T_2^*$ respectively. As T_2^*-weighted images are more sensitive to susceptibility effects due to iron deposition, signal will decrease more rapidly than in T_2 images. In PD, T_2^* is decreased and R_2^* is increased as a consequence of increased iron load (not shown).

measurements of the cortical differences can be calculated, such as thickness, surface area, and curvature. These measurements are regionally specific and the cortex is parceled out into gyral-based parcels [19, 24, 25]. Other structural methods are based on shape features. Shape features are extracted using spherical harmonics, a parametric description approach of structure boundaries [26, 27], or invariant moments [28].

Quantitative MRI techniques

Quantitative MRI is increasingly used to investigate the physical properties of water that generate the MRI contrast. Quantitative MRI provides markers that characterize tissue properties [29]. These markers can be used as surrogate parameters for diagnosis, prognosis, and monitoring of disease progression. Major contrast parameters include relaxation times and rates, magnetization transfer ratio (MTR), and diffusion parameters, including fractional anisotropy (FA) and mean diffusivity (MD). Despite their high

sensitivity to tissue differences, FA and MD are most often not specific to the underlying tissue microstructure, and consequently provide limited insights about the pathophysiology. Quantitative imaging provides parameter maps that can be analyzed using the ROI method or voxel by voxel in the entire image.

Relaxometry

The contrast underlying structural MRI results from T_1 and T_2 relaxation times. During the acquisition of an MR image, a radiofrequency pulse is used to modify the longitudinal (T_1) and transversal (T_2) components of the MR signal (Figure 3.2). Following the radiofrequency pulse, the T_1 and T_2 components return to equilibrium via exponential increase (for T_1 relaxation) and decrease (for T_2 relaxation). T_1 and T_2 relaxation times correspond to the time constant of this exponential function, and characterize how fast water magnetization returns to equilibrium after perturbation by a radiofrequency pulse. R_1 and R_2 relaxation rates correspond to $1/T_1$ and $1/T_2$ respectively.

29

T_1 relaxation time reflects interactions between protons and the lattice and behaves like the "magnetic plasticity" of the tissue. T_2 relaxation time reflects interactions between protons themselves. Relaxation times are therefore characteristic of tissue composition and depend on its molecular structure. The apparent transverse relaxation time T_2^* (T_2 star) takes into account the contribution of the macroscopic (linked to hardware imperfection or to the presence of tissue interfaces characterized by a significant gradient of susceptibility) and microscopic (linked to the tissue microstructure) inhomogeneities of the magnetic field. Structures which accumulate iron appear hypointense on T_2- and T_2^*-weighted MR images, and many experiments have shown that the relaxation rates R_2 and R_2^* are non-invasive estimates of iron content [30–32]. Methods have been described to obtain rapid determination of the T_1 relaxation time such as the driven equilibrium single pulse observation of T_1 (DESPOT1) which provides better delineation of the SN [22, 33, 34]. Improved relaxation measurement techniques have recently been proposed based on adiabatic pulse sequences, known as $T1_\rho$ and $T_{2\rho}$ [22, 35, 36]. $T_{2\rho}$ may be sensitive to iron content whereas $T_{1\rho}$ may provide an indication of neuronal loss [37]. Susceptibility-weighted imaging (SWI) uses the magnetic susceptibility differences in brain tissues. Changes in iron concentration result in changes in the phase of the tissue relative to its surroundings that can be used to quantify iron load [4, 7, 8, 38].

Magnetization transfer

MT imaging relies on the transfer of energy between highly bound protons and mobile protons of free water [39]. In the basal ganglia and brainstem nuclei, MT imaging increases contrast with the surrounding white matter, resulting in more accurate delineation and improved visualization of these structures [22, 40]. MT is a quantitative imaging technique allowing calculation of the MTR, which is expressed by the difference between the signal intensity of the images before (M_0) and after (M_T) the MT saturation pulse divided by the baseline signal (MTR = $M_0 - M_T/M_0$) [41]. Highly bound protons linked to macromolecules are present within structures such as myelin and the amount of MT is thought to correlate with the degree of myelination [42] and axonal density [43]. MT is therefore considered a quantitative measure of myelin content.

Diffusion imaging

Molecular diffusion refers to the random translational motion of molecules that results from their natural thermal energy. Diffusion-weighted imaging (DWI) is an MRI technique rendered sensitive to water diffusion through the application of magnetic field gradient pulses [44]. Diffusion tensor imaging (DTI) requires the application of strong diffusion gradients in at least six directions. Diffusion imaging allows the calculation of several indexes that characterize the overall displacement of molecules and presence of obstacles to diffusion (i.e., MD), the orientation of diffusion (i.e., FA), and the diffusion directions along the main direction of diffusion (axial or longitudinal diffusivity) and perpendicular to it (radial or transverse diffusivity) [44]. The directional dependence of diffusion is a property called anisotropy, which describes the spatial variations of water molecular displacements. Anisotropy relates to the presence of oriented structures such as axons in fiber bundles. At the cellular level, factors such as membrane, myelin, longitudinal filaments, and cytoskeleton contribute to anisotropy, with membrane properties being probably the main contributor [44]. It is generally accepted that changes in axial diffusivity mainly reflect axonal damage whereas changes in radial diffusivity reflect myelin damage. Because of the lack of specificity of the anisotropy and diffusivities, diffusion microscopy techniques were developed to probe directly tissue features such as mean axon radius and neurite density. Similar methodological developments are conducted to characterize cell size and density within the gray matter [45–47] and to quantify non-Gaussian water diffusion using diffusion kurtosis imaging [48].

Anatomical and functional connectivity
Anatomical connectivity

Anatomical connectivity can be assessed using tractography, a method that allows tracking of fiber bundles in the brain using dedicated software. Fiber tracts are reconstructed by assuming that the main direction of diffusion in a voxel indicates the local orientation of white matter fibers. Tractography algorithms have been proposed, including deterministic algorithms [49] and probabilistic algorithms which provide statistical indexes of tract probability [50]. Diffusion measures can be obtained within the specific fiber tracts as well as various measures of connectivity,

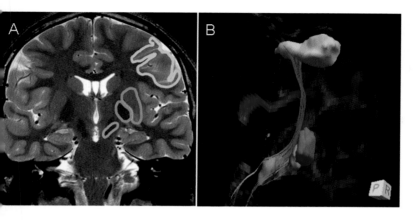

Figure 3.3 Tractography of the substantia nigra. (A) Coronal T$_2$-weighted image showing the SN (orange), the putamen (pink), the globus pallidus (green) and the motor cortex (yellow). (B) Fibers connecting the SN and the lenticular nucleus and the lenticular nucleus to the sensorimimotor cortex are superimposed on color-coded multiplanar FA maps.

including the number of tracts or connection probability between brain regions. This approach has been used successfully for the nigrostriatal and nigrothalamic fiber tracts (Figure 3.3) [51]. Tractography has also been successfully used to parcel out the basal ganglia into specific territories [20, 22, 52].

Functional connectivity

Functional connectivity (FC) between brain regions refers to temporal correlations between spatially remote neurophysiological events, as measured by fMRI blood oxygen level-dependent (BOLD) signal [53]. At rest, BOLD signal presents low frequency, spontaneous, and in some cases coherent signal fluctuations [54]. rs-fMRI studies have thus revealed correlations or "synchrony" of BOLD signal fluctuations in distributed cortical and subcortical functional brain networks (Figure 3.4). Such connectivity may or may not also involve a structural connection [55]. Several methods have been proposed to extract these networks from rs-fMRI data [56, 57].

MR imaging of the substantia nigra in PD

The SN is divided into two functionally and anatomically distinct regions, the SNc and the SN pars reticulata (SNr). The SNc neurons project to the striatum, the globus pallidus, the subthalamic nucleus, the anterior thalamic nuclei, and the prefrontal cortex. The SNr neurons predominantly project to the ventral thalamic nuclei and prefrontal cortex and receive afferents from the striatum, external globus pallidus, and STN [58, 59]. In the classical model of PD, motor features appear as a result of preferential degeneration in the sensorimotor

territory of the basal ganglia [60]. This model is supported by postmortem data, showing that a loss of dopaminergic cells predominates in the ventrolateral SNc [1, 61] with a corresponding loss of dopaminergic innervation in the posterior putamen [62].

MR imaging changes are summarized in Figure 3.5. Most studies using conventional T$_1$-weighted and T$_2$-weighted imaging and voxel-based types of analysis have been unsuccessful for detecting changes in the SN of PD patients [63, 64]. Recent developments in MR techniques have improved the visualization of the SN and detecting quantitative changes in the structure and signal within the structure. These changes include reduced T$_2$ and T$_2^*$ relaxation times, indicating increased iron load, reduced FA, reduced probability of connection between the SN and the striatum and thalamus, as well as abnormal shape at higher field strength.

New contrasts have provided better results for the detection of changes in the SN of PD patients. Inversion recovery images allowed accurate classification of PD patients from controls [10, 11]. Changes predominated in the lateral segments of the SN [10, 11] in line with the preferential degeneration of dopaminergic neurons in the caudal and lateral SN [60]. Using MT contrast, reduced SN volume was detected in PD patients compared with control subjects [22]. The MTR was also significantly reduced in the SN as well as other basal ganglia (globus pallidus, putamen, caudate nucleus) in PD patients [65, 66].

Using the neuromelanin-sensitive technique, reduced signal intensity was evidenced in the SNc of PD patients, suggesting depletion of neuromelanin-containing neurons [15].

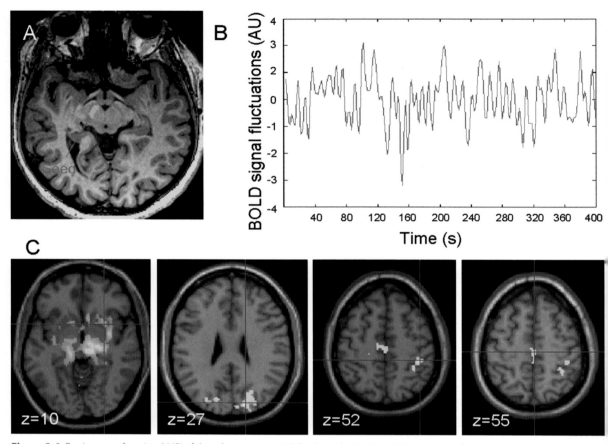

Figure 3.4 Resting-state functional MRI of the substantia nigra. (A) Seed voxel in the SN. (B) Time course of resting BOLD signal change in the SN of a control subject. (C) Statistical parametric mapping map of basal ganglia and cortical regions in which BOLD signal fluctuations were significantly correlated with signal fluctuations in the SN. Yellow color indicates greater correlations.

In the SN of PD patients, T_2/T_2^* relaxation times are decreased and R_2/R_2^* relaxation rates are increased [31, 38, 67–73]. Changes were interpreted as reflecting increased iron content. R_2^* changes predominated in the lateral SNc [68], in line with the predominance of cell loss that has been reported in the lateral part of the SN in histological studies [1]. Changes in R_2^* correlated with the motor score of the Unified Parkinson's Disease Rating Scale (UPDRS) [68]. However, some studies did not find any change in T_2 in PD patients [36] or observed a change only in a particular subgroup [31]. Reduced T_1 was also measured in the SN of PD patients [73]. Better results may be obtained using adiabatic T2ρ for detecting iron-related changes in the SN of PD patients and T1ρ also indicated neuronal loss in the SN in these patients [36].

Changes in diffusion have been reported in the SN of PD patients. Most studies reported reduced anisotropy in early PD patients (Hoehn and Yahr 1–2) [69, 70, 74–77], others did not [22, 51]. Using R_2^* and FA changes in the SN, PD patients were discriminated from control subjects with 95% global accuracy using logistic regression and receiver operating characteristic (ROC) curves [69]. Diffusion kurtosis was also increased in PD patients [78]. In contrast, diffusivity was mostly unchanged in the SN and the basal ganglia of PD patients using either ROI measurements or VBM [79, 80].

Using tractography, reduced connectivity was observed in PD patients between the SN and ipsilateral putamen and thalamus, as well as a trend towards reduced connectivity of the SN with the left caudate and globus pallidus [51]. Automated diffusion-based parcellation of SN subregions showed that the SNr and SNc in PD patients showed a general atrophy [22]. These data suggest that tractography has the

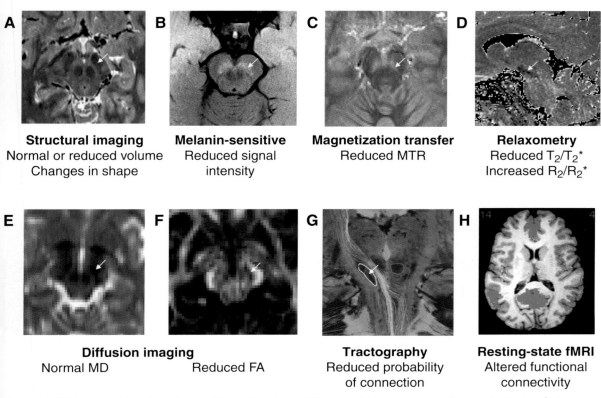

Figure 3.5 MR imaging of the substantia nigra. (A) Axial T_2-weighted, (B) neuromelanin-sensitive, and (C) magnetization transfer images, (D) sagittal T_2 relaxation time map, (E) axial mean diffusivity, and (F) fractional anisotropy maps, (G) coronal tractography image, and (H) functional connectivity map. The main results obtained with each one of the techniques is presented below each image. The SN is shown using arrows.

potential to investigate anatomical connection probability between basal ganglia regions in PD patients [22, 51].

Ultra-high-field MRI such as 7T offers improved contrast and increased spatial resolution (Figure 3.6). At higher field strength, the T_2^* effect due to iron deposition is greatly increased, allowing better visualization of basal ganglia contours and shapes. In PD, changes in the shape of the SN were reported [5, 81]. The boundary between the SN and crus cerebri had lost its smoothness and presented undulation in PD subjects that was confirmed using shape analysis [5]. Another difference with control subjects was that the brighter signal region observed along the dorsomedial surface of the lateral portion of SN in control subjects presented abnormal hypointensity in T_2^*-weighted images in PD subjects. It is therefore expected that the increased spatial resolution and new contrasts provided by 7T will further improve detection of anatomical alterations in PD.

Other brainstem nuclei

In idiopathic PD, there is extensive extranigral pathology in histological studies [3]. This extranigral pathology has been observed in the medulla oblongata, the reticular formation, and the pontine tegmentum; the coeruleus–subcoeruleus complex; the basal forebrain; and nuclei of the thalamus and amygdala. Cases with severe damage usually show lesions reaching the neocortex. MRI has been successful in detecting neurodegeneration in some of these nuclei.

The locus coeruleus

In PD patients, neuromelanin-sensitive images have shown reduced signal intensity in the LC compared with controls (Figure 3.7) [15]. Reduced signal intensity may reflect a loss of neuromelanin-containing neurons and a decrease in intracellular neuromelanin

33

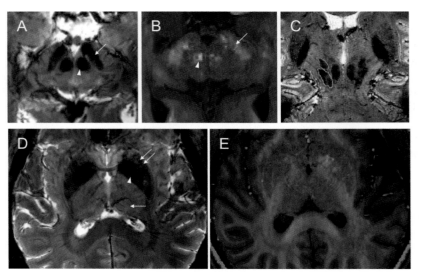

Figure 3.6 7T MRI of the substantia nigra. (A) Axial gradient echo T$_2$-weighted image of the midbrain passing at the level of the SN (arrow) and the red nucleus (arrowhead), (B) FA map passing at the same level. High FA values (in yellow colors) are observed in the cerebral peduncles (arrow) and the decussation of the superior cerebellar peduncles (arrowhead), (C) coronal gradient echo T$_2$-weighted image of the basal ganglia and thalamus. The SN is outlined in yellow, the red nucleus in pink, and the subthalamic nucleus in green. (D) Axial gradient echo T$_2$-weighted image of the midbrain passing at the level of the putamen (double arrows), globus pallidus (arrowhead), and and the thalamus (arrow), E) color-coded FA map at the same level.

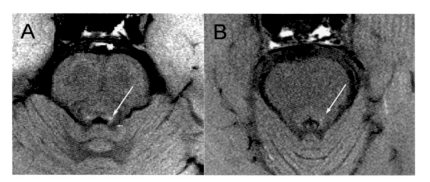

Figure 3.7 Neuromelanin-sensitive imaging of the locus coeruleus. Axial neuromelanin-sensitive T$_1$-weighted images of the LC in a control subject (A) and a patient with PD (B). The LC (arrow) is visible as areas of increased signal intensity (repetition time[TR]/echo time [TE]/flip angle: 600 ms/15/90°, voxel size: $0.4 \times 0.4 \times 3mm^3$).

content. Further studies are needed to confirm this finding and correlate it with clinical signs such as sleep, attention, or cognitive disorders.

Pontine reticular formation

Diffusion changes have been evidenced in patients with idiopathic rapid eye movement (REM) sleep behavior disorder (RBD). RBD is a sleep disorder characterized by the loss of normal skeletal muscle atonia during REM sleep with prominent motor activity accompanying dreaming [82]. RBD can be idiopathic (iRBD), that is, in the absence of any other neurological disorders, or secondary, that is, associated with other neurological illnesses such as PD [83, 84]. RBD is considered as an early premotor

condition in PD as RBD subjects commonly develop parkinsonism and cognitive impairment with time [83, 84]. iRBD patients showed decreases in FA in the tegmentum of the midbrain and rostral pons and increases of MD within the pontine reticular formation and midbrain [85]. Microstructural changes were also reported in the white matter of the brainstem, and the SN as well as other cortical regions, including the right visual stream, in patients with iRBD [86].

Cortical lesions

Using voxel-based or ROI methods, brain structure was often normal in PD [79, 87–92]. Volumetric studies of the brainstem reported normal volumes

[93, 94] and rate of atrophy [88]. Some studies reported decreased cortical volumes or thickness in cognitively intact PD patients mainly in frontal regions [95–97], but also in more widespread cortical areas [98–101]. Most often, reported changes were mild in cognitively intact patients. However, cortical atrophy accelerates with disease progression in frontotemporal regions [102].

The neuroanatomical correlates of various motor and non-motor dysfunctions were also investigated in PD patients. Depression in PD patients was associated with white matter loss in the right anterior cingulate bundle and orbitofrontal regions [103], gray matter loss in orbitofrontal regions and the right superior temporal pole [89], and increased gray matter in the mediodorsal region of the thalamus [104]. Scores on the Depression Rating Scale correlated with white matter [103] or gray matter loss in these regions [89]. In some studies, visual hallucinations were observed in patients with widespread atrophy in limbic, paralimbic, and neocortical areas [105, 106] whereas others did not find any gray matter differences between patients with and without visual hallucinations [98]. Freezing of gait was associated with reduced gray matter in posterior cortical regions that correlated with severity [90]. Increased prefrontal volume was reported in patients with levodopa-induced dyskinesias that may indicate aberrant neural plasticity [91]. Cognitive symptoms were also related to specific neurodegenerative changes (reviewed in [107, 108]). Recognition of facial emotion was found to be impaired in PD patients and was accompanied by degeneration of the orbitofrontal cortex and the amygdala and an altered decision-making in PD correlated with gray matter loss in the left lateral orbitofrontal cortex [109]. Olfactory dysfunction, a frequent non-motor symptom in idiopathic PD, was related to gray matter atrophy in olfactory regions including the piriform and amygdala [110], suggesting that this early symptom may be associated with extranigral pathology. Impaired cognition and dementia in PD were associated with more severe patterns of cortical atrophy [95, 111]. Regions predictive of cognitive decline included the hippocampus and parietotemporal regions suggesting that an Alzheimer's disease pattern of brain atrophy may be a preclinical biomarker of impaired cognition in PD patients [112].

Functional connectivity

Functional connectivity (FC) methods that take advantage of intrinsic signal fluctuations have demonstrated that the interactions of brain networks are abnormal in PD at the resting state. Resting-state BOLD fluctuations were successfully used to predict the presence of PD [113]. In one study, PD patients showed decreased coupling between the posterior putamen and the inferior parietal cortex [9], with thalamus, midbrain, pons, and cerebellum [114], and between the SN, putamen, and thalamus [115]. In contrast, the anterior putamen showed increased connectivity with the inferior parietal cortex – a finding that was interpreted as compensatory [9]. Reduction in striatal FC with the brainstem predominated in the posterior putamen as compared with the anterior striatum in line with the known gradient of striatal dopaminergic loss in PD [114]. The pattern of connectivity with both the pre-supplementary motor area (pre-SMA) and the motor cortex was changed in PD [116]. Increased FC was also reported between the STN and cortical motor and premotor areas in PD patients that may reflect increased STN–motor cortex synchronicity in the hyperdirect pathway [117]. Changes in FC varied in relation to symptoms in PD. In tremor patients, increased FC in the STN was specifically found with the hand area of M1 and the primary sensory cortex whereas in non-tremor patients, increased FC values were also found between the STN and the SMA [117]. In another study, tremor-dominant PD patients showed increased FC of the internal globus pallidus and putamen within the cerebellothalamic circuit. Also, pallidal (but not striatal) dopamine depletion correlated with clinical tremor severity [118]. These results suggested that resting tremor may result from pathological interactions between the basal ganglia and the cerebellothalamic circuit [118]. Non-motor symptoms had also distinct resting activity patterns in PD. The apathy score was best predicted by signals in the left supplementary motor cortex, the right orbitofrontal cortex, and the right middle frontal cortex, whereas depression score was best predicted by signals in the right subgenual cingulate [119]. Overall, findings with resting-state fMRI suggest that dopamine depletion in PD leads to a remapping of cerebral connectivity that affects predominantly the sensorimotor circuit and sensorimotor integration and that is differently associated with motor and non-motor symptoms.

Differential diagnosis of parkinsonian syndromes

MRI has proven useful in the differential diagnosis of the various atypical parkinsonian disorders such as progressive supranuclear palsy (PSP) and the Parkinson variant of multiple system atrophy (MSA-P). At the early stage, differentiation of these clinical entities may be difficult, and overlapping clinical presentations can lead to misdiagnosis. In PD, changes in the basal ganglia and brainstem are subtle and restricted to nuclei such as the SN and LC. Most studies did not find any global volumetric changes in the brainstem or the basal ganglia [64, 88, 93] or diffusion changes in the brainstem, putamen, and caudate nucleus in idiopathic PD [120–123]. However, a few studies reported changes in the basal ganglia of PD patients, including increased diffusivity in the striatum and thalamus [69, 77], reduced MTR in the globus pallidus [65], increased thalamic gray matter in depressed PD patients [104], or changes in susceptibility values [38].

In contrast, PSP patients present extensive changes in the brainstem, basal ganglia, and cortical regions (Figure 3.8). Midbrain atrophy is prominent in PSP, with a characteristic shape including a concave superior profile described as the "penguin" or "hummingbird" sign [124, 125]. Atrophy has been quantified in numerous ROI studies using variable indexes such as the midbrain/pons ratio, anteroposterior midbrain diameter [88, 93, 124, 126], or the MR parkinsonism index (MRPI), an index obtained by calculating pons/midbrain × MCP/SCP (middle cerebellar peduncle/superior cerebellar peduncle) ratio [126]. Using VBM, gray and white matter reductions have been constantly reported in PSP in the midbrain and more variably in the basal ganglia, the frontal cortex, the insula, and the thalamus (Figure 3.9) [92, 127–132]. Increased diffusivity has been reported in the basal ganglia [87, 133], the midbrain [79, 80, 120], the SCP [134], the precentral white matter [135], and the white matter of PSP patients [129]. PSP patients had widespread changes in T_2 relaxometry values in the caudate nucleus, putamen, and globus pallidus compared with PD patients and control subjects [136]. PSP patients also present reduced signal intensity in the putamen on gradient echo T_2 images [137].

In MSA-P, structural changes have been described that are evocative of the disease. These signs include atrophy and signal changes in the putamen (hypointensity in the dorsolateral part and hyperintense rim around the putamen), the pons (with the "hot cross bun" sign), the MCP (with atrophy and T_2 hyperintensity), as well as atrophy of the cerebellum (Figure 3.10) [79].

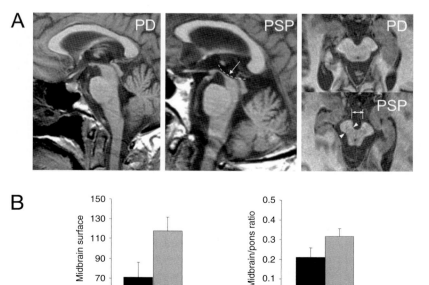

Figure 3.8 MRI in progressive supranuclear palsy. (A) Midsagittal three-dimensional T_1-weighted images (left and middle) and axial three-dimensional T_1-weighted images (right). The brainstem has a normal aspect in PD. In PSP, there is a typical hummingbird sign (arrow) with a concave superior profile of the midbrain (dashed line). On axial images, midbrain atrophy is visible as thinning of the cerebral peduncles (arrowheads), reduced anteroposterior diameter and enlarged interpeduncular cistern (double arrow). (B) Bar graphs showing reduced midbrain surface and midbrain/pons ratio in patients with PSP. (Adapted from [131].).

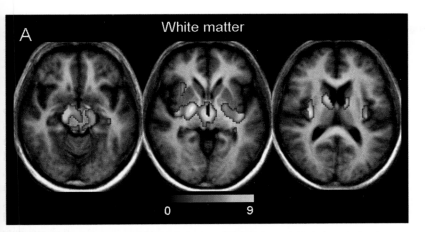

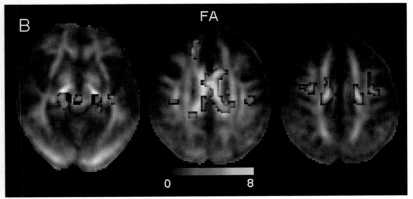

Figure 3.9 Voxel-based methods in PSP. Reduced white matter (A) and reduced FA (B) in patients with PSP is observed in the brainstem, basal ganglia, and frontal regions. (Adapted from [131].). Color bar indicates z-score.

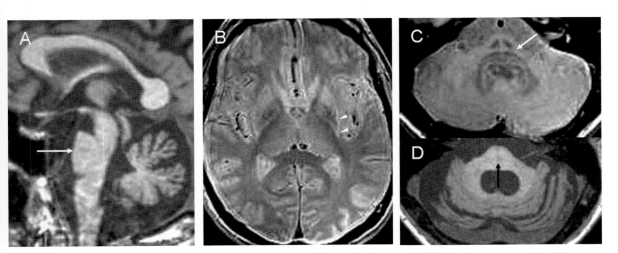

Figure 3.10 Multiple system atrophy. (A) Midsagittal three-dimensional T_1-weighted images in MSA showing severe atrophy of the pons (arrow), (B) axial proton density-weighted images showing hyperintense rim lateral to the putamen (arrowheads), (C) axial proton density-weighted image showing the "hot cross bun" sign in the pons (white arrow), (D) axial T_1-weighted image showing atrophy of the pons (arrow).

Compared with PSP, MSA-P patients have relatively greater pontine and MCP atrophy whereas PSP patients have greater atrophy of the midbrain and SCP [88, 93, 124, 126]. Using voxel-based techniques, atrophy was evidenced in the basal ganglia, cerebellum, brainstem, particularly the pons and MCP, as well as in the cortex [138, 139]. As a consequence, various quantitative measures of pontine and midbrain areas or volumes, including the pontine/midbrain areas [93] and the MRPI [126], have been suggested to discriminate accurately PSP and MSA-P from PD patients or healthy controls. Other changes include increased MD and reduced FA in the putamen, pons, and MCP [120–123], and reduced MTR in the putamen [65]. Greater iron deposition was also demonstrated in the putamen of MSA-P patients using phase-contrast susceptibility imaging [38] or relaxometry [136, 140].

In summary, MRI has shown sensitivity and specificity in distinguishing PD from other parkinsonian syndromes as well as between other causes of parkinsonism (PSP and MSA-P).

Conclusion

Research in neuroimaging has demonstrated that neuro-degeneration in parkinsonian syndromes is accessible to MRI. In particular, biomarkers were obtained in the SN of PD patients. New structural imaging contrasts provide better delineation of the SN and other brainstem nuclei. Ultra-high-field 7T MRI has shown morphological changes in the SN that were not visible at lower field. Quantitative MRI, such as MT, diffusion imaging, and relaxometry, provided markers that can be used for differential and early diagnosis of PD, and to monitor disease progression. rs-fMRI was used to investigate functional changes and pathophysiological correlates. These new imaging techniques and markers are still being evaluated and are not yet used in clinical practice. Studies are needed to assess the reproducibility of results. Increased spatial resolution and new contrasts provided by ultra-high-field MRI (7T and above) raise hope that SN imaging will further improve in the future.

Disclosures/conflict of interest

All authors report no disclosures.

References

1. Damier P, Hirsch EC, Agid Y, et al. The substantia nigra of the human brain. II. Patterns of loss of dopamine-containing neurons in Parkinson's disease. Brain. 1999;122(Pt 8):1437–48.

2. Gibb WR, Lees AJ. Anatomy, pigmentation, ventral and dorsal subpopulations of the substantia nigra, and differential cell death in Parkinson's disease. J Neurol Neurosurg Psychiatry. 1991;54:388–96.

3. Braak H, Del Tredici K, Rub U, et al. Staging of brain pathology related to sporadic Parkinson's disease. Neurobiol Aging. 2003;24:197–211.

4. Haacke EM, Cheng NY, House MJ, et al. Imaging iron stores in the brain using magnetic resonance imaging. Magn Reson Imaging. 2005;23:1–25.

5. Kwon DH, Kim JM, Oh SH, et al. Seven-Tesla magnetic resonance images of the substantia nigra in Parkinson disease. Ann Neurol. 2012;71:267–77.

6. Eapen M, Zald DH, Gatenby JC, et al. Using high-resolution MR imaging at 7T to evaluate the anatomy of the midbrain dopaminergic system. AJNR Am J Neuroradiol. 2011;32:688–94.

7. Schafer A, Forstmann BU, Neumann J, et al. Direct visualization of the subthalamic nucleus and its iron distribution using high-resolution susceptibility mapping. Hum Brain Mapp. 2012;33:2831–42.

8. Lotfipour AK, Wharton S, Schwarz ST, et al. High resolution magnetic susceptibility mapping of the substantia nigra in Parkinson's disease. J Magn Reson Imaging. 2012;35:48–55.

9. Helmich RC, Derikx LC, Bakker M, et al. Spatial remapping of cortico-striatal connectivity in Parkinson's disease. Cereb Cortex. 2009;20:1175–86.

10. Hutchinson M, Raff U, Lebedev S. MRI correlates of pathology in parkinsonism: segmented inversion recovery ratio imaging (SIRRIM). Neuroimage. 2003;20:1899–902.

11. Minati L, Grisoli M, Carella F, et al. Imaging degeneration of the substantia nigra in Parkinson disease with inversion-recovery MR imaging. AJNR Am J Neuroradiol. 2007;28:309–13.

12. Enochs WS, Petherick P, Bogdanova A, et al. Paramagnetic metal scavenging by melanin: MR imaging. Radiology. 1997;204:417–23.

13. Bazelon M, Fenichel GM, Randall J. Studies on neuromelanin. I. A melanin system in the human adult brainstem. Neurology. 1967;17:512–19.

14. Zecca L, Zucca FA, Wilms H, et al. Neuromelanin of the substantia nigra: a neuronal black hole with protective and toxic

characteristics. *Trends Neurosci.* 2003;**26**:578–80.

15. Sasaki M, Shibata E, Tohyama K, *et al.* Neuromelanin magnetic resonance imaging of locus ceruleus and substantia nigra in Parkinson's disease. *Neuroreport.* 2006;**17**:1215–18.

16. Shibata E, Sasaki M, Tohyama K, *et al.* Age-related changes in locus ceruleus on neuromelanin magnetic resonance imaging at 3 Tesla. *Magn Reson Med Sci.* 2006;**5**:197–200.

17. Keren NI, Lozar CT, Harris KC, *et al.* In vivo mapping of the human locus coeruleus. *Neuroimage.* 2009; **47**:1261–7.

18. Marrakchi-Kacem L, Delmaire C, Tucholka A, *et al.* Analysis of the striato-thalamo-cortical connectivity on the cortical surface to infer biomarkers of Huntington's disease. *Med Image Comput Comput Assist Interv.* 2011;**13**:217–24.

19. Dale AM, Fischl B, Sereno MI. Cortical surface-based analysis. I. Segmentation and surface reconstruction. *Neuroimage.* 1999;**9**:179–94.

20. Lehericy S, Ducros M, Van de Moortele PF, *et al.* Diffusion tensor fiber tracking shows distinct corticostriatal circuits in humans. *Ann Neurol.* 2004;**55**:522–9.

21. Behrens TE, Johansen-Berg H, Woolrich MW, *et al.* Non-invasive mapping of connections between human thalamus and cortex using diffusion imaging. *Nat Neurosci.* 2003;**6**:750–7.

22. Menke RA, Jbabdi S, Miller KL, *et al.* Connectivity-based segmentation of the substantia nigra in human and its implications in Parkinson's disease. *Neuroimage.* 2010; [Epub ahead of print].

23. Ashburner J, Friston KJ. Voxel-based morphometry–the methods. *NeuroImage.* 2000;**11**:805–21.

24. Makris N, Schlerf JE, Hodge SM, *et al.* MRI-based surface-assisted parcellation of human cerebellar cortex: an anatomically specified method with estimate of reliability. *Neuroimage.* 2005;**25**:1146–60.

25. Fischl B, Sereno MI, Dale AM. Cortical surface-based analysis. II: Inflation, flattening, and a surface-based coordinate system. *Neuroimage.* 1999;**9**:195–207.

26. Gerardin E, Chetelat G, Chupin M, *et al.* Multidimensional classification of hippocampal shape features discriminates Alzheimer's disease and mild cognitive impairment from normal aging. *Neuroimage.* 2009;**47**:1476–86.

27. Styner M, Lieberman JA, Pantazis D, *et al.* Boundary and medial shape analysis of the hippocampus in schizophrenia. *Med Image Anal.* 2004;**8**:197–203.

28. Sun ZY, Riviere D, Poupon F, *et al.* Automatic inference of sulcus patterns using 3D moment invariants. *Med Image Comput Comput Assist Interv.* 2007;**10**:515–22.

29. Tofts PS, editor. *Quantitative MRI of the Brain: Measuring Changes Caused by Disease.* Chichester: John Wiley & Sons Ltd.; 2003.

30. Hardy PA, Gash D, Yokel R, *et al.* Correlation of R2 with total iron concentration in the brains of rhesus monkeys. *J Magn Reson Imaging.* 2005;**21**:118–27.

31. Ordidge RJ, Gorell JM, Deniau JC, *et al.* Assessment of relative brain iron concentrations using T2-weighted and T2*-weighted MRI at 3 Tesla. *Magn Reson Med.* 1994;**32**:335–41.

32. Langkammer C, Krebs N, Goessler W, *et al.* Quantitative MR imaging of brain iron: a postmortem validation study. *Radiology.* 2010;**257**:455–62.

33. Deoni SC, Rutt BK, Peters TM. Rapid combined T1 and T2 mapping using gradient recalled acquisition in the steady state. *Magn Reson Med.* 2003;**49**: 515–26.

34. Deoni SC. High-resolution T1 mapping of the brain at 3T with driven equilibrium single pulse observation of T1 with high-speed incorporation of RF field inhomogeneities (DESPOT1-HIFI). *J Magn Reson Imaging.* 2007;**26**:1106–11.

35. Michaeli S, Grohn H, Grohn O, *et al.* Exchange-influenced T2rho contrast in human brain images measured with adiabatic radio frequency pulses. *Magn Reson Med.* 2005;**53**:823–9.

36. Michaeli S, Oz G, Sorce DJ, *et al.* Assessment of brain iron and neuronal integrity in patients with Parkinson's disease using novel MRI contrasts. *Mov Disord.* 2007;**22**:334–40.

37. Michaeli S, Sorce DJ, Springer CS, Jr., *et al.* T1rho MRI contrast in the human brain: modulation of the longitudinal rotating frame relaxation shutter-speed during an adiabatic RF pulse. *J Magn Reson.* 2006;**181**:135–47.

38. Wang Y, Butros SR, Shuai X, *et al.* Different iron-deposition patterns of multiple system atrophy with predominant parkinsonism and idiopathic Parkinson diseases demonstrated by phase-corrected susceptibility-weighted imaging. *AJNR Am J Neuroradiol.* 2012;**33**:266–73.

39. Wolff SD, Balaban RS. Magnetization transfer contrast (MTC) and tissue water proton relaxation in vivo. *Magn Reson Med.* 1989;**10**:135–44.

40. Helms G, Draganski B, Frackowiak R, *et al.* Improved segmentation of deep brain grey matter structures using magnetization transfer (MT) parameter maps. *Neuroimage.* 2009;**47**:194–8.

41. Dousset V, Grossman RI, Ramer KN, *et al.* Experimental allergic

encephalomyelitis and multiple sclerosis: lesion characterization with magnetization transfer imaging. *Radiology.* 1992;**182**:483–91.

42. Rademacher J, Engelbrecht V, Burgel U, *et al.* Measuring in vivo myelination of human white matter fiber tracts with magnetization transfer MR. *Neuroimage.* 1999;**9**:393–406.

43. van Waesberghe JH, Kamphorst W, De Groot CJ, *et al.* Axonal loss in multiple sclerosis lesions: magnetic resonance imaging insights into substrates of disability. *Ann Neurol.* 1999;**46**:747–54.

44. Le Bihan D. Looking into the functional architecture of the brain with diffusion MRI. *Nat Rev.* 2003;**4**:469–80.

45. Assaf Y, Blumenfeld-Katzir T, Yovel Y, *et al.* AxCaliber: a method for measuring axon diameter distribution from diffusion MRI. *Magn Reson Med.* 2008;**59**:1347–54.

46. Alexander DC. A general framework for experiment design in diffusion MRI and its application in measuring direct tissue-microstructure features. *Magn Reson Med.* 2008;**60**:439–48.

47. Zhang H, Schneider T, Wheeler-Kingshott CA, *et al.* NODDI: practical in vivo neurite orientation dispersion and density imaging of the human brain. *Neuroimage.* 2012;**61**:1000–16.

48. Jensen JH, Helpern JA, Ramani A, *et al.* Diffusional kurtosis imaging: the quantification of non-gaussian water diffusion by means of magnetic resonance imaging. *Magn Reson Med.* 2005;**53**: 1432–40.

49. Mori S, Crain BJ, Chacko VP, *et al.* Three-dimensional tracking of axonal projections in the brain by magnetic resonance imaging. *Ann Neurol.* 1999;**45**:265–9.

50. Dell'acqua F, Catani M. Structural human brain networks: hot topics in diffusion tractography. *Curr Opin Neurol.* 2012;**25**:375–83.

51. Menke RA, Scholz J, Miller KL, *et al.* MRI characteristics of the substantia nigra in Parkinson's disease: a combined quantitative T1 and DTI study. *Neuroimage.* 2009;**47**:435–41.

52. Draganski B, Kherif F, Kloppel S, *et al.* Evidence for segregated and integrative connectivity patterns in the human basal ganglia. *J Neurosci.* 2008;**28**:7143–52.

53. Friston KJ, Frith CD, Liddle PF, *et al.* Functional connectivity: the principal-component analysis of large (PET) data sets. *J Cereb Blood Flow Metab.* 1993;**13**:5–14.

54. Biswal B, Yetkin FZ, Haughton VM, *et al.* Functional connectivity in the motor cortex of resting human brain using echo-planar MRI. *Magn Reson Med.* 1995;**34**:537–41.

55. Honey CJ, Sporns O, Cammoun L, *et al.* Predicting human resting-state functional connectivity from structural connectivity. *Proc Natl Acad Sci U S A.* 2009;**106**:2035–40.

56. Ramnani N, Behrens TE, Penny W, *et al.* New approaches for exploring anatomical and functional connectivity in the human brain. *Biol Psychiatry.* 2004;**56**:613–19.

57. Bullmore E, Sporns O. Complex brain networks: graph theoretical analysis of structural and functional systems. *Nat Rev Neurosci.* 2009;**10**:186–98.

58. Beckstead RM, Domesick VB, Nauta WJ. Efferent connections of the substantia nigra and ventral tegmental area in the rat. *Brain Res.* 1979;**175**:191–217.

59. Haber SN. The primate basal ganglia: parallel and integrative networks. *J Chemical Neuroanat.* 2003;**26**:317–30.

60. Redgrave P, Rodriguez M, Smith Y, *et al.* Goal-directed and habitual control in the basal ganglia: implications for Parkinson's disease. *Nat Rev Neurosci.* 2010;**11**:760–72.

61. Fearnley JM, Lees AJ. Ageing and Parkinson's disease: substantia nigra regional selectivity. *Brain.* 1991;**114**(Pt 5):2283–301.

62. Kish SJ, Shannak K, Hornykiewicz O. Uneven pattern of dopamine loss in the striatum of patients with idiopathic Parkinson's disease. Pathophysiologic and clinical implications. *N Engl J Med.* 1988;**318**:876–80.

63. Oikawa H, Sasaki M, Tamakawa Y, *et al.* The substantia nigra in Parkinson disease: proton density-weighted spin-echo and fast short inversion time inversion-recovery MR findings. *AJNR Am J Neuroradiol.* 2002;**23**:1747–56.

64. Bonneville F, Welter ML, Elie C, *et al.* Parkinson disease, brain volumes, and subthalamic nucleus stimulation. *Neurology.* 2005;**64**:1598–604.

65. Eckert T, Sailer M, Kaufmann J, *et al.* Differentiation of idiopathic Parkinson's disease, multiple system atrophy, progressive supranuclear palsy, and healthy controls using magnetization transfer imaging. *Neuroimage.* 2004;**21**:229–35.

66. Tambasco N, Belcastro V, Sarchielli P, *et al.* A magnetization transfer study of mild and advanced Parkinson's disease. *Eur J Neurol.* 2011;**18**:471–7.

67. Dexter DT, Wells FR, Lees AJ, *et al.* Increased nigral iron content and alterations in other metal ions occurring in brain in Parkinson's disease. *J Neurochem.* 1989;**52**:1830–6.

68. Martin WR, Wieler M, Gee M. Midbrain iron content in early Parkinson disease: a potential biomarker of disease status. *Neurology.* 2008;**70**:1411–17.

69. Peran P, Cherubini A, Assogna F, *et al.* Magnetic resonance imaging markers of Parkinson's disease

nigrostriatal signature. *Brain.* 2010;**133**:3423–33.

70. Du G, Lewis MM, Styner M, *et al.* Combined R2* and diffusion tensor imaging changes in the substantia nigra in Parkinson's disease. *Mov Disord.* 2011;**26**:1627–32.

71. Zhang J, Zhang Y, Wang J, *et al.* Characterizing iron deposition in Parkinson's disease using susceptibility-weighted imaging: an in vivo MR study. *Brain Res.* 2010;**1330**:124–30.

72. Graham JM, Paley MN, Grunewald RA, *et al.* Brain iron deposition in Parkinson's disease imaged using the PRIME magnetic resonance sequence. *Brain.* 2000;**123**(Pt 12):2423–31.

73. Baudrexel S, Nurnberger L, Rub U, *et al.* Quantitative mapping of T1 and T2* discloses nigral and brainstem pathology in early Parkinson's disease. *Neuroimage.* 2010;**51**:512–20.

74. Yoshikawa K, Nakata Y, Yamada K, *et al.* Early pathological changes in the parkinsonian brain demonstrated by diffusion tensor MRI. *J Neurol Neurosurg Psychiatry* 2004;**75**:481–4.

75. Chan LL, Rumpel H, Yap K, *et al.* Case control study of diffusion tensor imaging in Parkinson's disease. *J Neurol Neurosurg Psychiatry* 2007;**78**:1383–6.

76. Vaillancourt DE, Spraker MB, Prodoehl J, *et al.* High-resolution diffusion tensor imaging in the substantia nigra of de novo Parkinson disease. *Neurology.* 2009;**72**:1378–84.

77. Zhan W, Kang GA, Glass GA, *et al.* Regional alterations of brain microstructure in Parkinson's disease using diffusion tensor imaging. *Mov Disord.* 2012;**27**:90–7.

78. Wang JJ, Lin WY, Lu CS, *et al.* Parkinson disease: diagnostic utility of diffusion kurtosis imaging. *Radiology* 2011;**261**:210–17.

79. Seppi K, Poewe W. Brain magnetic resonance imaging techniques in the diagnosis of parkinsonian syndromes. *Neuroimaging Clin N Am.* 2010;**20**:29–55.

80. Seppi K, Schocke MF. An update on conventional and advanced magnetic resonance imaging techniques in the differential diagnosis of neurodegenerative parkinsonism. *Curr Opin Neurol.* 2005;**18**:370–5.

81. Cho ZH, Oh SH, Kim JM, *et al.* Direct visualization of Parkinson's disease by in vivo human brain imaging using 7.0T magnetic resonance imaging. *Mov Disord.* 2011;**26**:713–18.

82. Schenck CH, Mahowald MW. REM sleep behavior disorder: clinical, developmental, and neuroscience perspectives 16 years after its formal identification in SLEEP. *Sleep.* 2002;**25**:120–38.

83. Iranzo A, Santamaria J, Rye DB, *et al.* Characteristics of idiopathic REM sleep behavior disorder and that associated with MSA and PD. *Neurology.* 2005;**65**:247–52.

84. Braak H, Del Tredici K. Invited Article: Nervous system pathology in sporadic Parkinson disease. *Neurology.* 2008;**70**:1916–25.

85. Scherfler C, Frauscher B, Schocke M, *et al.* White and gray matter abnormalities in idiopathic rapid eye movement sleep behavior disorder: a diffusion-tensor imaging and voxel-based morphometry study. *Ann Neurol.* 2010;**69**:400–7.

86. Unger MM, Belke M, Menzler K, *et al.* Diffusion tensor imaging in idiopathic REM sleep behavior disorder reveals microstructural changes in the brainstem, substantia nigra, olfactory region, and other brain regions. *Sleep.* 2010;**33**:767–73.

87. Rizzo G, Martinelli P, Manners D, *et al.* Diffusion-weighted brain imaging study of patients with clinical diagnosis of corticobasal degeneration, progressive supranuclear palsy and Parkinson's disease. *Brain.* 2008;**131**:2690–700.

88. Paviour DC, Price SL, Jahanshahi M, *et al.* Longitudinal MRI in progressive supranuclear palsy and multiple system atrophy: rates and regions of atrophy. *Brain.* 2006;**129**:1040–9.

89. Feldmann A, Illes Z, Kosztolanyi P, *et al.* Morphometric changes of gray matter in Parkinson's disease with depression: a voxel-based morphometry study. *Mov Disord.* 2008;**23**:42–6.

90. Tessitore A, Amboni M, Cirillo G, *et al.* Regional gray matter atrophy in patients with Parkinson disease and freezing of gait. *AJNR Am J Neuroradiol.* 2012;**33**:1804–9.

91. Cerasa A, Messina D, Pugliese P, *et al.* Increased prefrontal volume in PD with levodopa-induced dyskinesias: a voxel-based morphometry study. *Mov Disord.* 2011;**26**:807–12.

92. Messina D, Cerasa A, Condino F, *et al.* Patterns of brain atrophy in Parkinson's disease, progressive supranuclear palsy and multiple system atrophy. *Parkinsonism Relat Disord.* 2011;**17**:172–6.

93. Oba H, Yagishita A, Terada H, *et al.* New and reliable MRI diagnosis for progressive supranuclear palsy. *Neurology.* 2005;**64**:2050–5.

94. Longoni G, Agosta F, Kostic VS, *et al.* MRI measurements of brainstem structures in patients with Richardson's syndrome, progressive supranuclear palsy-parkinsonism, and Parkinson's disease. *Mov Disord.* 2011;**26**:247–55.

95. Burton EJ, McKeith IG, Burn DJ, *et al.* Cerebral atrophy in Parkinson's disease with and without dementia: a comparison with Alzheimer's disease, dementia with Lewy

bodies and controls. *Brain.* 2004;**127**:791–800.

96. Karagulle Kendi AT, Lehericy S, Luciana M, *et al.* Altered diffusion in the frontal lobe in Parkinson disease. *AJNR Am J Neuroradiol.* 2008;**29**:501–5.

97. Biundo R, Formento-Dojot P, Facchini S, *et al.* Brain volume changes in Parkinson's disease and their relationship with cognitive and behavioural abnormalities. *J Neurol Sci.* 2011;**310**:64–9.

98. Meppelink AM, de Jong BM, Teune LK, *et al.* Regional cortical grey matter loss in Parkinson's disease without dementia is independent from visual hallucinations. *Mov Disord.* 2010;**26**:142–7.

99. Lyoo CH, Ryu YH, Lee MS. Topographical distribution of cerebral cortical thinning in patients with mild Parkinson's disease without dementia. *Mov Disord.* 2010;**25**:496–9.

100. Tinaz S, Courtney MG, Stern CE. Focal cortical and subcortical atrophy in early Parkinson's disease. *Mov Disord.* 2011;**26**:436–41.

101. Jubault T, Gagnon JF, Karama S, *et al.* Patterns of cortical thickness and surface area in early Parkinson's disease. *Neuroimage.* 2011;**55**:462–7.

102. Ibarretxe-Bilbao N, Junque C, Segura B, *et al.* Progression of cortical thinning in early Parkinson's disease. *Mov Disord.* 2012;**27**:1746–53.

103. Kostic VS, Agosta F, Petrovic I, *et al.* Regional patterns of brain tissue loss associated with depression in Parkinson disease. *Neurology.* 2010;**75**:857–63.

104. Cardoso EF, Maia FM, Fregni F, *et al.* Depression in Parkinson's disease: convergence from voxel-based morphometry and functional magnetic resonance imaging in the limbic thalamus. *Neuroimage.* 2009;**47**:467–72.

105. Ibarretxe-Bilbao N, Junque C, Marti MJ, *et al.* Cerebral basis of visual hallucinations in Parkinson's disease: structural and functional MRI studies. *J Neurol Sci.* 2011;**310**:79–81.

106. Ibarretxe-Bilbao N, Ramirez-Ruiz B, Junque C, *et al.* Differential progression of brain atrophy in Parkinson's disease with and without visual hallucinations. *J Neurol Neurosurg Psychiatry.* 2010;**81**:650–7.

107. Ibarretxe-Bilbao N, Junque C, Marti MJ, *et al.* Brain structural MRI correlates of cognitive dysfunctions in Parkinson's disease. *J Neurol Sci.* 2011;**310**:70–4.

108. Ibarretxe-Bilbao N, Tolosa E, Junque C, *et al.* MRI and cognitive impairment in Parkinson's disease. *Mov Disord.* 2009;**24** Suppl 2:S748–53.

109. Ibarretxe-Bilbao N, Junque C, Tolosa E, *et al.* Neuroanatomical correlates of impaired decision-making and facial emotion recognition in early Parkinson's disease. *Eur J Neurosci.* 2009;**30**:1162–71.

110. Wattendorf E, Welge-Lussen A, Fiedler K, *et al.* Olfactory impairment predicts brain atrophy in Parkinson's disease. *J Neurosci.* 2009;**29**:15410–13.

111. Beyer MK, Janvin CC, Larsen JP, *et al.* A magnetic resonance imaging study of patients with Parkinson's disease with mild cognitive impairment and dementia using voxel-based morphometry. *J Neurol Neurosurg Psychiatry.* 2007;**78**: 254–9.

112. Weintraub D, Dietz N, Duda JE, *et al.* Alzheimer's disease pattern of brain atrophy predicts cognitive decline in Parkinson's disease. *Brain* 2012;**135**:170–80.

113. Skidmore FM, Yang M, Baxter L, *et al.* Reliability analysis of the resting state can sensitively and specifically identify the presence

of Parkinson disease. *Neuroimage.* 2013;**75**:249–61.

114. Hacker CD, Perlmutter JS, Criswell SR, *et al.* Resting state functional connectivity of the striatum in Parkinson's disease. *Brain* 2012;**135**:3699–711.

115. Sharman M, Valabregue R, Perlbarg V, *et al.* Parkinson's disease patients show reduced cortical-subcortical sensorimotor connectivity. *Mov Disord.* 2013;**28**:447–54.

116. Wu T, Long X, Wang L, *et al.* Functional connectivity of cortical motor areas in the resting state in Parkinson's disease. *Hum Brain Mapp.* 2011;**32**:1443–57.

117. Baudrexel S, Witte T, Seifried C, *et al.* Resting state fMRI reveals increased subthalamic nucleus-motor cortex connectivity in Parkinson's disease. *Neuroimage.* 2011;**55**:1728–38.

118. Helmich RC, Janssen MJ, Oyen WJ, *et al.* Pallidal dysfunction drives a cerebellothalamic circuit into Parkinson tremor. *Ann Neurol.* 2011;**69**:269–81.

119. Skidmore FM, Yang M, Baxter L, *et al.* Apathy, depression, and motor symptoms have distinct and separable resting activity patterns in idiopathic Parkinson disease. *Neuroimage.* 2011; [Epub ahead of press].

120. Blain CR, Barker GJ, Jarosz JM, *et al.* Measuring brain stem and cerebellar damage in parkinsonian syndromes using diffusion tensor MRI. *Neurology.* 2006;**67**:2199–205.

121. Schocke MF, Seppi K, Esterhammer R, *et al.* Trace of diffusion tensor differentiates the Parkinson variant of multiple system atrophy and Parkinson's disease. *Neuroimage.* 2004;**21**:1443–51.

122. Paviour DC, Thornton JS, Lees AJ, *et al.* Diffusion-weighted magnetic resonance imaging differentiates Parkinsonian

variant of multiple-system atrophy from progressive supranuclear palsy. *Mov Disord.* 2007;**22**:68–74.

123. Nicoletti G, Lodi R, Condino F, *et al.* Apparent diffusion coefficient measurements of the middle cerebellar peduncle differentiate the Parkinson variant of MSA from Parkinson's disease and progressive supranuclear palsy. *Brain.* 2006;**129**:2679–87.

124. Righini A, Antonini A, De Notaris R, *et al.* MR imaging of the superior profile of the midbrain: differential diagnosis between progressive supranuclear palsy and Parkinson disease. *AJNR Am J Neuroradiol.* 2004;**25**:927–32.

125. Kato N, Arai K, Hattori T. Study of the rostral midbrain atrophy in progressive supranuclear palsy. *J Neurol Sci.* 2003;**210**:57–60.

126. Quattrone A, Nicoletti G, Messina D, *et al.* MR imaging index for differentiation of progressive supranuclear palsy from Parkinson disease and the Parkinson variant of multiple system atrophy. *Radiology.* 2008;**246**:214–21.

127. Brenneis C, Seppi K, Schocke M, *et al.* Voxel based morphometry reveals a distinct pattern of frontal atrophy in progressive supranuclear palsy. *J Neurol Neurosurg Psychiatry.* 2004;**75**:246–9.

128. Cordato NJ, Duggins AJ, Halliday GM, *et al.* Clinical deficits correlate with regional cerebral atrophy in progressive supranuclear palsy. *Brain.* 2005;**128**:1259–66.

129. Padovani A, Borroni B, Brambati SM, *et al.* Diffusion tensor imaging and voxel based morphometry study in early progressive supranuclear palsy. *J Neurol Neurosurg Psychiatry.* 2006;**77**:457–63.

130. Boxer AL, Geschwind MD, Belfor N, *et al.* Patterns of brain atrophy that differentiate corticobasal degeneration syndrome from progressive supranuclear palsy. *Arch Neurol.* 2006;**63**:81–6.

131. Lehericy S, Hartmann A, Lannuzel A, *et al.* Magnetic resonance imaging lesion pattern in Guadeloupean parkinsonism is distinct from progressive supranuclear palsy. *Brain.* 2010;**133**:2410–25.

132. Josephs KA, Whitwell JL, Dickson DW, *et al.* Voxel-based morphometry in autopsy proven PSP and CBD. *Neurobiol Aging* 2008;**29**:280–9.

133. Seppi K, Schocke MF, Esterhammer R, *et al.* Diffusion-weighted imaging discriminates progressive supranuclear palsy from PD, but not from the parkinson variant of multiple system atrophy. *Neurology.* 2003;**60**:922–7.

134. Nicoletti G, Tonon C, Lodi R, *et al.* Apparent diffusion coefficient of the superior cerebellar peduncle differentiates progressive supranuclear palsy from Parkinson's disease. *Mov Disord.* 2008;**23**:2370–6.

135. Ohshita T, Oka M, Imon Y, *et al.* Apparent diffusion coefficient measurements in progressive supranuclear palsy. *Neuroradiology.* 2000;**42**:643–7.

136. Boelmans K, Holst B, Hackius M, *et al.* Brain iron deposition fingerprints in Parkinson's disease and progressive supranuclear palsy. *Mov Disord.* 2012;**27**:421–7.

137. Arabia G, Quattrone A. MRI measurements of brainstem structures in patients with Richardson's syndrome, progressive supranuclear palsy-parkinsonism, and Parkinson's disease. *Mov Disord.* 2011;**26**:1575–6; author reply 1576.

138. Minnerop M, Specht K, Ruhlmann J, *et al.* Voxel-based morphometry and voxel-based relaxometry in multiple system atrophy – a comparison between clinical subtypes and correlations with clinical parameters. *Neuroimage.* 2007;**36**:1086–95.

139. Brenneis C, Seppi K, Schocke MF, *et al.* Voxel-based morphometry detects cortical atrophy in the Parkinson variant of multiple system atrophy. *Mov Disord.* 2003;**18**:1132–8.

140. Arabia G, Morelli M, Paglionico S, *et al.* A magnetic resonance imaging T2*-weighted sequence at short echo time to detect putaminal hypointensity in Parkinsonisms. *Mov Disord.* 2010;**25**:2728–34.

141. Bardinet E, Bhattacharjee M, Dormont D, *et al.* A three-dimensional histological atlas of the human basal ganglia. II. Atlas deformation strategy and evaluation in deep brain stimulation for Parkinson disease. *J Neurosurg.* 2009;**110**:208–19.

Chapter 4

MR imaging of Parkinson's disease with cognitive impairment and dementia

Richard Camicioli

Background

Dementia, which is defined as a multidomain cognitive impairment affecting everyday function, is a major public health problem. Though less common than Alzheimer's disease (AD), dementia with Lewy bodies (DLB) and Parkinson's disease with dementia (PDD) together, which share Lewy body pathology, represent the second most common cause of degenerative dementia [1]. These conditions form a spectrum, distinguished clinically by the relative timing of onset of parkinsonism (tremor, rigidity, and bradykinesia) and dementia. In PDD parkinsonism precedes dementia by at least a year (with some studies stipulating 2 years to assure separation from DLB) [2, 3], while parkinsonism and dementia occur within a year of each other in DLB [4]. Both disorders commonly are associated with the presence of cognitive fluctuations, hallucinations, and other neuropsychiatric features. Cognitive impairment is among the common and important non-motor features seen in Lewy body disorders [5].

Pathologically, the substrates for cognitive impairment in DLB and PDD are not fully established. Both cortical Lewy bodies and Alzheimer changes (neurofibrillary tangles and neuritic plaques) are found and correlate with dementia [6]; however, the relationship between pathology and magnetic resonance imaging (MRI) measures of regional brain atrophy was less precise in one study [7]. Mild cognitive impairment (MCI), defined as cognitive decline without associated functional impairment on a cognitive basis [8], occurs in 25% of Parkinson's diease (PD) patients and is likely associated with the pathology seen in DLB and PDD [9, 10]. Cerebrovascular disease is another cause of cognitive impairment in parkinsonian disorders, but its role

is less prominent than Lewy body and Alzheimer pathology. While neurotransmitter deficits, especially dopaminergic and cholinergic, and possibly noradrenergic, serotonergic, and glutaminergic, likely also contribute to cognitive deficits in Lewy body-related disorders [11], structural changes, evident with MRI, have been associated with cognitive impairment. Brain changes might be influenced by genetic polymorphisms that can affect pathology in sporadic PD [12] as well as by causal genes in familial PD.

In this chapter we review structural MRI studies that examine cognitively impaired individuals with PD. Given their wide availability, and relative safety, MRI techniques have been applied clinically and in research studies to assist with differential diagnosis and to track progression of disease. While MRI is not currently able to examine neurotransmitter deficits, which can be examined using complementary imaging tools, it may still provide insight into the topology and pathophysiology of neurodegeneration. MRI-based methods may be helpful in tracking the progression of some aspects of cognitive decline, and may potentially be useful as surrogate markers in clinical trials. We will not examine functional imaging using MRI or positron emission tomography.

This chapter will review relevant imaging methods and their application to various stages of disease including early or incident PD, treated patients, including those with MCI, and those with PDD and DLB. Additionally, we will review longitudinal studies and the impact of white matter pathology. This chapter will focus on studies since 2010 except for older studies that cover relevant research and that highlight important landmarks. Much of the older literature has been considered in recent reviews [13–15].

Magnetic resonance imaging: overview

MRI is a powerful technique for examining brain structure and function. Image acquisition and image processing are separate steps, each of which is subject to different approaches. Generally, structural measurements are done using volumetric T_1-weighted imaging, which provides accurate anatomical information. MRI centers may use unique protocols with different specified voxel sizes and low or high magnetic field strengths that can alter the contrast between gray and white matter, which may affect results. As a result the differences between MRI methods may be one explanation for discrepancies in findings between studies [13].

While visual inspection of images can be useful, and is the basis of clinical neuroradiology, image processing is a critical step in MRI image analysis in research. At the simplest level, manual tracing methods are used to determine volumes of structures such as the hippocampus. Since these are time consuming and require considerable training in order to achieve accuracy and reliability for complex structures, fully and semi-automated techniques that employ computer programs are available to extract volumes in regions of interest for individual scans, as well as across groups of subjects. This approach still may be prone to systematic error and still requires validation. Specific statistical approaches are available to examine cross-sectional or longitudinal structural changes. Voxel-based morphometry (VBM) is the most commonly used approach, which is statistically based, unbiased, and does not specifically require selection of the region of interest, but other methods are becoming available [16, 17]. VBM involves several pre-processing steps, including spatial normalization with linear and non-linear mapping of images for each subject to a standard template, segmentation, with subsequent modulation and smoothing, followed by statistical inferences. Although individual gray and white matter volumes can be extracted, generally VBM is used for group comparisons or correlations. Related to VBM is deformation-based morphometry (DBM) [18], where the non-linear mapping rather than the resulting image is the focus of statistical analysis. The non-linear mapping captures information about global structural differences and provides information that is complementary to VBM. Another automated method for structural analysis is the measurement of cortical thickness [19–21].

Imaging techniques sensitive to white matter changes include FLAIR (fluid-attenuated inversion recovery), T_2- and proton-weighted images. These methods are ideal for identifying signal change within the white matter, which can be due to pathological processes, such as strokes or demyelination, but are not optimal for structural definition. In recent years diffusion-weighted imaging (DWI), which is sensitive to the movement of water molecules, has become available [22]. DWI is routinely used clinically to identify pathological processes, such as ischemic disease, that locally restrict diffusion of water molecules. Post-processing techniques can quantify diffusion and directionality of diffusion, yielding measures such as overall diffusivity (termed mean diffusivity, MD) and fractional anisotropy (FA), which are representative measures of diffusion tensor imaging (DTI). Reconstruction of white matter pathways can be performed using diffusion tensor tractography. There are several studies using DTI in PD and they will be discussed. Additional techniques are available in the literature that can use the biophysical properties of tissue to accentuate the detection of normal and abnormal white matter and gray matter.

As with volumes, methods are available for automated rating of white matter lesions as well as for their quantitative measurement. These have the advantage of greater accuracy compared to visual methods, and are hence more amenable to longitudinal studies [23]. It should be noted that diffusion changes may be present independent of the presence of obvious white matter lesions.

Incident or early PD and MRI

Cognitive changes are evident from the earliest stages of PD, which has led to stratification of patients into those with and without cognitive impairment in recent studies. One large multicenter study examined 100 cognitively normal subjects, 127 cognitively normal PD (PD-CN) patients, and 31 PD patients with MCI (PD-MCI) and found that PD-CN had smaller hippocampal radial distances, but that overall volumes were unchanged [24]. This group then subdivided the PD-MCI into amnestic and non-amnestic MCI groups. The non-amnestic PD-MCI patients who had deficits on neuropsychological domains other than memory (for example in attention, executive function, or visuospatial function) had smaller right hippocampal radial distance with lateral ventricular enlargement compared to normal controls and bilateral temporal, occipital, and left frontal dilation compared to PD-CN patients. Compared to controls, non-amnestic PD-MCI subjects had global ventricular dilation while amnestic PD-MCI had left occipital expansion.

Another cross-sectional study used VBM to evaluate a subgroup of the above subjects from one site and compared 42 incident PD cases, including 11 patients with PD-MCI, with 37 controls but did not find gray matter atrophy in patients as compared to controls [25]. In contrast, using an automated neuroanatomical labeling approach (available in the program FreeSurfer) on essentially the same sample a larger left lateral and third ventricle was found in PD-MCI compared to PD-CN [26]. Another group that also used VBM also did not demonstrate gray matter atrophy, but identified temporal lobe volume loss in white matter involving the right anterior fusiform gyrus and superior temporal gyrus in 24 untreated PD patients compared with 14 healthy controls. These findings did not correlate with cognitive deficits (verbal memory, executive function, visuospatial function) [27]. In contrast to these, an older study that used a visual rating showed hippocampal and prefrontal atrophy in a group of 20 untreated PD patients [28]. Thus, there remain discrepancies in the literature regarding volumetric changes in early, untreated PD, which to some extent might be related to sample size, inclusion criteria, duration of disease, the recognition of patients with MCI and its subtypes, as well as the imaging approach. Larger samples and novel analysis techniques such as radial measures or gray matter measurements using FreeSurfer noted above may be more sensitive to early changes. Techniques that identify focal atrophy (or focal dilation in the case of cerebrospinal fluid [CSF] space measures) are particularly relevant, given that global measures may miss significant focal atrophy.

Prevalent PD and cognitive impairment

A much larger number of studies have examined treated patients, which may reflect the relative ease and speed of recruiting and scanning a population of treated patients who are receiving their care at movement disorders centers where imaging studies are conducted (as opposed to untreated patients in the community). Typically these studies include those who are in the mild to moderate stages of disease and may include individuals with varying degrees of cognitive impairment. Hence, these enrollees most likely have a greater degree of dopamine denervation than untreated patients as well as a greater extent of Lewy body pathology involving non-motor areas, including those affecting cognition. Present structural imaging is unable to resolve the various subtleties of synuclein aggregation or neurochemical depletion and primarily reflects neuronal loss and gliosis when the changes are detectable at a macroscopic level. Microscopic alterations may be detectable using extremely high-field magnetic strengths in models of PD but these methods have not yet made their way onto clinical platforms and therefore will not be discussed herein.

The PD cognitive spectrum

A recent study evaluated 57 PD-CN, 23 PD-MCI, defined by performance on neuropsychological tests, and 16 with PDD [29]. The authors found no atrophy in the PD-CN group. They did find changes in multiple cortical areas, as well as the hippocampus and putamen in PD-MCI, which were more extensively involved in PDD patients, who had additional changes in intracalcarine and lingual gyri, posterior cingulate, and caudate. These investigators found that gray matter atrophy was correlated with cognitive decline. Other studies have included those with PD-CN, PD-MCI, and PDD and suggest that there is increasing and more widespread atrophy across this spectrum, with PD-MCI patients intermediate between PD-CN and PDD [30]. PDD patients tended to show temporal lobe atrophy compared to PD-MCI, along with increasing frontal atrophy and more global atrophy. Another group used VBM to compare cognitively impaired PD subjects (as defined by the Clinical Dementia Rating [CDR] Scale, a composite index that provides an integrated rating of cognitive and functional change [CDR = 0.5]) with intact PD patients and found gray matter loss in PD-CN, with more perisylvian change in the PD-MCI group [31]. Additionally, those who were cognitively impaired had cortical gray matter changes in the lateral and orbitofrontal, medial and lateral temporal, medial and lateral parietal, and lateral occipital cortices and cerebellum.

MCI subgroups

In addition to the studies examining amnestic versus non-amnestic MCI, another research group used VBM to examine two groups of PD patients with MCI: earlier onset of MCI (MCI onset < 1 year of PD symptoms) versus later onset (≥ 1 year of PD symptoms). They showed left inferior parietal and right orbitofrontal atrophy was greater in those with early- compared to late-onset cognitive impairment [32]. Superior temporal atrophy correlated with timing of cognitive decline, while anterior and posterior cingulate gyrus atrophy correlated negatively with timing. This group also compared PD patients with amnestic MCI with non-PD patients with amnestic MCI [33]. They found that gray matter density in the right temporal and posterior cingulate cortices was lower in the non-PD MCI subjects compared to controls. In the PD subjects there was lower gray matter density in the precuneus and left prefrontal and primary motor areas compared to controls. Differences between groups were also evident, highlighting different anatomical bases for amnestic MCI in PD versus non-PD subjects. Pathologically in non-PD MCI the ultimate cause of dementia in general is AD, whereas the pathological substrate for PDD is generally diffuse Lewy body change, with varying amounts of Alzheimer pathology.

Correlation with cognitive measures

Imaging correlates of cognitive tests have been examined by some investigators. These studies have generally used VBM. Pereira *et al.* have shown volumetric correlates of visuospatial and visuoperceptual function [34] as well as verbal fluency [35]. Visuospatial tests correlated with gray matter density in the superior parietal lobule and superior occipital gyrus while visuoperceptual tests correlated with the fusiform, parahippocampus, and superior occipital gyri. Semantic fluency correlated with the inferior and middle frontal gyri, temporal lobe, cerebellum and parahippocampus, caudate and anterior thalamus. In another group of PD subjects verbal memory scores correlated with the left middle temporal gyrus, fusiform gyrus, uncus, and putamen, and right temporal lobe [36]. A composite index of executive function (sum of Stroop, Trail Making, and digit ordering tests) correlated with the left middle temporal gyrus, right middle temporal gyrus, right and left caudate, left precuneus, and the left cerebellum. In another

study of cognitively normal subjects, memory scores correlated with hippocampal atrophy [37]. A group that examined PD, divided into early and advanced PD patients, using VBM found no difference between PD-CN and controls, but was able to show correlations between performance on the Raven's Colored Progressive Matrices Test, a test that involves both visuospatial processing and executive function, and dorsolateral prefrontal and parahippocampal volumes [38]. In PDD, limbic and paralimbic changes were observed, including anterior cingulate, hippocampus, temporal lobe, dorsolateral frontal lobe, thalamus, and caudate nucleus. Another older study showed that ventricular enlargement correlated with performance on the Stroop test and with verbal memory [39]. Focal hippocampal volume (measured using manual segmentation) has been associated with verbal and visual memory, and not measures of executive function [40].

Novel approaches

Studies using novel analysis of cortical thinning have shown focal changes in small samples, which will have to be confirmed in larger samples. One study found that cortical thickness in the left fusiform cortex correlated with verbal memory [41]. Another group examined early-stage PD patients and showed frontal and occipitoparietal as well as subcortical thinning [42]. While some of these studies have not included patients with cognitive impairment and some have not specifically examined cognitive correlates, it has been noted that changes may follow the distribution of Lewy body changes seen at autopsy [43]. Another study that used a novel approach termed corticography, an approach that decouples cortical thickness from local surface measurements, found in a group of 49 PD subjects compared with 33 controls that thickness did not differ between groups, but that surface area was larger in PD in specific brain areas (parietal lobules, right superior frontal gyrus, left cingulate cortex, left insula) while focal areas showed thinning (left medial supplementary motor area [SMA] and right dorsal pre-SMA) [44]. Thus, cortical thickness and related measures may allow for earlier detection of brain changes in the gray matter and may be more sensitive to focal changes, and are thus well suited to be applied to patients early in the course of disease and to patients with mild cognitive deficits. The current limitations include image acquisition, which continues to be optimized to account for tissue content, and computer processing time.

A study that used radial distance mapping of the hippocampus, caudate, and ventricles found that, while there were no differences between PD-CN, PD-MCI, and PDD in the hippocampus, there were differences in the caudate and ventricles in PD-MCI and PDD [45]. Another technique worth noting is DBM, which does not rely on a-priori knowledge of gray and white matter distributions, but uses contrasts as explicit representations of these regions. The authors of one study postulate that this approach may allow better detection of subtle differences [46]. Early non-demented, but treated PD-CN subjects, who had a thorough cognitive assessment, had decreased cerebellar volume compared to controls; correlations with the Unified Parkinson's Disease Rating Scale (UPDRS) were identified.

Structural imaging in PDD

Patients with dementia are a natural focus of structural imaging studies. Initially studies focused on global changes and atrophy in limbic structures, in part motivated by findings in AD as well as by pathological knowledge that limbic structures are affected in autopsy studies of PDD. In PD pathological changes have been found in the hippocampus, parahippocampus, amygdala, and the entorhinal cortex [47–50].

Global MRI measures

A recent study compared patients across the cognitive spectrum using an automated classification approach [51]. These researchers identified a pattern of changes specific to PDD, which they term the Spatial Pattern of Abnormalities for Recognition (SPARE-PDD). Their PD-CN subjects did not show atrophy compared to controls. The 11 PDD patients had significant hippocampal and mediotemporal atrophy, with PD-MCI subjects showing a similar pattern. PD-MCI subjects had atrophy in the basal ganglia, amygdala, and insula. It should be noted that because of image acquisition and analysis methods, deep gray matter structures may not always be reliably measured. Sanchez-Castaneda et al. compared PDD and DLB using VBM and found greater atrophy in DLB [52]. A study that compared PDD subjects with early versus later onset of cognitive decline (using a cutoff of 8 years to dementia) found that the early dementia

group had more atrophy than the late group in the medial frontal gyrus and right precuneus as well as the left inferior parietal lobule, superior frontal gyrus, and middle temporal gyrus. The late group had symmetrical reduction in both inferior frontal gyri [53]. The same group of researchers also showed more generalized atrophy in DLB compared to PDD. They found that DLB patients showed medial temporal atrophy compared to PDD [54]. Another group that compared PDD versus controls, using VBM, found atrophy in the putamen, nucleus accumbens, left thalamus, hippocampi, left parahippocampal gyrus, and the anterior cingulate [55]. PD subjects showed changes in the right hippocampus, left anterior cingulate, and left superior temporal gyri, with PDD subjects showing greater left superior temporal gyrus and right hippocampal changes compared with PD. In an early VBM study Burton et al. [56] found medial temporal atrophy in PDD compared to controls, including the hippocampus and parahippocampus. There was also frontal, parietal, thalamic, and basal ganglia atrophy in PDD. Compared to PD-CN, PDD patients had greater occipital atrophy. This study also compared patients with DLB and AD to those with PD and PDD and found that AD patients had more medial temporal atrophy, while DLB and PDD had similar changes. PD-CN in this study showed frontal atrophy compared to controls. One study that examined caudate volume loss in AD, PD, DLB, and controls, found that it was proportionate to generalized brain atrophy [57].

Hippocampus and related structures

In a seminal study, Laakso et al. compared hippocampal volumes measured, using tracing methods, across various groups that included patients with AD, vascular dementia, and PD [58]. They found hippocampal volume loss in PD and PDD, with the PDD patients showing even more atrophy than AD patients. This finding was confirmed in a study showing a gradient of atrophy with volumes being largest in controls > PD > PDD > AD [59]. The PDD group in the latter study included mainly patients with milder cognitive impairment (most had CDR = 0.5), which could represent MCI, or early dementia, depending on the degree of functional impairment based on cognitive decline. Another study using visual rating measures identified prominent volume loss in DLB and PDD that was comparable with that n AD; PD subjects had less atrophy [60]. The majority of studies in the literature have confirmed the finding of hippocampal atrophy in PDD. What isn't known is whether the patterns of atrophy are identical in various dementing conditions and the precise timing of hippocampal atrophy in PD. Findings in PD-CN and PD-MCI have not been as consistent. Novel imaging techniques may be able to identify change in the hippocampus prior to obvious structural changes, as evidenced by a study that examined $T_{1\rho}$ values, which were found to be elevated in the hippocampus in both patients with AD and those with PDD [61].

The effect of age and neuropsychiatric factors

A study of younger non-demented cognitively intact PD patients found no atrophy [62], which led to the hypothesis that age-related atrophy might be accelerated in PD. This was supported by a follow-up study on an independent sample, which showed that HC atrophy was present in older (age > 70 years) compared to younger subjects (aged 65–75) [63]. Longitudinal follow-up would be necessary to confirm this. This study suggested that atrophy may predominate in the hippocampal head; a finding also observed in another study that included PD patients with visual hallucinations, a subgroup at particularly high risk for later conversion to dementia [64]. A recent paper using VBM showed changes in the thalamus and the pedunculopontine nucleus in PD patients with hallucinations [65].

Amygdala

One gray matter structure of particular interest is the amygdala. Amydgala atrophy is important since it is pathologically involved with Lewy bodies, but it is difficult to measure, because of its proximity to the hippocampus and other gray matter structures. Nevertheless several studies have identified amygdala atrophy in PDD or PD-MCI patients using tracing methods [66]. This finding is consistent with studies using VBM [67] and other automated methods [51] as well as with a study that examined atrophy in autopsied PD, PSP, and DLB that showed amygdala atrophy in PD [68]. In contrast to this autopsy study, this group of researchers showed minimal change in

living PD patients, with atrophy in the intraparietal sulcus, using VBM [69].

Entorhinal cortex

Some studies have specifically addressed the entorhinal cortex, which is prominently affected in AD, but also shows autopsy changes that correlate with the presence of dementia in PD [49]. In one recent study, where the hippocampus and entorhinal cortex were both traced, while both PD-CN and PDD had hippocampal atrophy, the entorhinal cortex had greater atrophy in patients with PDD [70]. In another study with a larger sample size and range of patients, but which did not separate PD-MCI (20 DLB, 26 AD, 30 PDD, 31 PD, and 37 controls) [71], there was entorhinal cortex atrophy in all the demented groups, which was slightly less prominent in PDD compared to DLB and AD.

Substantia innominata

Several groups of investigators have shown that the substantia innominata is atrophic in PD, with progressive loss in PD-MCI and PDD [72, 73]. The substantia innominata size correlated with the Mini-Mental State Examination (MMSE) score, a global cognitive measure [74]. This area is one origin of cortical cholinergic projections, and has early Lewy body involvement in PD; hence these findings are of interest. Together with the above studies, it can be concluded that limbic changes occur in PD patients and that they appear to progress across the spectrum of PD patients.

Longitudinal studies

The majority of studies performed thus far have been cross-sectional, though methods for longitudinal studies have been developed [75]. Cross-sectional studies necessarily enroll heterogeneous populations of patients at different stages of disease, since group matching is usually imperfect and timing the onset of cognitive impairment may be challenging. Different levels of cognitive dysfunction, as found in these studies, may partially contribute to the discrepancies between imaging results. To address this, researchers would need to attempt to evaluate a cohort of similarly affected individuals and follow them prospectively for changes in an outcome of interest, for example cognitive decline.

49

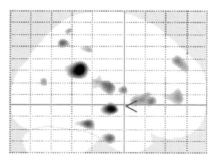
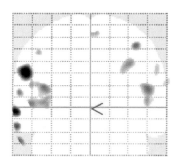
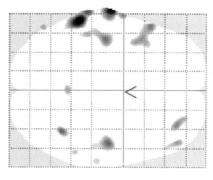
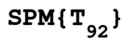

Figure 4.1 Longitudinal comparison of PD patients with and without dementia (see [83] for patient details) illustrating VBM results. A group of PD subjects without dementia (n = 22) was compared to a group of PD subjects with a dementia diagnosis or significant cognitive impairment at 36 months after the baseline scan (n = 10) using VBM in statistical parametric mapping (SPM). The model used dementia classification and scan as the main factors, with intracranial volume (ICV) included as a covariate. Regions where the PD subjects without dementia had higher gray matter tissue volume compared to PD subjects with dementia are show below (p-values are corrected using peak family-wise error [FWE]). The regions of note include clusters in the left and right insula (peak FWE-corrected p-values of 0.004 and 0.003, respectively), as well as a large cluster in the left parietal lobe (peak FWE corrected p-value < 0.001). Illustrated is a glass brain depiction of the significant differences. (Images courtesy of Dr. Myrlene Gee, unpublished data, 2012).

Some studies have used baseline scan patterns to predict future decline. One found those participants with an atrophy pattern derived from patients with AD had cognitive decline [76]. Another group evaluated a cohort of PD patients undergoing deep brain stimulation (DBS) surgery and showed those with smaller hippocampal volumes preoperatively had a greater chance of developing dementia after surgery [77]. Other researchers have performed scans at various intervals. One showed an increased rate of atrophy in PDD with no difference in the rate of atrophy between cognitively intact PD patients and controls [78]. Another study found atrophy in both PD and PDD using VBM [79], consistent with an earlier study of PD patients that showed that global atrophy correlated with cognitive decline on neuropsychological testing [80].

A recent study stratified patients by the presence or absence of visual hallucinations and showed a greater rate of atrophy in PD subjects with visual hallucinations, who also were more likely to develop dementia [81]. Another study performing longitudinal volumetric scans grouped patients according to olfactory abnormalities rather than cognitive decline [82]. Changes in olfactory ability might reflect progressive Lewy body pathology, which affects the olfactory bulbs. These workers found that patients with olfactory abnormalities had global atrophy at baseline involving the amygdalae; frontal, temporal, and occipital lobes; and cingulate cortex. The group with normal olfactory perception, who had larger starting volumes, showed progressive changes in the right amygdala and bilateral temporal lobes. We prospectively examined older PD patients (65 years of age and older) who were initially non-demented and found that patients who developed significant cognitive impairment (including dementia) over 3 years of follow-up showed increased atrophy (reflected in global brain volumes and ventricular dilation) over time (Figure 4.1). Those who did not have any cognitive decline did not differ from controls, indicating that global atrophy was a marker of cognitive decline [83].

White matter changes

In a large sample of 155 untreated PD patients compared with 101 controls there were no white matter high-signal change differences in early PD compared to controls, which was confirmed using different methods [84, 85]. As PD patients age white matter changes may become more prominent just as in normal aging and in relation to vascular risk factors (e.g., hypertension, diabetes, smoking, hypercholesterolemia, body mass index). Studies that include patients with PDD have inconsistently shown increased high-signal changes in PDD [86]. One study showed no relationship between visually rated changes and cognitive status [87]. In contrast, a recent study examining a range of PD subjects (PD-CN, PD-MCI, PDD) [88] showed that cognitive change in PD subjects was related to white matter hyperintensities as well as supine hypertension and orthostatic hypotension. Another recent study suggested that white matter high-signal changes along cholinergic cortical projection pathways are associated with cognitive decline [89]. These signal changes might reflect Wallerian degeneration or direct ischemic pathology. A study that compared progression of white matter changes between AD, PDD, and DLB and older controls found that AD patients had more white matter changes than controls; there was no difference in progression of white matter changes between the dementia groups [90].

Multimodal imaging methods, including DTI, have started to shed light on brain changes in PD. One study using both DTI and structural imaging found that increased diffusivity of the hippocampus was associated with memory scores in PD-CN subjects, in whom there was no hippocampal atrophy compared to controls [91]. Another study compared patients with PD-CN with patients with PD-MCI, PDD, and DLB [92]. While PD-CN did not show differences in FA, the cognitively impaired groups showed differences, which correlated with global cognitive function (MMSE). Several DTI studies have included patients with PDD. One found that there were changes in FA in the cingulate gyrus that were predominantly anterior in PD, but more widespread in PDD [93]. These findings were consistent with a study that compared PDD with PD [94], but contrasted with a study that included a smaller number of PDD subjects that showed a correlation between

MMSE scores and transcallosal tractography, but did not find a significant association with changes along the cingulum [95]. Likely the latter study lacked the power of the former study to show group differences. In another publication Matsui *et al.* found that PD patients with impaired performance on the Wisconsin Card Sorting Test, a test of executive function, had decreased left parietal white matter FA [96]. Another group that compared PDD and DLB found that FA was more widely affected in DLB [97]. Table 4.1 summarizes the MRI findings in PD from this chapter.

Summary

It is clear that structural changes occur in gray and white matter in PD. These findings are most evident in patients with cognitive impairment and, based on the few prospective studies, may represent a useful surrogate for tracking cognitive decline. The timing of the changes in imaging parameters and clinical correlates will be better understood as additional longitudinal studies using ever improving approaches are completed. Novel imaging techniques may be able to identify changes from the earliest stages of PD.

Acknowledgements

I thank Drs. Wendy Johnston and Myrlene Gee for helpful comments on the manuscript. I also thank my collaborators at the Peter Allen MRI Research Centre and the Movement Disorders Program at the University of Alberta for their support. Our imaging research has been funded by the Alzheimer Research Alliance (Oregon, USA), the Medical Research Foundation (Oregon Health and Sciences University, USA), the Department of Veterans Affairs (USA), the National Institutes on Aging (USA), Canadian Institutes for Health Research, and the University of Alberta Hospital Foundation. Pfizer Canada and Johnson and Johnson Canada helped support some of our studies in PDD.

PubMed search terms

Parkinson's disease and magnetic resonance imaging/ MRI and cognitive impairment/cognition/dementia/ neuropsychology/neuropsychological and added incident/early/mild.

Table 4.1. Summary of some of the brain regions affected as evidenced by MRI in Parkinson's disease with normal cognition (PD-CN), mild cognitive impairment (PD-MCI), and dementia (PDD) in studies comparing across these levels of severity. See text for details and additional references

Brain region	PD-CN	PD-MCI	PDD
Limbic regions			
Hippocampus	VR [28, 37] MS [58, 59, 63, 70] VBM [55] RD [24]	MS [40] VBM [29, 51] RD [24]	VR [60] MS [58, 59, 63, 66, 70] VBM [29, 38, 51, 55, 56, 67]
Entorhinal cortex			MS [70, 71] VBM [51]
Parahippocampus	VBM [38]		VBM [29, 51, 55, 56]
Amygdala	MS [63]	VBM [29, 51]	MS [66] VBM [29, 67]
Substantia innominata	MS [73, 74]	MS [73]	MS [72, 73]
Anterior cingulate	VBM [55] CG [44]		VBM [38, 55]
Posterior cingulate			VBM [29]
Insula	CG [44]	VBM [29, 30, 51]	VBM [29, 30]
Cortical			
Frontal	VR [28, 37] VBM [31, 38, 55, 56, 67] CT [42–44] CG [44]	VBM [29–31]	VBM [29, 30, 38, 56, 67]
Temporal	VBM [27, 31, 55] CT [41–43]	VBM [29–31, 51]	VBM [29, 30, 38, 51, 55, 56, 67]
Parietal	VBM [31, 69] CT [42, 43] CG [44]	VBM [29–31]	VBM [29, 30, 56, 67]
Occipital	VBM [30, 31, 38] CT [42, 43]	VBM [29–31]	VBM [29, 30, 56, 67]
Subcortical			
Caudate		RD [45]	VBM [29, 38, 56, 67] RD [45]
Putamen	CT [42]	VBM [29, 51]	VBM [29, 30, 55, 56]
Nucleus accumbens			VBM [55]
Thalamus			VBM [38, 55, 56, 67]
Cerebellum	VBM [36] DBM [46]	VBM [31]	
Ventricular			
Lateral (global)		RD [24] FS [26]	RD [45]
Frontal		RD [24]	

Table 4.1. (cont.)

Brain region	PD-CN	PD-MCI	PDD
Temporal		RD [24]	
Parietal		RD [24]	
Occipital		RD [24]	
Third ventricle		FS [26]	
Fourth ventricle		FS [26]	

CG, corticography; CT, cortical thickness; DBM, deformation-based morphometry; FS, FreeSurfer; MS, manual segmentation; RD, radial distance measurements; VBM, voxel-based morphometry; VR, visual rating

References

1. Rahkonen T, Eloniemi-Sulkava U, Rissanen S, et al. Dementia with Lewy bodies according to the consensus criteria in a general population aged 75 years or older. *J Neurol Neurosurg Psychiatry*. 2003;**74**(6):720–4.

2. Dubois B, Burn D, Goetz C, et al. Diagnostic procedures for Parkinson's disease dementia: recommendations from the Movement Disorder Society task force. *Mov Disord*. 2007;**22**(16):2314–24.

3. Emre M, Aarsland D, Brown R, et al. Clinical diagnostic criteria for dementia associated with Parkinson's disease. *Mov Disord*. 2007;**22**(12):1689–707.

4. McKeith IG, Dickson DW, Lowe J, et al. Diagnosis and management of dementia with Lewy bodies: third report of the DLB Consortium. *Neurology*. 2005;**65**(12):1863–72.

5. Romenets S, Wolfson C, Galatasm C, et al. Validation of the non-motor symptoms questionnaire (NMS-Quest). *Parkinsonism Relat Disord*. 2012;**18**(1):54–8.

6. Compta Y, Parkkinen L, O'Sullivan SS, et al. Lewy- and Alzheimer-type pathologies in Parkinson's disease dementia: which is more important? *Brain*. 2011;**134**(Pt 5):1493–505.

7. Burton EJ, Mukaetova-Ladinska EB, Perry RH, et al. Neuropathological correlates of volumetric MRI in autopsy-confirmed Lewy body dementia. *Neurobiol Aging*. 2012;**33**(7):1228–36.

8. Petersen RC. Clinical practice. Mild cognitive impairment. *N Engl J Med*. 2011; **364**(23):2227–34.

9. Aarsland D, Bronnick K, Williams-Gray C, et al. Mild cognitive impairment in Parkinson disease: a multicenter pooled analysis. *Neurology*. 2010;**75**(12):1062–9.

10. Molano J, Boeve B, Ferman T, et al. Mild cognitive impairment associated with limbic and neocortical Lewy body disease: a clinicopathological study. *Brain*. 2010;**133**(Pt 2):540–56.

11. Stoessl AJ, Martin WW, McKeown MJ, Sossi V. Advances in imaging in Parkinson's disease. *Lancet Neurol*. 2011;**10**(11): 987–1001.

12. Wider C, Ross OA, Nishioka K, et al. An evaluation of the impact of MAPT, SNCA and APOE on the burden of Alzheimer's and Lewy body pathology. *J Neurol Neurosurg Psychiatry*. 2012; **83**(4):424–9.

13. Draganski B, Bhatia KP. Brain structure in movement disorders: a neuroimaging perspective. *Curr Opin Neurol*. 2010;**23**(4):413–19.

14. Silbert LC, Kaye J. Neuroimaging and cognition in Parkinson's disease dementia. *Brain Pathol*. 2010;**20**(3):646–53.

15. Ibarretxe-Bilbao N, Junque C, Marti MJ, Tolosa E. Brain structural MRI correlates of cognitive dysfunctions in Parkinson's disease. *J Neurol Sci*. 2011;**310**(1–2):70–4.

16. Ashburner J, Friston KJ. Unified segmentation. *Neuroimage*. 2005;**26**(3):839–51.

17. Ashburner J, Friston KJ. Voxel-based morphometry – the methods. *Neuroimage*. 2000; **11**(6 Pt 1):805–21.

18. Ashburner J, Hutton C, Frackowiak R, et al. Identifying global anatomical differences: deformation-based morphometry. *Hum Brain Mapp*. 1998; **6**(5–6):348–57.

19. Fischl B, Dale AM. Measuring the thickness of the human cerebral cortex from magnetic resonance images. *Proc Natl Acad Sci U S A*. 2000;**97**(20):11050–5.

20. Kim JS, Singh V, Lee JK, et al. Automated 3-D extraction and evaluation of the inner and outer cortical surfaces using a Laplacian map and partial volume effect classification. *Neuroimage*. 2005;**27**(1):210–21.

21. Lerch JP, Evans AC. Cortical thickness analysis examined through power analysis and a

population simulation. *Neuroimage.* 2005;**24**(1):163–73.

22. Beaulieu C. The basis of anisotropic water diffusion in the nervous system – a technical review. *NMR Biomed* 2002; **15**(7–8):435–55.

23. van den Heuvel DM, ten Dam VH, de Craen AJ, *et al.* Measuring longitudinal white matter changes: comparison of a visual rating scale with a volumetric measurement. *AJNR Am J Neuroradiol.* 2006;**27**(4):875–8.

24. Apostolova L, Alves G, Hwang KS, *et al.* Hippocampal and ventricular changes in Parkinson's disease mild cognitive impairment. *Neurobiol Aging.* 2012;**33**(9):2113–24.

25. Dalaker TO, Zivadinov R, Larsen JP, *et al.* Gray matter correlations of cognition in incident Parkinson's disease. *Mov Disord.* 2010;**25**(5):629–33.

26. Dalaker TO, Zivadinov R, Ramasamy DP, *et al.* Ventricular enlargement and mild cognitive impairment in early Parkinson's disease. *Mov Disord.* 2011; **26**(2):297–301.

27. Martin WR, Wieler M, Gee M, Camicioli R. Temporal lobe changes in early, untreated Parkinson's disease. *Mov Disord.* 2009;**24**(13):1949–54.

28. Bruck A, Kurki T, Kaasinen V, Vahlberg T, Rinne JO. Hippocampal and prefrontal atrophy in patients with early non-demented Parkinson's disease is related to cognitive impairment. *J Neurol Neurosurg Psychiatry.* 2004;**75**(10):1467–9.

29. Melzer TR, Watts R, MacAskill MR, *et al.* Grey matter atrophy in cognitively impaired Parkinson's disease. *J Neurol Neurosurg Psychiatry.* 2012;**83**(2):188–94.

30. Song SK, Lee JE, Park HJ, *et al.* The pattern of cortical atrophy in patients with Parkinson's disease according to cognitive status. *Mov Disord.* 2011;**26**(2):289–96.

31. Nishio Y, Hirayama K, Takeda A, *et al.* Corticolimbic gray matter loss in Parkinson's disease without dementia. *Eur J Neurol.* 2010;**17**(8):1090–7.

32. Lee JE, Cho KH, Kim M, Sohn YH, Lee PH. The pattern of cortical atrophy in Parkinson's disease with mild cognitive impairment according to the timing of cognitive dysfunction. *J Neurol.* 2012;**259**(3):469–73.

33. Lee JE, Park HJ, Song SK, *et al.* Neuroanatomic basis of amnestic MCI differs in patients with and without Parkinson disease. *Neurology.* 2010;**75**(22):2009–16.

34. Pereira JB, Junque C, Marti MJ, *et al.* Neuroanatomical substrate of visuospatial and visuoperceptual impairment in Parkinson's disease. *Mov Disord.* 2009;**24**(8):1193–9.

35. Pereira JB, Junque C, Marti MJ, *et al.* Structural brain correlates of verbal fluency in Parkinson's disease. *Neuroreport.* 2009;**20**(8):741–4.

36. Camicioli R, Gee M, Bouchard TP, *et al.* Voxel-based morphometry reveals extra-nigral atrophy patterns associated with dopamine refractory cognitive and motor impairment in parkinsonism. *Parkinsonism Relat Disord.* 2009;**15**(3):187–95.

37. Jokinen P, Bruck A, Aalto S, *et al.* Impaired cognitive performance in Parkinson's disease is related to caudate dopaminergic hypofunction and hippocampal atrophy. *Parkinsonism Relat Disord.* 2009;**15**(2):88–93.

38. Nagano-Saito A, Washimi Y, Arahata Y, *et al.* Cerebral atrophy and its relation to cognitive impairment in Parkinson disease. *Neurology.* 2005;**64**(2):224–9.

39. Alegret M, Junque C, Pueyo R, *et al.* MRI atrophy parameters related to cognitive and motor impairment in Parkinson's disease. *Neurologia.* 2001;**16**(2):63–9.

40. Riekkinen P, Jr., Kejonen K, Laakso MP, *et al.* Hippocampal atrophy is related to impaired memory, but not frontal function in non-demented Parkinson's disease patients. *Neuroreport.* 1998;**9**(7):1507–11.

41. Pellicano C, Assogna F, Piras F, *et al.* Regional cortical thickness and cognitive functions in non-demented Parkinson's disease patients: a pilot study. *Eur J Neurol.* 2012;**19**(1):172–5.

42. Tinaz S, Courtney MG, Stern CE. Focal cortical and subcortical atrophy in early Parkinson's disease. *Mov Disord.* 2011;**26**(3):436–41.

43. Lyoo CH, Ryu YH, Lee MS. Topographical distribution of cerebral cortical thinning in patients with mild Parkinson's disease without dementia. *Mov Disord.* 2010;**25**(4):496–9.

44. Jubault T, Gagnon JF, Karama S, *et al.* Patterns of cortical thickness and surface area in early Parkinson's disease. *Neuroimage.* 2011;**55**(2):462–7.

45. Apostolova LG, Beyer M, Green AE, *et al.* Hippocampal, caudate, and ventricular changes in Parkinson's disease with and without dementia. *Mov Disord.* 2010;**25**(6):687–8.

46. Borghammer P, Ostergaard K, Cumming P, *et al.* A deformation based morphometry study of patients with early-stage Parkinson's disease. *Eur J Neurol.* 2010;**17**(2):314–20.

47. Churchyard A, Lees AJ. The relationship between dementia and direct involvement of the hippocampus and amygdala in Parkinson's disease. *Neurology.* 1997;**49**(6):1570–6.

48. Harding AJ, Halliday GM. Cortical Lewy body pathology in the diagnosis of dementia. *Acta Neuropathol.* 2001;**102**(4):355–63.

49. Kovari E, Gold G, Herrmann FR, *et al.* Lewy body densities in the entorhinal and anterior cingulate

cortex predict cognitive deficits in Parkinson's disease. *Acta Neuropathol.* 2003;**106**(1):83–8.

60. Braak H, Rub U, Jansen Steur ENH, Del Tredici K, de Vos RAI. Cognitive status correlates with neuropathologic stage in Parkinson's disease. *Neurology.* 2005;**64**:1404–10.

61. Weintraub D, Doshi J, Koka D, *et al.* Neurodegeneration across stages of cognitive decline in Parkinson disease. *Arch Neurol.* 2011;**68**(12):1562–8.

62. Sanchez-Castaneda C, Rene R, Ramirez-Ruiz B, *et al.* Correlations between gray matter reductions and cognitive deficits in dementia with Lewy bodies and Parkinson's disease with dementia. *Mov Disord.* 2009;**24**(12):1740–6.

63. Beyer MK, Aarsland D. Grey matter atrophy in early versus late dementia in Parkinson's disease. *Parkinsonism Relat Disord.* 2008;**14**(8):620–5.

64. Beyer MK, Larsen JP, Aarsland D. Gray matter atrophy in Parkinson disease with dementia and dementia with Lewy bodies. *Neurology.* 2007;**69**(8):747–54.

65. Summerfield C, Junque C, Tolosa E, *et al.* Structural brain changes in Parkinson disease with dementia: a voxel-based morphometry study. *Arch Neurol.* 2005;**62**(2):281–5.

66. Burton EJ, McKeith IG, Burn DJ, Williams ED, O'Brien JT. Cerebral atrophy in Parkinson's disease with and without dementia: a comparison with Alzheimer's disease, dementia with Lewy bodies and controls. *Brain.* 2004;**127**:791–800.

67. Almeida OP, Burton EJ, McKeith I, *et al.* MRI study of caudate nucleus volume in Parkinson's disease with and without dementia with Lewy bodies and Alzheimer's disease. *Dement Geriatr Cogn Disord.* 2003;**16**(2):57–63.

58. Laakso MP, Partanen K, Riekkinen P, *et al.* Hippocampal volumes in Alzheimer's disease, Parkinson's disease with and without dementia, and in vascular dementia: an MRI study. *Neurology.* 1996;**46**(3):678–81.

59. Camicioli R, Moore MM, Kinney A, *et al.* Parkinson's disease is associated with hippocampal atrophy. *Mov Disord.* 2003;**18**(7):784–90.

60. Tam CW, Burton EJ, McKeith IG, Burn DJ, O'Brien JT. Temporal lobe atrophy on MRI in Parkinson disease with dementia: a comparison with Alzheimer disease and dementia with Lewy bodies. *Neurology.* 2005;**64**(5):861–5.

61. Haris M, Singh A, Cai K, *et al.* T1rho (T1ρ) MR imaging in Alzheimer's disease and Parkinson's disease with and without dementia. *J Neurol.* 2011;**258**(3):380–5.

62. Camicioli RM, Korzan JR, Foster SL, *et al.* Posterior cingulate metabolic changes occur in Parkinson's disease patients without dementia. *Neurosci Lett.* 2004;**354**(3):177–80.

63. Bouchard TP, Malykhin N, Martin WR, *et al.* Age and dementia-associated atrophy predominates in the hippocampal head and amygdala in Parkinson's disease. *Neurobiol Aging.* 2008;**29**(7):1027–39.

64. Ibarretxe-Bilbao N, Ramirez-Ruiz B, Tolosa E, *et al.* Hippocampal head atrophy predominance in Parkinson's disease with hallucinations and with dementia. *J Neurol.* 2008;**255**(9):1324–31.

65. Janzen J, van 't Ent D, Lemstra AW, *et al.* The pedunculopontine nucleus is related to visual hallucinations in Parkinson's disease: preliminary results of a voxel-based morphometry study. *J Neurol.* 2012;**259**(1):147–54.

66. Junque C, Ramirez-Ruiz B, Tolosa E, *et al.* Amygdalar and

hippocampal MRI volumetric reductions in Parkinson's disease with dementia. *Mov Disord.* 2005;**20**(5):540–4.

67. Beyer MK, Janvin CC, Larsen JP, Aarsland D. A magnetic resonance imaging study of patients with Parkinson's disease with mild cognitive impairment and dementia using voxel-based morphometry. *J Neurol Neurosurg Psychiatry.* 2007;**78**(3):254–9.

68. Cordato NJ, Halliday GM, Harding AJ, Hely MA, Morris JG. Regional brain atrophy in progressive supranuclear palsy and Lewy body disease. *Ann Neurol.* 2000;**47**(6):718–28.

69. Cordato NJ, Duggins AJ, Halliday GM, Morris JG, Pantelis C. Clinical deficits correlate with regional cerebral atrophy in progressive supranuclear palsy. *Brain.* 2005;**128**(Pt 6):1259–66.

70. Goldman JG, Stebbins GT, Bernard B, *et al.* Entorhinal cortex atrophy differentiates Parkinson's disease patients with and without dementia. *Mov Disord.* 2012;**27**(6):727–34.

71. Kenny ER, Burton EJ, O'Brien JT. A volumetric magnetic resonance imaging study of entorhinal cortex volume in dementia with Lewy bodies. A comparison with Alzheimer's disease and Parkinson's disease with and without dementia. *Dement Geriatr Cogn Disord.* 2008;**26**(3):218–25.

72. Hanyu H, Asano T, Sakurai H, *et al.* MR analysis of the substantia innominata in normal aging, Alzheimer disease, and other types of dementia. *AJNR Am J Neuroradiol.* 2002;**23**(1):27–32.

73. Choi SH, Jung TM, Lee JE, *et al.* Volumetric analysis of the substantia innominata in patients with Parkinson's disease according to cognitive status. *Neurobiol Aging.* 2012;**33**(7):1265–72.

74. Oikawa H, Sasaki M, Ehara S, Abe T. Substantia innominata:

MR findings in Parkinson's disease. *Neuroradiology* 2004;**46**(10):817–21.

75. Wild EJ, Fox NC. Serial volumetric MRI in Parkinsonian disorders. *Mov Disord.* 2009;**24** Suppl 2:S691–8.

76. Weintraub D, Dietz N, Duda JE, *et al.* Alzheimer's disease pattern of brain atrophy predicts cognitive decline in Parkinson's disease. *Brain.* 2012;**135**(Pt 1): 170–80.

77. Aybek S, Lazeyras F, Gronchi-Perrin A, *et al.* Hippocampal atrophy predicts conversion to dementia after STN-DBS in Parkinson's disease. *Parkinsonism Relat Disord.* 2009;**15**(7):521–4.

78. Burton EJ, McKeith IG, Burn DJ, O'Brien JT. Brain atrophy rates in Parkinson's disease with and without dementia using serial magnetic resonance imaging. *Mov Disord.* 2005;**29**(12):1571–6.

79. Ramirez-Ruiz B, Marti MJ, Tolosa E, *et al.* Longitudinal evaluation of cerebral morphological changes in Parkinson's disease with and without dementia. *J Neurol.* 2005;**252**(11):1345–52.

80. Hu MT, White SJ, Chaudhuri KR, *et al.* Correlating rates of cerebral atrophy in Parkinson's disease with measures of cognitive decline. *J Neural Transm.* 2001;**108**(5):571–80.

81. Ibarretxe-Bilbao N, Ramirez-Ruiz B, Junque C, *et al.* Differential progression of brain atrophy in Parkinson's disease with and without visual hallucinations. *J Neurol Neurosurg Psychiatry.* 2010;**81**(6):650–7.

82. Baba T, Kikuchi A, Hirayama K, *et al.* Severe olfactory dysfunction is a prodromal symptom of dementia associated with Parkinson's disease: a 3 year longitudinal study. *Brain.* 2012;**135**(Pt 1):161–9.

83. Camicioli R, Sabino J, Gee M, *et al.* Ventricular dilatation and brain atrophy in patients with Parkinson's disease with incipient dementia. *Mov Disord.* 2011;**26**(8):1443–50.

84. Dalaker TO, Larsen JP, Bergsland N, *et al.* Brain atrophy and white matter hyperintensities in early Parkinson's disease(a). *Mov Disord.* 2009;**24**(15):2233–41.

85. Dalaker TO, Larsen JP, Dwyer MG, *et al.* White matter hyperintensities do not impact cognitive function in patients with newly diagnosed Parkinson's disease. *Neuroimage.* 2009;**47**(4):2083–9.

86. Slawek J, Roszmann A, Robowski P, *et al.* The impact of MRI white matter hyperintensities on dementia in Parkinson's disease in relation to the homocysteine level and other vascular risk factors. *Neurodegener Dis.* 2012; [Epub ahead of print].

87. Rodriguez-Oroz MC, Lage PM, Sanchez-Mut J, *et al.* Homocysteine and cognitive impairment in Parkinson's disease: a biochemical, neuroimaging, and genetic study. *Mov Disord.* 2009;**24**(10):1437–44.

88. Kim JS, Oh YS, Lee KS, *et al.* Association of cognitive dysfunction with neurocirculatory abnormalities in early Parkinson disease. *Neurology* 2012;**79**(13):1323–31.

89. Shin J, Choi S, Lee JE, *et al.* Subcortical white matter hyperintensities within the cholinergic pathways of Parkinson's disease patients according to cognitive status. *J Neurol Neurosurg Psychiatry.* 2012;**83**(3):315–21.

90. Burton EJ, McKeith IG, Burn DJ, Firbank MJ, O'Brien JT. Progression of white matter hyperintensities in Alzheimer disease, dementia with Lewy bodies, and Parkinson disease dementia: a comparison with normal aging. *Am J Geriatr Psychiatry.* 2006;**14**(10):842–9.

91. Carlesimo GA, Piras F, Assogna F *et al.* Hippocampal abnormalities and memory deficits in Parkinson disease: a multimodal imaging study. *Neurology.* 2012;**78**(24):1939–45.

92. Hattori T, Orimo S, Aoki S, *et al.* Cognitive status correlates with white matter alteration in Parkinson's disease. *Hum Brain Mapp.* 2012;**33**(3):727–39.

93. Kamagata K, Motoi Y, Abe O, *et al.* White matter alteration of the cingulum in Parkinson disease with and without dementia: evaluation by diffusion tensor tract-specific analysis. *AJNR Am J Neuroradiol.* 2012;**33**(5):890–5.

94. Matsui H, Nishinaka K, Oda M, *et al.* Dementia in Parkinson's disease: diffusion tensor imaging. *Acta Neurol Scand.* 2007; **116**(3):177–81.

95. Wiltshire K, Concha L, Gee M, *et al.* Corpus callosum and cingulum tractography in Parkinson's disease. *Can J Neurol Sci.* 2010;**37**(5):595–600.

96. Matsui H, Nishinaka K, Oda M, *et al.* Wisconsin Card Sorting Test in Parkinson's disease: diffusion tensor imaging. *Acta Neurol Scand.* 2007;**116**(2):108–12.

97. Lee JE, Park HJ, Park B, *et al.* A comparative analysis of cognitive profiles and white-matter alterations using voxel-based diffusion tensor imaging between patients with Parkinson's disease dementia and dementia with Lewy bodies. *J Neurol Neurosurg Psychiatry.* 2010;**81**(3):320–6.

Chapter 5

Functional MRI of motor signs in Parkinson's disease

Tobias Wächter

Introduction

Greater understanding of the motor features of Parkinson's disease (PD) is clearly needed. Researchers have focused on motor signs such as tremor, rigidity, bradykinesia, and postural instability and evaluated for functional cortical and subcortical imaging correlates of these features as well as the associated brain imaging changes that result with treatments. This chapter will review functional imaging studies, including those with functional magnetic resonance imaging (fMRI), and nuclear tracing studies such as positron emission tomography (PET) and single-photon emission computed tomography (SPECT) scanning as they relate to motor signs of PD.

Underlying the clinical features of PD is the loss of the dopamineric neurons in the substantia nigra pars compacta, which results in a dopaminergic deficit in projecting fibers to the dorsolateral prefrontal cortex and the striatum. The dorsal region of the striatum, namely the putamen, functions as a relay within the motor basal ganglia, connecting the motor cortex to the globus pallidus, with further connections through the thalamus back to cortical motor areas. Within the putamen, dopaminergic cells function like a relay, as GABAergic spiny neurons with inhibitory connections project to the globus pallidus internus containing excitatory D1 receptors whereas spiny neurons of the excitatory pathway project to the globus pallidus externus and the subthalamic nucleus containing inhibitory D2 receptors. Therefore, a dopaminergic deficiency in the dorsal striatum results in increased inhibitory input to the thalamus and therefore reduced output to the motor cortex, mainly the supplementary motor area (SMA) [1, 2]. In accordance with this pathological concept, early functional imaging studies using PET or SPECT studies in

patients with PD found decreased neuronal activation in the putamen, the dorsolateral prefrontal cortex (DLPFC), the anterior cingulate, and the SMA [3–7]. Areas with increased neuronal activation in PD were found in the lateral premotor cortex [7], the cerebellum [6], and the parietal cortex [4, 7].

Functional MRI correlates of hand movements in PD and changes with disease progression

fMRI of healthy controls (HC) performing unilateral hand movements typically identifies cerebral correlates in the motor system, for example the contralateral primary sensorimotor cortex, premotor cortex, SMA, DLPFC, right inferior frontal gyrus, bilateral insula, bilateral basal ganglia, and bilateral cerebellum [8]. When evaluating PD and HC participants during hand movements, fMRI studies revealed findings similar to those seen with PET described below (Table 5.1) [3–7]. Sabatini et al. [9] had akinetic PD subjects perform sequential finger movements and showed alterations in the blood oxygen level dependent (BOLD) signal of the motor system compared to HC. However, the higher spatial resolution of fMRI allowed Sabatini et al. to demonstrate the heterogeneity of changes in the SMA; with decreased activation in the rostral SMA and hyperactivity in the caudal SMA. Also, varied findings were noted in the inferior parietal cortex with regions of increased and areas of decreased activation. In keeping with PET, there was hypoactivation of the DLPFC, bilateral hyperactivation in the primary sensorimotor cortex, the premotor cortex as well as the contralateral cingulum. Interestingly, there was also a region with hypoactivation within the contralateral premotor cortex. A study

Table 5.1. Characteristics of studies on fMRI of movements in PD

Citation	MR system	Number of PD	Disease stage	Disease duration (years)	Type of PD	Medication	Movement	Pacing
Sabatini et al., 2000 [9]	Siemens (1.5T) EPI: 9 slices of 5 mm	6	H & Y = 2.7 ± 0.5	5 ± 2	Akinetic-rigid	Off	Sequential finger	None
Haslinger et al., 2001 [10]	Philips (1.5T) EPI: 6 slices of 6 mm	8	H & Y = 1.5 ± 0.7	1.9 ± 1.3	Akinetic-rigid	Off and on	Joystick	Auditory pacing
Rowe et al., 2002 [29]	(2T) EPI: ? slices of 3 mm	12	H & Y = 2.5 ± 0.5	5.3 ± 3.5	Not stated	Off	Sequential finger	Auditory and visual pacing
Buhmann et al., 2003 [13]	Siemens (1.5T) EPI: 26 slices of 3 mm	8	H & Y ≤ 1.5	1.2 ± 0.5	Akinetic-rigid	Off (de novo) and on	Random finger opposition	Auditory pacing
Wu et al., 2005 [16] 2008 [22] 2010 [21]	GRE (1.5T) EPI: 21 slices of 5 mm	12	H & Y = 2.0 ± 0.6	6.3 ± 2.8	Akinetic-rigid and tremor	Off	Sequential finger + distraction	None
Cerasa et al., 2006 [17]	Siemens (1.5T) EPI: 32 slices of 3 mm	10	H & Y = 2.5 ± 0.6	7.2 ± 3.5	Akinetic-rigid	Off	Rhythmic taping of index finger	With and without visual pacing
Eckert et al., 2006 [15]	GRE (1.5T) EPI: 23 slices of 5 mm	9	H & Y = 1.3 ± 0.4	1.7 ± 0.7	Akinetic-rigid	Off (de novo) and on	Fist opening–closing	None
Lewis et al., 2007 [32]	Siemens (3T) EPI: 49 slices of 3 mm	1		2	Tremor + rigidity	Off and on	Sequential finger	With and without visual pacing
Yu et al., 2007 [14]	GRE (3T) EPI: 25 slices of 5 mm	8	UPDRS III = 29.5 ± 13.6	5.9 ± 2.6	Akinetic-rigid	Off	Thumb button-press	Auditory pacing
Foki et al., 2010 [34]	Siemens (3T) EPI: 34 slices of 3 mm	10	H & Y = 2.3 ± 0.5	7.0 ± 4.9	Akinetic-rigid	Off	Finger tapping and coin rotation	None
Ng et al., 2010 [43]	Philips (3T) EPI: 36 slices of 3 mm	10	H & Y = 2–3	5.8 ± 3	Not stated	Off and on	Bulb-squeezing	Not stated
Sen et al. 2010 [18]	Siemens (3T) EPI: slices of 3 mm	5	UPDRS III = 4.4 ± 2.1 UPDRS III = 5.7 ± 3.3	Not given 21.6 months later	3 Akinetic-rigid 2 Tremor	Off	Sequential finger	With and without visual pacing

Table 5.1. (cont.)

Citation	MR system	Number of PD	Disease stage	Disease duration (years)	Type of PD	Medication	Movement	Pacing
Wu et al., 2010 [8]	Siemens (1.5T) EPI: 20 slices of 5 mm	15	H & Y = 1.7 ± 0.4	3.5 ± 1.6		Off	Finger flexion–extension	None
Lewis et al., 2011 [35]	Siemens (3T) EPI: 49 slices of 3 mm	8	H & Y = 1.3 ± 0.5	1.3 ± 2.0	Akinetic-rigid	Off	Sequential finger	Only without pacing analyzed
		9	H & Y = 1.3 ± 0.4	0.3 ± 0.4	Tremor			
Snijders et al., 2011 [40]	Siemens Trio (3T) EPI: 35 slices of 3 mm	12 with freezing	UPDRS III = 34.6 ± 9.6	9.8 ± 4.6	Patients with severe tremor excluded	Off	Motor imagery of walking	None
		12 without freezing	UPDRS III = 28.6 ± 12.2	7.1 ± 3.0				
Wu et al., 2011 [19]	Siemens (1.5T) EPI: 20 slices of 5 mm	18	H & Y = 1.7 ± 0.5	4.2 ± 1.6	Most akinetic-rigid	Off	Finger tapping	None

EPI, echo-planar imaging; GRE, gradient echo; H & Y, Hoehn and Yahr Scale; UPDRS, Unified Parkinson's Disease Rating Scale.

by Haslinger et al. [10] with akinetic PD patients off medication performing joystick movements confirmed the decreased BOLD signal in the rostral SMA and adjacent lateral premotor areas bilaterally and an increased activation in the primary sensorimotor cortex and a trend towards increased activation in more distal regions of the lateral premotor cortex on both sides as well as in the ipsilateral superior parietal cortex.

The decrease in BOLD signal in the SMA and premotor areas seen in both fMRI studies [9, 10] is in accordance with the hypothesis that there is functional cortical deafferentation after dopaminergic depletion in the basal ganglia loops of the motor system. However, the increase in BOLD signal in areas of the primary motor as well as more lateral areas of the premotor cortex seen in both these studies [9, 10] and previous PET studies [7] cannot easily be explained by this model. The authors interpreted the increase in neuronal activation in the primary motor cortex as uncontrolled afferent noise caused by defective cortico-cortical inhibition in PD as demonstrated earlier in studies using transcranial magnetic stimulation [11, 12]. In contrast, the increased activation in the lateral premotor cortex and

concomitantly in the parietal cortex was postulated to be caused by increased parietal–premotor connectivity. Therefore, hyperactivation of lateral motor areas was suggested to represent neuronal reorganization in which cortical motor areas compensate for the impaired subcortical motor system.

To investigate further the BOLD signal change in the primary motor cortex of PD, Buhmann et al. [13] performed fMRI during paced finger movements in a group of patients with unilateral symptoms in a very early stage of PD (Hoehn and Yahr ≤ 1.5) who had never been exposed to dopaminergic medication. As seen in the previous fMRI studies [9, 10] there was hypoactivation of the SMA. However, in contrast to these former studies, the BOLD signal in the primary motor cortex contralateral to the affected side was reduced rather than increased. As this finding is in accordance with the hypothesis of a functional cortical deafferentation in PD the authors suggested that the exposure to dopaminergic medication accounted for the increased BOLD signal in the primary motor areas in prior studies on previously treated PD. However, as Buhmann et al. examined individuals not only untreated but also very early in the disease, it cannot be determined if the increased BOLD signal in the motor cortex seen in prior studies on PD with longer disease duration and dopaminergic treatment [9, 10] is actually caused by the exposure to dopaminergic treatment, or due to disease progression [14]. As Buhmann et al. examined individuals primarily with unilateral signs they also compared both hemispheres within subjects and found decreased activation in the primary motor cortex contralateral to the affected hand more pronounced than contralateral to the less affected hand, supporting the underlying hypothesis of functional deafferentation of the motor system.

A very similar cohort of early untreated patients with PD was evaluated in an fMRI study of hand movements by Eckert et al. [15]. In contrast to Buhmann et al., patients in this study performed hand-opening and -closing instead of finger movements. Furthermore, the movements in the study by Eckert et al. were self-paced and not externally triggered as they were in the study by Buhmann et al. The results differed as there was hyperactivation of the pre-SMA, but no hypoactivation of the SMA. Interestingly, a previous fMRI study [9] testing finger movements of PD without external pacing also found increased activation of the SMA and therefore Eckert et al. attributed this finding to the internal generation of the movement. It must, however, be noted that the hyperactivation found by Sabatini et al. was in a more caudal region of the SMA than the activation found in the PD group by Eckert et al. and that other studies testing self-paced movements could not replicate this finding [16] or only found increased activation in a between-group comparison between HC and PD but not when comparing externally paced with self-initiated movements within the PD group [17]. Furthermore, even in early untreated PD subjects, increased activation both in the premotor and primary motor cortices challenges the assumption that the enhanced activation of motor areas is secondary to medication treatment [13]. Additionally, the study by Eckert et al. found areas with increased and decreased activation of the parietal cortex and hyperactivation in the cerebellum during finger movements in PD (Figure 5.1).

The effect of disease progression on cerebral correlates of movements was studied by Sen et al. [18]. This group evaluated individuals with early PD and then approximately 2 years later by evaluating visually paced and self-generated sequential finger movements. Neuronal activity in predefined neuronal

circuits was analyzed with BOLD signal changes over time as the multivariate dependent variable. A comparison to HC over the first 2 years of disease progression found no change within the striato-thalamo-cortical circuit (putamen/globus pallidus, thalamus, SMA, primary motor cortex) in PD subjects. However, the ipsilateral cerebellar/vermis-thalamo-cortical circuit (cerebellar vermis/paravermis/dentate nuclei, thalamus, lateral premotor cortex, somatosensory cortex) in PD showed a significant increase in activation and the ipsilateral cerebellar hemisphere-thalamo-cortical circuit (cerebellar hemisphere, thalamus, lateral premotor cortex, somatosensory cortex) suggested a trend towards increased activation for the less affected hand when performing self-generated movements. In contrast, a within-group comparison found that after 2 years movements with the more affected hand revealed a significant increase in BOLD signal in the contralateral neuronal circuit deriving from the thalamus when performing self-generated movements and in the ipsilateral neuronal circuit deriving from the cerebellar hemisphere when performing visually triggered movements. The authors explain these findings as a result of compensatory recruitment of cerebellar-thalamo-cortical circuits for decompensation of initial functional striato-thalamo-cortical circuits, which the authors claimed were not due to remaining drug effects. While the longitudinal design of the study is very interesting, the interpretation of the heterogeneous findings remains difficult; important questions remain such as the finding of BOLD signal changes in premotor and primary motor areas with disease progression. The small sample size of five PD and five HC as well as the heterogeneity of the disease with akinesia and tremor subtypes of PD certainly account for the low statistical power of this interesting scientific approach.

To investigate further the underlying pathological changes at the level of neuronal networks, Wu et al [19] performed an analysis of effective connectivity using the method of psychophysiological interaction during finger tapping movements [20]. Effective connections were found in PD and HC during self-initiated finger tapping movements between neuronal activation of the primary motor, lateral premotor and parietal cortices as well as the pre-SMA and the cerebellum. However, effective connectivity in PD from the putamen to the primary motor and lateral premotor cortices as well as to the SMA and cerebellum was decreased, while the connectivity between the

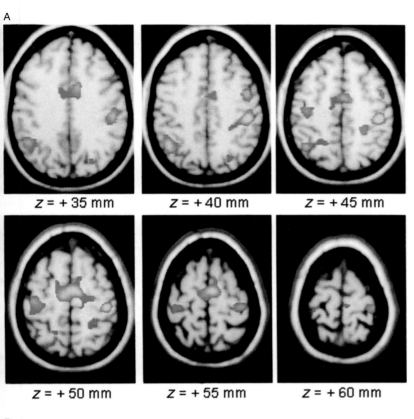

z = +35 mm   z = +40 mm   z = +45 mm

z = +50 mm   z = +55 mm   z = +60 mm

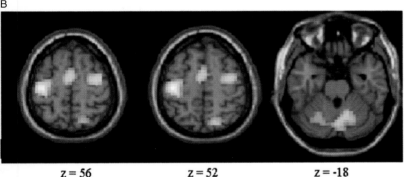

z = 56   z = 52   z = -18

Figure 5.1 Area of relative hyperactivity in PD compared to HC during right hand movement (A = sequential finger movements; B = fist opening and closing movements): both studies with self-initiated movements find increased activation in the SMA in contrast to several other fMRI studies of externally triggered movements. Z = location of area of activation above commissural plane. (Part A from Sabatini *et al. Brain.* 2000;**123**:394–403, with kind permission of Oxford University Press [9]; part B from Eckert *et al. J Neurol.* 2006;**253**:199–207, with kind permission of Springer Science+Business Media [15].)

primary motor cortex and the lateral premotor cortex, pre-SMA, and cerebellum was increased compared to HC. Moreover, the connection of the DLPFC to the primary motor and lateral premotor cortices as well as the pre-SMA and cerebellum are weaker in PD. This study demonstrates that in PD not only the activity of certain brain regions but also the pattern of interacting brain networks is disrupted. While striato-cortical and striato-cerebellar connections are

weakened, there is a most likely compensatory increase of the cortico-cerebellar connections, and correlations of these changes in connectivity with disease severity indicate that these changes progress with the disease (Figure 5.2).

Findings of fMRI studies investigating hand movements of PD in comparison to HC are summarized in Table 5.2. Most fMRI studies of simple hand movements find hypoactivity in the SMA with

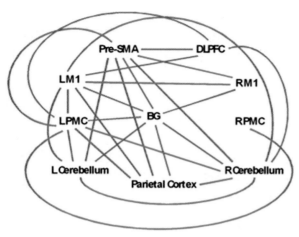

Figure 5.2 Differences of effective connectivity between PD and HC among the basal ganglia, pre-SMA, bilateral M1, bilateral PMC (= premotor cortex), bilateral cerebellum, DLPFC (= dorsolateral prefrontal cortex), and parietal cortex. Red/blue lines indicate increased/decreased connectivity between the two brain regions in PD patients compared to HC. (From Wu *et al. Neuroimage.* 2011;**55**:204–15, with kind permission of Elsevier [19].)

externally triggered movements, while some studies investigating self-paced movements also find regions with hyperactivation in rostral areas of the SMA. Furthermore, in PD there is decreased activation of the striatum and thalamus as well as in the DLPFC. Increased activation is generally found in the premotor region and in most studies also in the primary motor cortex. Meanwhile some studies report additional hypoactivation in lateral areas of the premotor cortex. Hypoactivation of the parietal cortex is reported in most studies, with some studies reporting additional hyperactivation of the superior parietal cortex. All studies find hyperactivation of the cerebellum, with only one study reporting an additional hypoactivation of the inferior hemisphere. Over the disease progression this pattern develops with a decrease of activation in striato-cortical and striato-cerebellar connections and a compensatory increase of cortico-cerebellar connections.

Complex hand movements; learning sequences, dual tasking, bimanual coordination

To examine the functional changes occurring with learning of automatic finger movements Wu and Hallett [16] performed fMRI on a group of individuals with moderate or advanced PD before and after practicing a finger-sequence. A comparison of BOLD signals between PD and HC confirmed hyperactivation of the bilateral premotor cortex as well as in the DLPFC, parietal cortex, and precuneus, but also in both cerebellar hemispheres, similar to previous studies (see Table 5.2). At the scanning session before practice, those with PD showed additional hypoactivation of the pre-SMA bilaterally similar to the previous studies [9, 10], but after training this difference from HC was no longer detectable, while the differences in BOLD signal in the other cerebral regions with hyperactivation in PD remained. Within-group analysis in PD found less activation in the superior parietal lobe bilaterally as well as in the contralateral insular cortex. Changes of the BOLD signal in the premotor cortex, SMA, and inferior parietal cortex demonstrated that learning in HC did not occur in PD. Therefore, the authors conclude that PD can achieve automaticity of movements only with heightened effort. To further investigate the underlying interaction of these pathological neuronal activations between these regions, Wu *et al.* [21] performed an additional effective connectivity analysis on the same data using the method of psychophysiological interaction [20]. Using this analysis they discovered that execution of automatic movements in PD and HC strengthens connectivity of the caudal SMA, bilateral cerebellum, and cingulum, but only in HC was the putamen found interconnected. Furthermore, an intergroup comparison found stronger connectivity of the caudal SMA, bilateral cerebellum, and cingulum in HC than in PD. HC also showed stronger integration of the DLPFC during novel movements, which was not found in PD. Therefore, the increased effort with learning of automatic movements in PD is not only explained by a less effective encoding, but might also be explained by a failure to shift execution of automatic movements to subcortical connections [21].

To study cerebral correlates of increasing demand by dual-task performance, Wu and Hallett [22] also introduced two secondary distractor tests (letter counting and finger tapping) in addition to the sequential finger movements during the same experimental session. Interestingly, there was no significant difference in the brain pattern of activation with the two different secondary tasks, indicating that various dual tasks might not necessarily involve different cerebral mechanisms. However, people with PD recruited more brain areas than HC when executing the dual task at a comparable behavioral level. Many movements, even if this was only the baseline condition and not the main comparison tested in the study

Citation	Prefrontal	Premotor	SMA	Sensorimotor	Parietal	Striatum	Cerebellum	Other
Sabatini et al., 2000 [9]	↓ (dorsolat.) ipsilat.	↓ (lateral) contralat. ↑ (bilat.)	↓ (rostral) contralat. ↑ (caudal) contralat.	↑ bilat.	↓ (inferior) contralat. ↑ (inferior) bilat.			↑ (Cingulum) contralat.
Haslinger et al., 2001 [10]		**↓ (lateral) bilat. (↑) (lateral) bilat.**	**↓ (rostral) bilat.**	**↑ (M1) bilat.**	**(↓) (superior) ipsilat.**			
Rowe et al., 2002 [29]			↑ ipsilat.			↓ (Putamen) contralat.		
Buhmann et al., 2003 [13]			↓ contralat.	↓ (M1) contralat.				
Wu et al., 2005 [16]	↑ (dorsolat.) bilat.	↑ bilat.	↓ (pre-SMA) bilat.		↑ bilat. ↑ (Precuneus) bilat.		↑ bilat.	
Cerasa et al., 2006 [17]							↑ ipsilat.	↑ (Thalamus) bilat.
Eckert et al., 2006 [15]		↑ (lateral) bilat.	↑ (pre-SMA) contralat.	↑ contralat.	↑ contralat. ↓ (superior) bilat.		↑ (superior) bilat. ↓ (inferior) ipsilat.	
Lewis et al., 2007 [32]			**↓ contralat.**	**↓ (primary motor) ipsilat.**		**↓ (Putamen) contralat.**	**↑ ipsilat.**	↓ (Thalamus) contralat. ↓ (Globus pallidum) contralat.
Yu et al., 2007 [14]	**↓ (dorsolat.) ipsilat.**		**↓ contralat. ↓ (pre-SMA) bilat.**	**↑ (M1) contralat.**		**↓ (Striatum) ipsilat. ↓ (Putamen) contralat.**	**↑ bilat.**	
Ng et al., 2010 [43]			↑ contralat.	↑ (M1) ipsilat.				
Wu et al., 2011 [19]		↑ (lateral) bilat.	↓ (pre-SMA) bilat.		↑ bilat.	↓ (Putamen) contralat.	↑ bilat.	

↓ = BOLD signal in PD decreased in comparison to HC, ↑ = BOLD signal in PD increased in comparison to HC during movement (arrows in brackets symbolize a reported trend). Areas are specified in brackets behind the arrows. Laterality given below the arrow.

63

of the following areas with increased activation in PD had been associated earlier with dual-task performance; DLPFC and parietal cortex with attention and executive processes [23, 24], as well as the primary motor cortex and cerebellum with temporal organization [25, 26]. During dual tasking additional over-activation in PD was also found in the middle frontal gyrus, the precuneus, the temporal and occipital lobes, the cerebellum, and thalamus, as well as the cingulum. In accordance with a capacity-sharing mode [19, 27], these findings suggest an increased attentional demand in PD compared to HC when executing dual tasks. However, in PD as well as in the age-matched elderly HC the only change in BOLD signal found when comparing single with dual task was in the precuneus bilaterally, which was not shown in younger subjects performing the same dual tasks in an earlier study by the same group [28]. Therefore, the authors discuss that the precuneus might serve as a central supervisor during the execution of dual tasks. The authors conclude that limited attentional resources and a deficient central executive function might explain the deficits in dual tasking in PD.

In a similar experiment, Rowe et al. [29] studied PD patients and HC performing overlearned sequential finger movements with and without an additional attentional task and applied structural equation modeling [30] to compare effective connectivity of activated brain areas in both groups. This study found increased activation in the ipsilateral SMA and decreased activation in the contralateral putamen during movement in PD patients. However, when subjects were instructed to attend to their action the BOLD signal in HC increased in the prefrontal, paracingulate region, and supplementary motor cortex similar to a comparable PET study [31], which was not seen in PD. Accordingly, a between-group comparison found reduced activation of the SMA and parietal cortex in PD during attention-related activation. Structural equation modeling found increased connectivity between prefrontal areas and premotor areas as well as the SMA in HC during attention-related activation, which was not seen in PD nor in HC performing an alternative visual attentional task. The authors conclude that a task-specific abnormality of the SMA, resulting at least partly from a functional disconnection of the SMA, accounts for movement deficits in PD.

The demand on neuronal processing increases with the complexity of movements. In a consecutive

study Wu et al. [8] investigated the changes of BOLD signal during in-phasic and anti-phasic bimanual movements in PD compared to age-matched HC. Within-group analysis in PD showed no increase in activation of the SMA during anti-phase movement compared to in-phase movements in PD, which was seen in the HC. Comparing BOLD signals between groups during in-phase bimanual movements found PD with increased activity in the right primary sensorimotor cortex, left premotor cortex, bilateral postcentral gyrus, left superior parietal lobe, right precuneus, and bilateral cerebellum, while the activation in the caudal SMA, bilateral thalamus, left putamen, and right globus pallidus was decreased. During anti-phasic movements activation in PD is greater than in HC in the left primary sensorimotor cortex, left premotor cortex, right inferior frontal gyrus, bilateral precentral and postcentral gyri, left superior and inferior parietal lobes, bilateral paracentral lobule, bilateral precuneus, and bilateral cerebellum, while activation is decreased in the caudal SMA, bilateral thalamus, and right globus pallidus. These findings by Wu et al. suggest not only an increase in neuronal demand in PD and HC with increasing complexity of movement coordination, but the difference in pattern of activation between both groups also mounts. This indicates that not only are certain regions deficient, but the entire network seems to be affected. To investigate further the psychophysiological interaction of cerebral regions Wu et al. subsequently performed an effective connectivity analysis of these regions with the caudal SMA as the index region. While performing in-phase movements PD showed greater connectivity of the caudal SMA to the left primary sensorimotor cortex, left postcentral gyrus, left precuneus, and bilateral cerebellum, while the connection to the right premotor cortex and right putamen was reduced in comparison to HC. During anti-phasic movements the caudal SMA of PD had stronger connection to the bilateral primary sensorimotor cortex, the bilateral superior parietal cortex, right precuneus, and bilateral cerebellum, while the connection of the caudal SMA to the left DLPFC and left putamen was weaker than in HC. These findings illustrate how complex motor behaviors on a dysfunctional basal ganglia lead to pathological activations in some areas and possibly compensatory changes in others.

To test the influence of an external trigger on simple index tapping movements in PD, Cerasa *et al.* [17] compared visual externally triggered movements with self-generated rhythmic movements in PD and HC while undergoing fMRI. Within-group comparison between visually triggered and self-generated movements in both groups found difference of the BOLD signal in visual areas but not in areas attributed to motor control, even though those with PD performed self-generated movements with increased movement latency. A between-group comparison of the BOLD signal during untriggered index-finger movement showed increased activation of the thalamus bilaterally and the ipsilateral cerebellum in PD, which was interpreted by the authors as an increased demand on the cerebello-thalamic pathway in accordance with former findings in a PET study [6] and fMRI studies [14, 16]. However, during visually paced movements the between-group comparison found hyperactivation in the PD group in several frontal areas (SMA, ipsilateral inferior frontal gyrus, contralateral frontal operculum, and lingual gyrus), in the ipsilateral insula, the ipsilateral putamen, and the thalamus as well as contralateral cerebellum. The authors attribute this broad extent of increased activation to involvement of three specific networks: the medial premotor pathway for timing representation, the inferior frontal gyrus and the insular for rehearsal and retrieval of time-related representation, and the cerebellum for greater control. These findings are difficult to reconcile with results of an earlier fMRI study by the same group [9] of a comparable sample of patients performing self-paced sequential finger movements, which led to changes of BOLD signal, with hypoactivation in the contralateral rostral SMA and premotor cortex as well as the ipsilateral DLPFC and hyperactivation in the bilateral sensorimotor, premotor, and inferior parietal cortices. The differences between these studies might partly be explained by greater imaging resolution in the later study. Nonetheless the findings in the SMA and premotor and primary motor areas demonstrated in several studies [4, 5, 9, 10, 13] during self-initiated as well as externally paced movements remain unexplained.

Lewis *et al.* [32] used a multivariate analysis of regions of interest (ROIs) constituting basal ganglia–cortical (globus pallidus/putamen, thalamus, SMA, and primary motor cortex) and cerebellar–cortical circuits (cerebellum, thalamus, somatosensory cortex, and lateral premotor cortex) to compare BOLD signals during sequential finger movements with and without visual pacing in a monozygotic twin pair

discordant for clinical PD. During self-initiated movements, activation was decreased in the basal ganglia–cortical as well as the cerebellar–cortical circuit bilaterally in the PD patient off medication; however, activation was increased in ROIs of both circuits (premotor cortex and sensorimotor cortex, thalamus, and cerebellum) when the patient with PD was on medication. During visually paced movements the difference between the twins was only found in increased BOLD signal in the bilateral cerebellar–cortical circuit (cerebellum and premotor cortex), only when the PD subject was off medication.

Functional MRI correlates of motor symptoms in PD

PD is characterized by the cardinal motor signs of tremor, rigidity, akinesia, and gait disorder; however, motor features such as apraxia and freezing are also common in the disease. Wu *et al.* [19] found positive correlations of motor signs with neuronal connectivity between the primary motor cortex, pre-SMA, premotor cortex, and cerebellum, while the effective connectivity of the putamen with the primary motor cortex, premotor cortex, SMA, and cerebellum correlated inversely with motor features of PD as ascertained through Unified Parkinson's Disease Rating Scale (UPDRS) scores. These findings demonstrate that with progression of PD the lateral network compensates for dysfunction of subcortical connections. However, differentiating neuronal correlates of defined motor features using fMRI would certainly contribute to the understanding of the pathophysiological mechanism resulting from the underlying neuroanatomical pathology. Functional imaging of neuronal correlates of characteristic motor signs might ultimately allow the development of new diagnostic methods and finally support the differential diagnosis or classification subtypes of PD.

The first fMRI studies in PD described increased activation in the primary motor cortex during finger movement [9, 10], which was attributed to signs of PD, most likely rigidity, as it could not be explained by the underlying striatal dopaminergic deafferentation and interconnected motor areas [10–12, 33]. To investigate further the correlation of hyperactivation in the motor system and motor signs Yu *et al.* [14] conducted an fMRI study in PD patients and HC performing thumb movements at two different frequencies – 0.9 Hz for automatic and 2.4 Hz for cognitively controlled

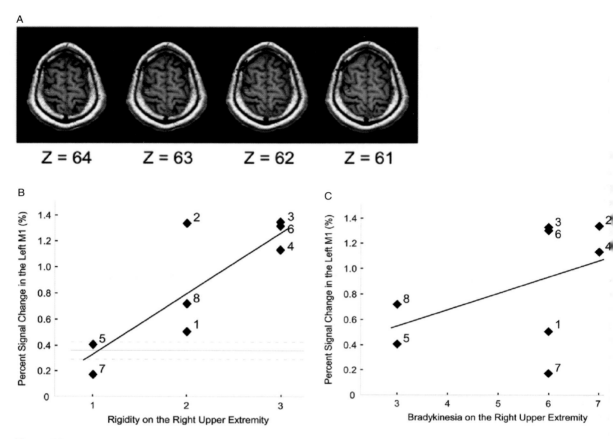

Figure 5.3 Correlation between hyperactivation in the left primary motor cortex with rigidity and bradykinesia in PD patients. (A) Regions of hyperactivation in the left primary motor cortex in PD. (B) The percent signal change in the left primary motor cortex against the rigidity score of the right upper limb in PD. The horizontal solid line represents the average percent signal change of the left primary motor cortex in healthy individuals with the dotted lines as standard error. The linear relation was significant (r = 0.85, p < 0.05). (C) The percent signal change in the left primary motor cortex against the bradykinesia score from the right upper limb in PD patients. There was no significant correlation (r = 0.48, p = 0.23). (From Yu *et al. Neuroimage.* 2007;**35**:222–33, with kind permission of Elsevier.)

timing movements. Both groups showed an increase of activation of the pre-SMA and SMA with slower, cognitively controlled movements, but only the HC additionally activated the DLPFC during 2.4 Hz movements. An intergroup comparison using an ROI analysis found, in accordance with previous studies, hypoactivation of the motor system [9, 10, 13] (contralateral SMA and putamen as well as pre-SMA bilaterally) in PD and a hyperactivation in the contralateral primary motor cortex [9, 10] and both cerebellar hemispheres, which was pronounced on the ipsilateral side [16, 17]. For further investigation of the functional impact of these findings the authors correlated BOLD signals in these regions with the BOLD signal of the putamen to detect pathological coherence and with

clinical symptoms to recognize the functional relevance of the increased neuronal activation of these regions. Interestingly, increased BOLD signals of the ipsilateral cerebellum and contralateral putamen correlated negatively, indicating an increased compensation by the cerebellum for progressive basal ganglia dysfunction. In contrast, the BOLD signal of the primary motor cortex correlated positively with the upper limb rigidity of the patients but not with bradykinesia, whereas a correlation of the cerebellar hyperactivation with clinical symptoms could not be found. These findings suggest that the hyperactivation of the primary motor cortex in PD directly relates to rigidity as suggested before [10–12, 33] and is not a compensatory response (Figure 5.3).

To investigate the neuronal correlates of apraxia in contrast to bradykinesia, Foki et al. [34] compared coin rotation to finger tapping in ten PD patients and ten HC while undergoing fMRI. When comparing the activation pattern of both groups, there was hyperactivation with impaired coin rotation as a sign of apraxia in the contralateral precentral perirolandic cortex and hypoactivation in the contralateral postcentral perirolandic cortex of PD compared to HC. Using individually defined ROIs Foki et al. calculated a "perirolandic index" as "peak t-value of postcentral perirolandic cortex"/"peak t-value of precentral perirolandic cortex." Using this index Foki et al. succeeded in significantly separating PD patients from HC, establishing the first attempt to create a diagnostic fMRI tool for movement disorder patients.

To differentiate functional cerebral correlates of akinesia-rigidity type of PD from those in tremor type of PD Lewis et al. [35] studied both types of PD as well as HC while performing sequential finger movements. As in a previous study by the same group [18] they used a multivariate analysis of variance of ROIs constituting striato-thalamo-cortical and cerebello-thalamo-cortical circuits to compare the activation patterns of these neuronal networks. The striato-thalamo-cortical circuit consisted of ROIs including the lentiform nucleus, thalamus, SMA, and primary motor cortex. The cerebellar pathway was divided into a hemispheric pathway with ROIs originating from the cerebellar hemisphere and including the thalamus, lateral premotor cortex, and somatosensory cortex as well as a pathway originating in the vermis, which consisted of ROIs over the vermis/paravermis including the bilateral dentate nuclei, thalamus, lateral premotor cortex, and somatosensory cortex. During self-initiated finger movements, both types of PD showed increased activation of the contralateral cerebello-thalamo-cortical circuits when compared with HC. Furthermore, the increased BOLD signal of the contralateral striato-thalamo-cortical circuits in tremor-predominant PD reached significance and a trend towards increased activation of this circuit was seen in the akinetic-rigid-type PD bilaterally. A direct comparison between both PD groups found significant differences in all circuits ipsilateral, but not contralateral, to the performing hand. Comparison of ROIs between both groups found BOLD signals increased in almost all cortical and subcortical regions, except for the vermis, contralateral cerebral hemisphere, and ipsilateral thalamus. From these comparisons between both types of PD, the authors conclude, that the akinetic-rigid type of PD might require additional recruitment including the ipsilateral hemisphere to compensate for motor deficits. Interestingly, similar to an fMRI study comparing twins of which one suffered from tremor-dominant PD [32], activation in the primary motor cortex in the tremor subtype of PD was also reduced in comparison to HC, rather than elevated as in several fMRI studies in the akinetic-rigid type of PD [9, 10, 14, 15], supporting the hypothesis that increased activation of the primary motor cortex can be interpreted as a correlate of rigidity. It must however be noted that, contrary to the akinetic-rigid type of PD, the group of tremor-predominant PD subjects examined by Lewis et al. was at a very early stage of the disease and some were de novo to dopaminergic treatment. These data are therefore also in accordance with a previous fMRI study [13] of akinetic-rigid de novo PD patients showing decreased activation of the primary motor cortex during finger movements. Therefore, the change in activation of the primary motor cortex could also be explained by the disease progression or the pharmacological status. Other patterns of fMRI activation in the tremor-type PD studied by Lewis et al. [35] are comparable to findings in previous studies on the akinetic-rigid type of PD with increased activation in the SMA and thalamus and decreased activation in the lentiform nucleus.

Gait is difficult to study using imaging techniques as movements are limited by the physical restrictions of imaging equipment and measures to avoid artifact. Functional emission tomography studies using nuclear tracers to examine PD patients with gait disturbances have shown cerebral correlates of gait disorders in the striatum [36] as well as in lateral premotor and parietal cortical areas dominantly on the right side [36, 37], while frontal involvement remains disputed [38, 39]. To study planning of gait with fMRI and avoid movement artifacts Snijders et al. [40] opted to use motor imagery of walking in people with PD and freezing of gait, PD without freezing of gait, and HC. All groups showed comparable behavioral performance as measured by the time required for imagined walking of paths with different widths and lengths. During imagined walking, both PD groups showed decreased activation of the right superior parietal lobule and anterior cingulate cortex using an ROI analysis. An ROI analysis comparing PD patients with those without freezing of gait showed only a trend towards decreased activation in the left SMA as well as the right superior parietal lobule. However, a whole brain analysis demonstrated a significant increase of the BOLD signal in the posterior mid-mesencephalon in PD with freezing. The BOLD signal increase had a maximum dorsomedial to the pedunculopontine nucleus also including several nuclei of the mesencephalic locomotor region, especially the cuneiform nucleus and the periaqueductal gray. Because the BOLD signal of the locomotor region correlated with disease duration and clinical measurements of gait disturbance, the authors conclude that the pathological activation of the mesencephalon might reflect a decreased inhibition from the basal ganglia to this mesencephalic region.

Effect of treatment on BOLD signal changes in PD

One would hope that functional imaging may be able to provide a correlate of treatment effects. For medications, this would provide a quantitative measurement of the response to symptomatic or disease altering treatments. For deep brain stimulation (DBS), the imaging findings may provide a surrogate that would help guide stimulator programming. To test the effect of dopaminergic medication on the BOLD signal Haslinger et al. [10] examined individuals with PD after they had been off dopaminergic medications for 12 hours and again after a 200 mg oral dose of levodopa. During joystick movements a similar pattern of cerebral activation was seen on as well as off medication – with activation in the primary sensorimotor and lateral premotor cortices bilaterally as well as the left superior parietal cortex, but additionally, activation in the mesial premotor cortex and SMA bilaterally. A direct comparison between both conditions found that levodopa increased BOLD signals in the bilateral pre-SMA and SMA proper as well as adjoining lateral premotor cortices, but decreased activation in the primary sensorimotor cortex bilaterally as well as the right lateral premotor cortex; there was also a trend of decreased activation in the left lateral premotor cortex as well as in both superior parietal cortices. The authors concluded that levodopa leads to a partial reversal of cortical hyperactivation in PD and to increased activation of the rostral and caudal SMA in accordance with previous emissions tomography studies [5, 41, 42]. Lewis et al. [32] used fMRI to test the effect of levodopa on the neuronal network of a single PD patient in comparison to his twin brother and confirmed after medication an increased activation in ROIs comprising the basal ganglia–cortical and cerebellar–cortical circuit. However, this pattern of activation was only found when movements were self-initiated and not when they were visually paced. Next, Ng et al. [43] examined the effect of dopaminergic medication on the amplitude and the spatial extend of the BOLD effect in predefined ROIs in PD during bulb-squeezing movements at three different frequencies. PD patients with their regular morning dose of medication showed a decrease in BOLD amplitude in the bilateral primary motor cortex and contralateral SMA over all frequencies, while at high frequencies there was an additional decrease of the BOLD amplitude in subcortical and cerebellar regions. Medication reduced the spatial extent of the BOLD signal in the bilateral cerebellar hemispheres, primary motor cortex, SMA and right prefrontal cortex. In comparison to HC dopaminergic medication normalized the BOLD signal in the examined ROIs (ipsilateral primary motor cortex and contralateral SMA). A study by Wu et al. [44] using the regional homogeneity method to examine the resting state in PD also found dopaminergic medication to decrease activation in the putamen, thalamus, and SMA, but to increase activation in the cerebellum, primary sensorimotor cortex, and premotor area. To exclude effects of long-term treatment, two studies examined cerebral activation in untreated individuals with early PD. Within-group comparisons between those off medication and patients after four weeks of treatment by Eckert et al. [15] found decreased activation in the contralateral superior parietal cortex and in the ipsilateral DLPFC during opening and closing of the fist. In contrast, a comparison of the BOLD signal during finger opposition movements by Buhmann et al. in previously untreated PD patients and in the same patients 45 minutes after first intake of 300 mg levodopa found an increase of activation in the contralateral primary motor cortex and the bilateral SMA [13]. Even though the effect of dopaminergic medication in both studies seems different, both represent a normalization relative to HC, as untreated PD examined by Eckert et al. showed hyperactivation of the primary motor cortex and SMA besides other areas with hyper- and hypoactivation, whereas Buhmann et al. showed hypoactivation in the same areas relative to HC. These data indicate that the BOLD signal depends on various factors, including the type of disease (akinetic-rigid or tremor-dominant), duration of disease and drug treatment, age, etc. Therefore, these data must be interpreted with caution and consideration of these various factors.

Two studies have used fMRI to study the effect of DBS of the subthalamic nucleus in PD [45, 46]. Both studies were designed to evaluate the feasibility rather than the effect of this treatment on functional cerebral correlates of movements. The studies showed an increase in activation of the ipsilateral basal ganglia and thalamus as well as the contralateral cerebellum with DBS turned on during rest [45], while the effect of DBS on neuronal activation during complex movements demonstrated in PET studies [47, 48] could not be replicated [46]. It must however be stated that fMRI does not comply with the safety recommendations of commercially available DBS systems.

Subramanian *et al.* [49] used biofeedback of the BOLD signal to train five PD patients to increase regional BOLD signal in the SMA by motor imagery. After two training sessions these patients showed increased movement speed and improvement in clinical symptoms compared to five matched PD without biofeedback training. This leaves biofeedback as an interesting intervention for scientific approaches.

Summary

To date fMRI studies have contributed to our understanding of the functional and structural pathology of PD as they relate motor symptoms of the disease to specific patterns of cerebral hypoactivation and hyperactivation and demonstrate changes in comparison to HC. Further studies using connectivity analysis have integrated these findings on a level of neuronal networks and demonstrated that motor deficits in PD not only result from pathological activation of certain areas, but also from changes in functional connectivity. In addition, fMRI studies on complex motor behavior demonstrate that the differences in activation patterns between PD and HC mount with increasing complexity of the movement coordination. Yet it must be realized that all these studies have been performed on relatively small samples of subjects that are not necessarily homogeneous, as findings might be influenced by clinical and genetic subtypes of the disease, disease duration, side of onset, handedness, and types of symptomatic treatments. Furthermore, so far there exist data almost only on finger movement, and we know very little about functional cerebral correlates of other movements.

fMRI studies in PD demonstrated cerebral correlates for rigidity, tremor, and apraxia as well as imaginary planning of gait, and several studies have shown a change of BOLD signal, mostly reversal of pathological activation, with dopaminergic medication. These findings represent a beginning in the clinical use for differentiating subtypes of PD or evaluating pharmacological effects. These techniques however are also not validated. Furthermore data are lacking demonstrating the ability of fMRI to separate PD from other Parkinsonian conditions or to distinguish genetic subtypes of PD. Therefore, the clinical use of fMRI for motor symptoms in PD is still limited.

References

1. Albin RL, Young AB, Penney JB. The functional anatomy of basal ganglia disorders. *Trends Neurosci.* 1989;12(10):366–75.

2. DeLong MR. Primate models of movement disorders of basal ganglia origin. *Trends Neurosci.* 1990;13(7):281–5.

3. Playford ED, Jenkins IH, Passingham RE, *et al.* Impaired mesial frontal and putamen activation in Parkinson's disease: a positron emission tomography study. *Ann Neurol.* 1992;32(2):151–61.

4. Jahanshahi M, Jenkins IH, Brown RG, *et al.* Self-initiated versus externally triggered movements. I. An investigation using measurement of regional cerebral blood flow with PET and movement-related potentials in normal and Parkinson's disease subjects. *Brain.* 1995;118(Pt 4):913–33.

5. Rascol O, Sabatini U, Chollet F, *et al.* Supplementary and primary sensory motor area activity in Parkinson's disease. Regional cerebral blood flow changes during finger movements and effects of apomorphine. *Arch Neurol.* 1992;49(2):144–8.

6. Rascol O, Sabatini U, Fabre N, *et al.* The ipsilateral cerebellar hemisphere is overactive during hand movements in akinetic parkinsonian patients. *Brain.* 1997; 120(Pt 1):103–10.

7. Samuel M, Ceballos-Baumann AO, Blin J, *et al.* Evidence for lateral premotor and parietal overactivity in Parkinson's disease during sequential and bimanual movements. A PET study. *Brain.* 1997; 120(Pt 6):963–76.

8. Wu T, Wang L, Hallett M, Li K, Chan P. Neural correlates of bimanual anti-phase and in-phase movements in Parkinson's disease. *Brain*. 2010;**133**(Pt 8):2394–409.

9. Sabatini U, Boulanouar K, Fabre N, *et al*. Cortical motor reorganization in akinetic patients with Parkinson's disease: a functional MRI study. *Brain*. 2000;**123**(Pt 2):394–403.

10. Haslinger B, Erhard P, Kampfe N, *et al*. Event-related functional magnetic resonance imaging in Parkinson's disease before and after levodopa. *Brain*. 2001;**124**(Pt 3):558–70.

11. Ridding MC, Inzelberg R, Rothwell JC. Changes in excitability of motor cortical circuitry in patients with Parkinson's disease. *Ann Neurol*. 1995;**37**(2):181–8.

12. Ziemann U, Bruns D, Paulus W. Enhancement of human motor cortex inhibition by the dopamine receptor agonist pergolide: evidence from transcranial magnetic stimulation. *Neurosci Lett*. 1996;**208**(3):187–90.

13. Buhmann C, Glauche V, Sturenburg HJ, *et al*. Pharmacologically modulated fMRI–cortical responsiveness to levodopa in drug-naive hemiparkinsonian patients. *Brain*. 2003;**126**(Pt 2):451–61.

14. Yu H, Sternad D, Corcos DM, Vaillancourt DE. Role of hyperactive cerebellum and motor cortex in Parkinson's disease. *Neuroimage*. 2007;**35**(1):222–33.

15. Eckert T, Peschel T, Heinze HJ, Rotte M. Increased pre-SMA activation in early PD patients during simple self-initiated hand movements. *J Neurol*. 2006;**253**(2):199–207.

16. Wu T, Hallett M. A functional MRI study of automatic movements in patients with Parkinson's disease. *Brain*. 2005;**128**(Pt 10):2250–9.

17. Cerasa A, Hagberg GE, Peppe A, *et al*. Functional changes in the activity of cerebellum and frontostriatal regions during externally and internally timed movement in Parkinson's disease. *Brain Res Bull*. 2006;**71**(1–3):259–69.

18. Sen S, Kawaguchi A, Truong Y, Lewis MM, Huang X. Dynamic changes in cerebello-thalamo-cortical motor circuitry during progression of Parkinson's disease. *Neuroscience*. 2010;**166**(2):712–19.

19. Wu T, Wang L, Hallett M, *et al*. Effective connectivity of brain networks during self-initiated movement in Parkinson's disease. *Neuroimage*. 2011;**55**(1):204–15.

20. Friston KJ, Buechel C, Fink GR, *et al*. Psychophysiological and modulatory interactions in neuroimaging. *Neuroimage*. 1997;**6**(3):218–29.

21. Wu T, Chan P, Hallett M. Effective connectivity of neural networks in automatic movements in Parkinson's disease. *Neuroimage*. 2010;**49**(3):2581–7.

22. Wu T, Hallett M. Neural correlates of dual task performance in patients with Parkinson's disease. *J Neurol Neurosurg Psychiatry*. 2008;**79**(7):760–6.

23. D'Esposito M, Detre JA, Alsop DC, *et al*. The neural basis of the central executive system of working memory. *Nature*. 1995;**378**(6554):279–81.

24. Corbetta M, Shulman GL. Control of goal-directed and stimulus-driven attention in the brain. *Nat Rev Neurosci*. 2002;**3**(3):201–15.

25. Halsband U, Ito N, Tanji J, Freund HJ. The role of premotor cortex and the supplementary motor area in the temporal control of movement in man. *Brain*. 1993;**116**(Pt 1):243–66.

26. Ivry RB. The representation of temporal information in perception and motor control. *Curr Opin Neurobiol*. 1996;**6**(6):851–7.

27. Pashler H. Dual-task interference in simple tasks: data and theory. *Psychol Bull*. 1994;**116**(2):220–44.

28. Collette F, Olivier L, Van der Linden M, *et al*. Involvement of both prefrontal and inferior parietal cortex in dual-task performance. *Brain Res Cogn Brain Res*. 2005;**24**(2):237–51.

29. Rowe J, Stephan KE, Friston K, *et al*. Attention to action in Parkinson's disease: impaired effective connectivity among frontal cortical regions. *Brain*. 2002;**125**(Pt 2):276–89.

30. Buchel C, Friston K. Assessing interactions among neuronal systems using functional neuroimaging. *Neural Netw*. 2000;**13**(8–9):871–82.

31. Jueptner M, Stephan KM, Frith CD, *et al*. Anatomy of motor learning. I. Frontal cortex and attention to action. *J Neurophysiol*. 1997;**77**(3):1313–24.

32. Lewis MM, Slagle CG, Smith AB, *et al*. Task specific influences of Parkinson's disease on the striato-thalamo-cortical and cerebello-thalamo-cortical motor circuitries. *Neuroscience*. 2007;**147**(1):224–35.

33. Pierantozzi M, Palmieri MG, Marciani MG, *et al*. Effect of apomorphine on cortical inhibition in Parkinson's disease patients: a transcranial magnetic stimulation study. *Exp Brain Res*. 2001;**141**(1):52–62.

34. Foki T, Pirker W, Klinger N, *et al*. FMRI correlates of apraxia in Parkinson's disease patients OFF medication. *Exp Neurol*. 2010;**225**(2):416–22.

35. Lewis MM, Du G, Sen S, *et al*. Differential involvement of striato- and cerebello-thalamo-cortical pathways in tremor- and akinetic/rigid-predominant Parkinson's disease. *Neuroscience*. 2011;**177**:230–9.

36. Bartels AL, de Jong BM, Giladi N, *et al*. Striatal dopa and glucose metabolism in PD patients with freezing of gait. *Mov Disord*. 2006;**21**(9):1326–32.

37. Hanakawa T, Fukuyama H, Katsumi Y, Honda M, Shibasaki H. Enhanced lateral premotor activity during paradoxical gait in Parkinson's disease. *Ann Neurol*. 1999;**45**(3):329–36.

38. Fabre N, Brefel C, Sabatini U, *et al*. Normal frontal perfusion in patients with frozen gait. *Mov Disord*. 1998;**13**(4):677–83.

39. Matsui H, Udaka F, Miyoshi T, *et al*. Three-dimensional stereotactic surface projection study of freezing of gait and brain perfusion image in Parkinson's disease. *Mov Disord*. 2005;**20**(10):1272–7.

40. Snijders AH, Leunissen I, Bakker M, *et al*. Gait-related cerebral alterations in patients with Parkinson's disease with freezing of gait. *Brain*. 2011;**134**(Pt 1):59–72.

41. Jenkins IH, Fernandez W, Playford ED, *et al*. Impaired activation of the supplementary motor area in Parkinson's disease is reversed when akinesia is treated with apomorphine. *Ann Neurol*. 1992;**32**(6):749–57.

42. Rascol O, Sabatini U, Chollet F, *et al*. Normal activation of the supplementary motor area in patients with Parkinson's disease undergoing long-term treatment with levodopa. *J Neurol Neurosurg Psychiatry*. 1994;**57**(5):567–71.

43. Ng B, Palmer S, Abugharbieh R, McKeown MJ. Focusing effects of L-dopa in Parkinson's disease. *Hum Brain Mapp*. 2010;**31**(1):88–97.

44. Wu T, Long X, Zang Y, *et al*. Regional homogeneity changes in patients with Parkinson's disease. *Hum Brain Mapp*. 2009;**30**(5):1502–10.

45. Phillips MD, Baker KB, Lowe MJ, *et al*. Parkinson disease: pattern of functional MR imaging activation during deep brain stimulation of subthalamic nucleus – initial experience. *Radiology*. 2006;**239**(1):209–16.

46. Arantes PR, Cardoso EF, Barreiros MA, *et al*. Performing functional magnetic resonance imaging in patients with Parkinson's disease treated with deep brain stimulation. *Mov Disord*. 2006;**21**(8):1154–62.

47. Ceballos-Baumann AO, Boecker H, Bartenstein P, *et al*. A positron emission tomographic study of subthalamic nucleus stimulation in Parkinson disease: enhanced movement-related activity of motor-association cortex and decreased motor cortex resting activity. *Arch Neurol*. 1999;**56**(8):997–1003.

48. Limousin P, Greene J, Pollak P, *et al*. Changes in cerebral activity pattern due to subthalamic nucleus or internal pallidum stimulation in Parkinson's disease. *Ann Neurol*. 1997;**42**(3):283–91.

49. Subramanian L, Hindle JV, Johnston S, *et al*. Real-time functional magnetic resonance imaging neurofeedback for treatment of Parkinson's disease. *J Neurosci*. 2011;**31**(45):16309–17.

Chapter 6

Functional MRI of cognition and mood in Parkinson's disease

Alison Simioni and Alain Dagher

Introduction

Although James Parkinson famously described Parkinson's disease (PD) as "leaving the senses and intellect unaffected," cognitive and mood disturbances are now recognized as an integral part of the disease. Indeed, with the amelioration in the treatment of motor symptoms over the past few decades, it is now the cognitive and mood disorders that most impair quality of life [1]. Pharmacological therapy relieves the motor deficits of PD consistently and rapidly, and for the entire duration of the illness, albeit with adverse side effects in the later stages. However, PD is also associated with cognitive and emotional disturbances (Figure 6.1), whose response to dopamine therapy is either absent or, occasionally, deleterious to the patient.

Dopamine deficiency in the striatum is the salient feature of PD and can be linked to many of the motor, cognitive, and emotional symptoms and signs of the disease. Because the striatum is part of neural networks involving the entire cortex, striatal dopamine deficiency has widespread functional effects. A systems neuroscience approach based on the circuitry of the cortico-striatal system [2–4] has influenced our understanding of the motor and cognitive symptoms and led to therapeutic advances such as deep brain stimulation. This understanding forms the basis of functional neuroimaging as applied to PD.

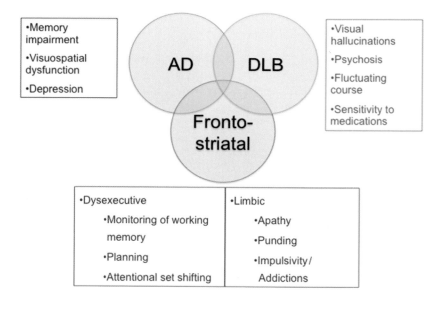

Figure 6.1 Cognitive dysfunction in PD. Cognitive impairment can be categorized into one of three potentially overlapping syndromes: one resembling Alzheimer's disease (AD), with prominent memory impairment and progressive dementia, another resembling dementia with Lewy bodies (DLB), with visual hallucinations and psychotic episodes, and finally a frontostriatal syndrome attributable to loss of dopamine signaling in the striatum. The frontostriatal syndrome can be further subdivided into a dysexecutive and a limbic component. Executive dysfunction involves attention, planning, and working memory, deficits also seen in patients with frontal lobe lesions and attributable to dysfunction within lateral prefrontal and dorsal striatal cortico-striatal loops. Abnormal mesolimbic dopamine signaling can lead to apathy or conversely to impulse control disorders such as pathological gambling. Both dopamine deficiency and dopamine excess due to overmedication can impair frontostriatal function.

Magnetic Resonance Imaging in Movement Disorders, ed. Paul Tuite and Alain Dagher. Published by Cambridge University Press. © Cambridge University Press 2013.

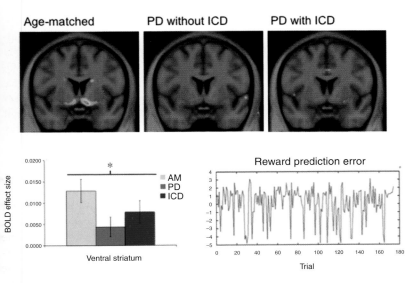

Figure 6.2 Reward prediction error (RPE) signal. Bottom right panel: trial-by-trial RPE taken from the subjects' gambles and the outcomes, during a simple gambling task. The RPE is the difference between expected reward and actual outcome. The expected reward here is simply p.w − (1 − p).w where p is the probability of winning and w the amount wagered. Top panel: fMRI t-map of the RPE in 12 age-matched elderly controls, 12 PD patients without impulse control disorders (ICD), and 12 PD patients with ICD. The RPE signal is introduced as a covariate in the general linear model of fMRI data analysis. The t-map is thresholded at t-stat > 3.0. This demonstrates, consistent with the extant literature, that the RPE is encoded by the ventral striatum, and most likely represents phasic dopamine release. The absence of an RPE signal in the two PD groups is likely due to degeneration of dopamine neurons. Bottom left: effect size from the ventral striatum. * p < 0.05.

By measuring cerebral blood flow (CBF), first with positron emission tomography (PET) and now with functional magnetic resonance imaging (fMRI), researchers have mapped the neurobiological substrates of cognitive and behavioral symptoms in PD.

The functional neuroanatomy of the dopamine system

Basal ganglia processing is based on the anatomy of parallel cortico-striatal loops [2], each of which has a functional role. Sensorimotor, cognitive, and limbic regions of the striatum can be distinguished [4, 5]: the posterior dorsal putamen (sensorimotor), caudate plus anterior putamen (cognitive), and ventral striatum or nucleus accumbens (limbic/affective) [4]. The dorsal striatum (caudate and putamen) receives input from motor, association, and prefrontal cortices, while the ventral striatum receives input from limbic areas such as the hippocampus, amygdala, and orbitofrontal cortex.

Dopamine neurons project to the basal ganglia and cerebral cortex. Different populations constitute the mesostriatal (to dorsal caudate and putamen), mesolimbic (to ventral striatum and other limbic areas such as amygdala), and mesocortical projections [6]. Dopamine neurons synapse on the dendrites of medium spiny neurons in the striatum close to glutamatergic cortical afferents [7]. Dopamine may act to increase the efficiency of active cortico-striatal synapses while suppressing inactive ones [8], and modulate synaptic plasticity in the direct and indirect pathways via D1 and D2 dopamine receptors [9].

Low dopamine levels due to neurodegeneration in PD lead to increased tonic firing of inhibitory output neurons in the globus pallidus internal segment (GPi), which is thought to lead to widespread cortical dysfunction [3]. This accounts for motor symptoms such as bradykinesia and dopamine-induced dyskinesias; however, it is more difficult to fit cognitive and mood symptoms in this model. Recently, the role of dopamine in reward, reinforcement, learning, and motivation has received more attention. Wolfram Schultz demonstrated that dopamine neuronal firing in monkeys undergoing classical conditioning appeared to reflect the changing reward value of conditioned stimuli [10]. It became apparent that dopamine neuron activity had a similar temporal pattern to a learning signal from machine learning algorithm [11]. This reward prediction error (RPE) signal is thought to promote learning, consistent with dopamine's role in synaptic plasticity [9]. The early observations from primate neurophysiology have been confirmed repeatedly in humans undergoing fMRI [12–14] (Figure 6.2). Important new theoretical models have shown that dopamine has a role in motivated behaviors that goes beyond learning: it also acts as a motivational signal, increasing an individual's drive and willingness to expend effort in the pursuit of rewards [15–18]. This may be of considerable relevance to our understanding of apathy and impulse control disorders (ICDs) in PD [19].

Functional imaging methods

Synaptic firing requires energy and therefore fairly rapid changes in local CBF and oxygen delivery [20]. Brain mapping is possible because synaptic neuronal activity leads to a proportionate increase in CBF [21]. Typically, data from multiple subjects are combined to overcome the relatively low signal-to-noise ratio of available CBF measurement methods. This requires spatially normalizing all subject data into a standard coordinate space. Most imaging studies use a commonly accepted coordinate space referred to as Montreal Neurological Institute space [22], based on the stereotaxic atlas of Talairach and Tournoux [23]. Statistical tests can be applied to each voxel of these spatially normalized brain maps, usually by applying a general linear model, to yield a z or t statistical map. One can then search this statistical parametric map, which is a three-dimensional Gaussian random field, for areas where z or t values exceed a certain statistical threshold [24, 25].

The development of fMRI has allowed brain mapping to be performed without the injection of radioactive tracers. fMRI is based on the blood oxygen level-dependent (BOLD) signal [26]. BOLD imaging uses pulse sequences sensitive to magnetic field inhomogeneities created by paramagnetic deoxyhemoglobin molecules. The mismatch between the increase in CBF and the increase in oxygen consumption in tissue causes a reduction in deoxyhemoglobin concentration, which is the basis of the BOLD signal. BOLD signal is a function of the synaptic inputs into a brain area, and of local neuronal processing, including the activity of excitatory and inhibitory interneurons [27–31]. Note however that, while reductions in neuronal activity coincide with reduced BOLD [32], neuronal inhibition per se may not always cause changes in BOLD [33].

Of relevance here is the relation between fMRI signal change and dopamine neuron activity. While BOLD is known to depend on CBF and oxygen metabolism, the relationship of these to dopamine release is not known. BOLD signal in the striatum, for example, could reflect the firing of plentiful cortical glutamatergic afferents and of the sparser dopaminergic afferents [4]. Animal experiments support the theory that extrasynaptic dopamine can augment BOLD signal [34]. Also, dopamine directly modulates excitatory postsynaptic potentials [35], which contribute to local field potentials and hence perhaps to BOLD. Dopamine also increases glutamate-induced dendritic currents in striatal medium spiny neurons [35–37], which require energy and hence increased CBF. It is therefore likely that an increase in phasic dopamine neuron firing leads to an increase in BOLD in the projection areas of the dopamine neurons, as noted earlier (and below) in the case of RPE signals. This is consistent with a fairly large number of fMRI and PET studies in PD demonstrating reduced striatal signal compared to age-matched controls (see below), presumably due to degeneration of dopamine nerve terminals.

Cortico-striatal network function and cognitive impairment in PD

Even in the absence of dementia, PD patients have cognitive deficits [38, 39], which are similar to those seen in patients with frontal lobe lesions [39], and involve the domains of attention, planning, and cognitive flexibility. Functional imaging studies in normal subjects have shown that tasks sensitive to both frontal lobe lesions and PD, such as the Wisconsin Card Sorting Test [40], a test of cognitive flexibility, and the Tower of London [41], a test of planning, appear to involve a network of regions that include the caudate nucleus, anterior cingulate cortex (ACC), lateral prefrontal cortex (PFC), and posterior parietal cortex, which make up the cognitive cortico-striatal loop [2].

The earliest PET CBF studies of cognition in PD suggested that the "frontal lobe" deficits could be explained by basal ganglia dysfunction. For example, during performance of the Tower of London planning task, PD patients showed normal activation of the lateral PFC but deficient CBF activation in basal ganglia [42, 43]. Two PET studies in PD showing a correlation between the degree of executive dysfunction and the reduction in caudate dopamine innervation [44, 45] also support attributing frontal lobe deficits to abnormal processing within basal ganglia. However, there is also evidence of abnormal cortical activity in PD during cognitive tasks. For example, Cools *et al.* [46] carried out CBF PET studies on PD patients on and off levodopa while they performed the

Tower of London planning task. Patients off medication, compared to controls, showed greater CBF activation in the lateral PFC during planning. This excessive activation disappeared when the patients were given levodopa, and the reduction in CBF correlated with the improvement in performance. Mattay *et al.* [47] replicated these findings using fMRI and a different test of frontal lobe function: the n-back task. They found greater BOLD activation in numerous cortical areas (including dorsolateral PFC, ACC, and posterior parietal cortex) when PD patients were off compared to on levodopa. Once again the relative increase in BOLD activation and the deterioration in performance while off medication were correlated. It is suggested that dopamine replacement may cause a beneficial reduction in frontal neuronal activity by a direct effect on cortical neurons. There is evidence to support such a role for dopamine, which could be acting by reducing unwanted neuronal activity [48], essentially by making neurons less sensitive to weak inputs and more sensitive to strong excitatory afferents [49]. Dopamine acting on the caudate nucleus could also lead to a focusing of cortical neuronal activity, via the cortico-striatal system [50]. It could do this by a direct gating of cortico-striatal inputs at the level of the striatal dendrite [7, 8], or by varying the balance of information flow between the direct and indirect pathways. The arrangement of the direct and indirect basal ganglia pathways, one designed for focused action selection and the other for broader inhibition [51], may result in a focusing of cortical activity [50].

The studies described above demonstrate that dopamine deficiency in PD can be associated with either absent or excessive cortical activation. In fact, both patterns may co-exist: during the Wisconsin Card Sorting Test, a frontal lobe test of flexibility and attention, PD patients displayed defective ventrolateral PFC activation and dorsolateral PFC hyperactivation [52]. The authors proposed that, in this task, the ventrolateral PFC was activated as part of a cortico-striatal loop, which explained why it demonstrated deficient activation in the PD patients, while the dorsolateral PFC was activated as part of a network that did not include the striatum, which explains why it showed hyperactivation in the PD group. Monchi *et al.* went on to test this theory further with a modified card sorting task that showed PFC underactivation, in PD compared to controls, only during those phases of the task that also recruited the caudate

[53]. During the task phases that do not normally involve the caudate, the PD patients showed cortical hyperactivation compared to controls.

The hyperactivation seen in the lateral PFC in PD patients consists of higher amplitude and greater spatial extent of BOLD signal change. Indeed, greater spatial extent of cortical activation is frequently reported in PD. Ng *et al.* [54] found that PD patients off medications showed more spatially extensive activation in the supplementary motor area (SMA) and M1, and this anomaly was reversed by levodopa, consistent with the theory that optimum dopamine levels reduce neuronal noise, leading to focusing of brain activity [49].

Not all PD patients demonstrate impaired executive function. Lewis *et al.* [55] compared two groups of PD patients with and without executive dysfunction, but matched for all other relevant criteria (disease duration, motor dysfunction, and Mini-Mental State Examination) to age-matched controls. Subjects performed a simple working memory task during fMRI. The PD group with executive dysfunction had deficient activation in the PFC and caudate bilaterally compared to the PD group without executive dysfunction. The degree of underactivation correlated with performance impairment. On the other hand, the unimpaired PD patients had an activation pattern no different than that of age-matched controls. This suggests that the cognitive cortico-striatal loop (PFC–caudate) may be affected in PD independently of the motor cortico-striatal loops (cortical motor areas–posterior putamen). Subsequent work by the same group showed that a polymorphism in the catechol-O-methyltransferase (COMT) gene predicted performance differences on the Tower of London task in PD [56]. COMT metabolizes dopamine and is the main regulator of dopamine levels in the frontal lobe (but not the striatum). Individuals with the low activity met/met *COMT* allele, and hence higher frontal dopamine levels, were impaired on the task (paradoxically, since in healthy subjects and patients with schizophrenia the exact opposite relationship holds; patients with met/met alleles perform better on most frontal lobe tasks). Moreover, the impairment was greater in patients taking dopaminergic medications, suggesting that excessive frontal dopamine stimulation may impair certain types of cognitive performance in PD. Imaging studies confirmed the COMT effect, with met/met PD patients demonstrating reduced lateral PFC activation, compared to val/val carriers, during the Tower of London task [57]. Similar findings were found with a set-shifting task [58]. In sum, it appears that excessive dopaminergic stimulation of the PFC can also cause frontal lobe dysfunction in PD. It may be that levodopa dosing adequate to restore motor function may, in vulnerable individuals, overdose the frontal cortex.

This overmedication hypothesis of cognitive deficits in PD was originally proposed by Gotham *et al.* [59]. It states that an optimum dosage of dopaminergic medications to treat a patient's motor symptoms may result in side effects in the cognitive or emotional domains. This may result if there is preservation of non-motor dopamine projections, relative to meso-striatal motor projections [60]. There is an optimum level of dopamine such that both deficiency and excess can lead to functional deficits. The relationship between frontal lobe function and dopaminergic stimulation thus has an inverted-U shape consistent with the proposal of Yerkes and Dodson, and supported by electrophysiology [61].

Cools *et al.* tested the overmedication theory using fMRI and a probabilistic reversal learning task previously shown to be sensitive to levodopa in PD [62]. Patients perform better at this task off medications than on. Previous work has implicated the ventral striatum and ventrolateral PFC in this task in normal subjects, and the ventral striatum has relatively preserved dopamine innervation in PD compared to the dorsal striatum [60]. An fMRI study in PD patients supports the overmedication hypothesis: levodopa inhibited activation in the ventral striatum during the reversal learning task. In sum, dopaminergic overmedication may lead to cognitive impairment via an action on the relatively preserved mesocortical or mesolimbic systems.

Cortico-striatal network function and disorders of motivation in PD

The overmedication hypothesis has been rekindled recently with the description of disorders of motivation and impulse control in PD. These disorders include ICDs such as pathological gambling, compulsive sexuality, and compulsive shopping, punding, which consists of compulsive engagement in repetitive behaviors, and dopamine dysregulation syndrome, which is essentially an addiction to dopaminergic medication. Dopamine replacement therapies, more specifically dopamine agonists, have

been implicated in the development of ICDs in a subset of people with PD [19, 63–66]. These disorders, described as "behavioral addictions," share a conceptual resemblance to drug addiction in that individuals pursue particular activities in a compulsive manner despite harmful consequences [19]. Although somewhat diverse, these behaviors are linked by their repetitive, reward- or incentive-based natures. It is hypothesized that some individuals are vulnerable to these addictive phenomena because dopaminergic stimulation that restores motor function overdoses the mesolimbic dopamine system, leading to pathological incentive behaviors.

To date, the largest epidemiological evaluation of ICDs in PD (n = 3090) reported at least one ICD in 13.6% of patients: compulsive buying in 5.7%, problem and pathological gambling in 5.0%, binge-eating disorder in 4.3%, and compulsive sexual behavior in 3.5%. Although single ICDs were more common, two or more ICDs were present in 3.9% (or 28.7% of patients with an ICD) [63]. It is thought that in the general population, the prevalence of ICDs in PD is likely to be grossly under-reported. Due to social conventions, people likely hesitate to tell their doctors that they gambled away the family savings or that their need for sexual behavior consumes so much money, time, concentration, and energy [67].

Although causality has yet to be unequivocally established, it is thought these disorders result from interactions between dopamine replacement therapy and intrinsic vulnerabilities to such behaviors in individual patients [68, 69]. Younger patients are at greater risk, as are males, current/former smokers, those with a history of ICD symptoms prior to development of PD, and those with a family history of gambling problems [63, 70, 71]. Consistent with the notion that PD patients who develop ICDs have an inherent vulnerability, Rao *et al.* [72] reported that PD patients with ICDs have reduced resting CBF in the ventral striatum compared to PD patients without ICDs. Although the functional significance of the resting blood flow differences is unclear, this does suggest an inherent difference between PD patients with and without ICD. Recall that the greatest risk factor for clinically evident ICDs in PD is dopaminergic drug use [63], which is thought to restore motor function, but overdose the mesolimbic dopaminergic system. Mesolimbic dopamine likely contributes to these behavioral addictions via its role in reward processing and learning, incentive salience, and risky decision-making. Here, we highlight evidence provided by fMRI.

Reward processing and learning

fMRI studies of healthy subjects consistently demonstrate that rewarding events increase activity in the medial orbitofrontal cortex, the amygdala, and the dopamine-rich ventral striatum [14, 73, 74]. Consistent with the primate work cited earlier, the striatal BOLD signal most consistently fits an RPE signal (Figure 6.2) [12]. Given that this signal likely depends on intact dopamine fibers, it is perhaps not surprising to find it reduced or absent in PD patients. Schonberg *et al.* found that, in relatively mildly affected PD patients, the RPE fMRI signal was absent in the dorsal striatum but preserved in the ventral striatum [75]. This finding is consistent with the known relative preservation of mesolimbic dopamine fibers in early PD, and supports the notion that this RPE signal measured by fMRI is indicative of dopamine neuron activity.

Reduced sensitivity to rewarding stimuli in the striatum has been described in non-parkinsonian addiction [76–78]. Dopamine's effect on reward-related circuitry was assessed by measuring the neural BOLD response to unexpected financial wins in a group of healthy subjects after the administration of the dopamine agonist pramipexole. Compared to a placebo-control group, those who had taken the dopamine agonist showed a blunted ventral striatal response [79]. The finding that dopamine altered ventral striatal activity during reward processing was later confirmed and extended by van Eimeren *et al.* [69] to PD. Using fMRI, they studied a single group of PD patients in three conditions: off dopaminergic medications, after levodopa, and after dopamine agonist (pramipexole) treatment, while the patients performed a "roulette" game. They found that both forms of dopaminergic medication equally diminished ventral striatal reward processing relative to the "off" condition. In the orbitofrontal cortex, however, it was only the dopamine agonist that reduced reward processing. The authors suggested that pramipexole diminished reward processing in the orbitofrontal cortex by relatively increasing activity during negative RPEs, and thus impaired negative reinforcement. Insensitivity to losses could lead to persistent gambling.

Dopamine replacement therapy has specific effects on reward-based learning. A computational modeling approach (Figure 6.3B) shows that unexpected rewards are associated with phasic increases in dopamine activity, leading to positive reinforcement via D1 receptor signaling (i.e., "Go" learning). Conversely, unexpected punishment or reward omission is associated with phasic dips in dopamine firing, leading to negative reinforcement via D2 receptor signaling (i.e., "No-Go" learning), thereby reducing the behavior after a negative outcome [80]. Through tonic stimulation of D2 receptors, dopamine agonists can interfere with reward-based learning by relatively enhancing "Go" learning (via D2 autoreceptors), while also preventing natural dips in dopamine firing, thereby impairing "No-Go" learning. Consistent with this model, PD patients show relatively impaired learning from positive outcomes when off medications, and enhanced learning from reward, compared to punishment, when on medications [81–83]. Indeed, it has been hypothesized that by impairing negative reinforcement learning, dopamine agonist therapies may facilitate the progression to compulsive behavior in those who are vulnerable [19].

To investigate potential differences in neural activity underlying reward-related learning in PD patients with ICDs, Voon *et al.* [68] performed fMRI on a group of PD patients with problem gambling or shopping and on a group of demographically matched PD controls, while they performed a monetary reward gambling task, off and on dopamine agonist therapy. To find neural signals related to learning about gains, the researchers modeled an RPE signal, and found that when tested "off" their dopaminergic medication, the PD ICD group had a reduced signal in the ventral striatum compared to the non-ICD PD group. The administration of a dopamine agonist reversed this effect and was associated with increased gain learning only in those PD patients with an ICD. This evidence further suggests that PD patients who develop behavioral addictions may have an inherent vulnerability, possibly due to relatively greater ventral striatal dopamine innervation, which makes them more sensitive to dopaminergic medication's effects on the mesolimbic system.

Incentive salience

fMRI also provides evidence that dopamine may contribute to ICDs in PD via its role as an energizing or activating agent that assigns incentive value to stimuli and actions [19]. This theory takes into account evidence that dopamine appears to have motivating and

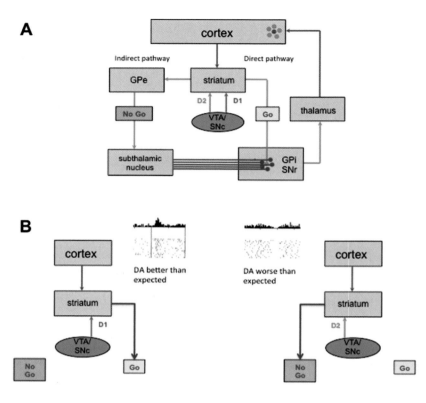

Figure 6.3 Organization of the basal ganglia. (A) Basal ganglia model (see [2, 3] for details). The basal ganglia are organized in a direct and an indirect pathway. Striatal projections to the GPi make up the direct pathway. These striatal neurons express dopamine D1 receptors and respond to phasic dopamine bursts. Information in the indirect pathway travels via the GPe and subthalamic nucleus. Indirect pathway striatal neurons express D2 receptors and respond to tonic dopamine. The center–surround arrangement in the GPi allows focused action selection. Connections are color-coded: red for inhibitory and green for excitatory. (B) The Go pathway responds to unexpected rewards with a phasic burst of dopamine neuron activity. This signals via the D1 system, which promotes long-term potentiation in the direct pathway (Go learning/action). Withheld rewards (or punishments) lead to a transient reduction in tonic firing of dopamine neurons. This is sensed by high affinity D2 receptors in the indirect pathway, which leads to long-term depression and No-Go learning/inhibition of action. See [79–81] for details. Abbreviations: DA, dopamine; GPe, globus pallidus external segment; GPi, globus pallidus internal segment; SNc, substantia nigra pars compacta; SNr, substantia nigra pars reticulata; VTA, ventral tegmental area.

activating effects independent of learning. In this case, the emphasis is on dopamine enhancing reward-seeking behaviors by acting on arousal, attention, movement, and effort [18, 84]. For example, dopamine may alter sensitivity to incentive processing so that motivation is assigned to the cues associated with the reward, turning the cues into "objects of desire" [85, 86]. Frosini *et al.* [87] provided evidence for this theory. They performed fMRI on medicated PD patients with pathological gambling, and on medicated PD patients without ICDs, while they were exposed to gambling-related visual cues. They found that compulsive gamblers had increased ventral striatal activity in response to gambling-related cues, in conjunction with a significantly higher level of gaming urge after viewing the cues. This assumes that the ventral striatal cue-response is a measure of incentive salience.

Risk-taking

Finally, changes secondary to dopamine's role in risk-taking may also contribute to ICDs in PD. fMRI studies have highlighted an important role for the ventral striatum and orbitofrontal cortex in risky decision-making. Pathological gamblers have reduced activity in these regions, compared to healthy controls when performing simulated gambling tasks [78]. In PD patients, dopaminergic drugs have been shown to increase risk-taking in those with [88] and without ICDs [89], although the effect may be more pronounced in those with ICDs [70]. Voon *et al.* [90] also showed that the enhanced sensitivity to risk in those with ICDs was associated with decreased ventral striatal activity. In the same vein, Rao *et al.* [72] performed fMRI on medicated PD patients with and without ICDs while the patients performed a risk-taking task that has shown real-world validity. They found that although both groups showed similar risk-taking performance on the task, the PD patients with ICDs showed reduced activity in the ventral striatum during risk-taking.

In summary, ICDs in PD are associated with functional changes in cortico-striatal circuitries that evaluate or mediate rewarding outcomes and evaluate risks during decision-making. Behavioral, epidemiological, and imaging evidence converge on a model whereby patients with an underlying, possibly hereditary, vulnerability develop ICDs when exposed to dopamine agonists, possibly through disruption of normal inhibitory mechanisms and enhancement of reward function. The ventral striatum and orbitofrontal cortex appear to play a role in this process.

Non-cortico-striatal mechanisms

PD may also lead to CBF changes in brain areas other than the striatum or connected cortical areas. In one study using the Tower of London task, PD patients had excessive activation of the hippocampus, whereas normal controls showed deactivation (reduced CBF) while performing the task [42], findings that were replicated using fMRI with an implicit learning task [91]. The excess hippocampal activity in PD could represent recruitment of the intact declarative memory system to overcome the deficits of the impaired frontostriatal (procedural) memory system. On the other hand, hippocampal activity during the performance of "frontostriatal" tasks may actually be deleterious and need to be suppressed [92]. Thus, the hippocampal recruitment seen in these PD patients could be contributing to the cognitive deficits. Grossman *et al.* [93] studied the processing of complex sentences in stage-I PD patients using fMRI. In healthy subjects, processing of long sentences requires working memory and grammatical processing, and involves the striatum, lateral temporal cortex, ACC, and left inferior frontal cortex. PD patients showed relatively impaired activation of these areas, but recruitment of other cortical areas (posterior parietal and ventrolateral PFC). Once again, it is unclear whether this represents compensation or deleterious activity by a non-essential area.

Finally, Gusnard and Raichle have demonstrated that deactivations (i.e., reductions in CBF compared to baseline) in certain areas are a consistent feature in a wide range of cognitive tasks [94]. These deactivated brain regions are referred to by Gusnard and Raichle as the default mode network (DMN) because they are found to have high resting activity and appear to form a functional network. The DMN includes the medial PFC and ACC, posterior cingulate cortex (PCC), precuneus, and lateral parietal and temporal cortices. DMN deactivation is usually proportional to task difficulty. Activity within the DMN is inversely correlated with that in the frontostriatal system, which is defective in PD. There is evidence that DMN deactivation may be under the control of dopamine, as reducing dopamine levels in healthy humans disrupts DMN deactivation during an executive task [95]. In PD, several studies have demonstrated deficient deactivation of the DMN [96, 97]. This deficiency is partially restored by apomorphine [98] and levodopa [99], although one study demonstrated impaired ventromedial PFC deactivation induced by levodopa administration [100].

In summary, functional brain imaging has consistently demonstrated abnormal cortico-striatal function associated with cognitive deficits in PD; however, several questions remain. Which deficits are due to dopamine loss in the striatum as opposed to extrastriatal (e.g., frontal) areas? Are some cognitive deficits worsened by dopaminergic medication? Moreover, what is the role of other neurotransmitter systems affected by the neurodegenerative process, such as acetylcholine, serotonin, and noradrenaline [101], all of which play a role in cognition? Acetylcholine loss is associated with cognitive impairment in PD [102–104]. Finally, it is possible that intrinsic cortical neurodegeneration plays a role in cognitive impairment [105, 106], independent of dopamine denervation.

References

1. Schrag A, Jahanshahi M, Quinn N. What contributes to quality of life in patients with Parkinson's disease? *J Neurol Neurosurg Psychiatry*. 2000;**69**(3):308–12.

2. Alexander GE, DeLong MR, Strick PL. Parallel organization of functionally segregated circuits linking basal ganglia and cortex. *Annu Rev Neurosci*. 1986;**9**:357–81.

3. Albin RL, Young AB, Penney JB. The functional anatomy of basal ganglia disorders [see comments]. *Trends Neurosci*. 1989;**12**(10):366–75.

4. Haber SN, Fudge JL, McFarland NR. Striatonigrostriatal pathways in primates form an ascending spiral from the shell to the dorsolateral striatum. *J Neurosci*. 2000;**20**(6):2369–82.

5. Parent A. Extrinsic connections of the basal ganglia. *Trends Neurosci*. 1990;**13**(7):254–8.

6. Moore RY, Bloom FE. Central catecholamine neuron systems: anatomy and physiology of the dopamine systems. *Annu Rev Neurosci*. 1978;**1**:129–69.

7. Sesack S.R, Pickel VM. Prefrontal cortical efferents in the rat synapse on unlabeled neuronal targets of

catecholamine terminals in the nucleus accumbens septi and on dopamine neurons in the ventral tegmental area. *J Comp Neurol.* 1992;**320**(2):145–60.

8. Wickens J, Kotter R. Cellular models of reinforcement. In: Houk JC, Davis JL, Beiser DG, editors. *Models of Information Processing in the Basal Ganglia.* Cambridge, MA: MIT Press; 1995. 187–214.

9. Shen W, Flajolet M, Greengard P, Surmeier DJ. Dichotomous dopaminergic control of striatal synaptic plasticity. *Science.* 2008;**321**(5890):848–51.

10. Schultz W. Predictive reward signal of dopamine neurons. *J Neurophysiol.* 1998;**80**(1):1–27.

11. Schultz W, Dayan P, Montague PR. A neural substrate of prediction and reward. *Science.* 1997;**275**(5306):1593–9.

12. Hare TA, O'Doherty J, Camerer CF, Schultz W, Rangel A. Dissociating the role of the orbitofrontal cortex and the striatum in the computation of goal values and prediction errors. *J Neurosci.* 2008; **28**(22):5623–30.

13. McClure SM, Berns GS, Montague PR. Temporal prediction errors in a passive learning task activate human striatum. *Neuron.* 2003;**38**(2):339–46.

14. O'Doherty JP, Dayan P, Friston K, Critchley H, Dolan RJ. Temporal difference models and reward-related learning in the human brain. *Neuron.* 2003; **38**(2):329–37.

15. McClure SM, Daw ND, Montague PR. A computational substrate for incentive salience. *Trends Neurosci.* 2003;**26**(8):423–8.

16. Niv Y, Daw ND, Joel D, Dayan P. Tonic dopamine: opportunity costs and the control of response vigor. *Psychopharmacology (Berl).* 2007;**191**(3):507–20.

17. Berridge KC. The debate over dopamine's role in reward: the case for incentive salience. *Psychopharmacology (Berl).* 2007;**191**(3):391–431.

18. Salamone JD, Correa M, Mingote SM, Weber SM. Beyond the reward hypothesis: alternative functions of nucleus accumbens dopamine. *Curr Opin Pharmacol.* 2005;**5**(1):34–41.

19. Dagher A, Robbins TW. Personality, addiction, dopamine: insights from Parkinson's disease. *Neuron.* 2009;**61**(4):502–10.

20. Attwell D, Buchan AM, Charpak S, *et al.* Glial and neuronal control of brain blood flow. *Nature,* 2010;**468**(7321):232–43.

21. Raichle ME. Circulatory and metabolic correlates of brain function in normal humans. In Mountcastle VB, editor. *Handbook of Physiology, Sect 1, Vol 5: The Nervous System.* Bethesda: American Physiological Society; 1987. 643–74.

22. Collins DL, Neelin P, Peters TM, Evans AC. Automatic 3D intersubject registration of MR volumetric data in standardized Talairach space. *J Comput Assist Tomogr.* 1994;**18**(2):192–205.

23. Talairach J, Tournoux P. *Co-planar Stereotaxic Atlas of the Human Brain.* Stuttgart: Thieme; 1988.

24. Worsley KJ, Liao CH, Aston J, *et al.* A general statistical analysis for fMRI data. *Neuroimage.* 2002;**15**(1):1–15.

25. Friston KJ. Models of brain function in neuroimaging. *Annu Rev of Psychol.* 2005;**56**(1):57–87.

26. Ogawa S, Lee TM, Kay AR, Tank DW. Brain magnetic resonance imaging with contrast dependent on blood oxygenation. *Proc Natl Acad Sci U S A.* 1990;**87**(24):9868–72.

27. Logothetis NK. The neural basis of the blood-oxygen-level-dependent functional magnetic resonance imaging signal. *Philos Trans R Soc Lond B Biol Sci.* 2002;**357**(1424):1003–37.

28. Logothetis NK, Pfeuffer J. On the nature of the BOLD fMRI contrast mechanism. *Magn Reson Imaging.* 2004;**22**(10):1517–31.

29. Lee JH, Durand R, Gradinaru V, *et al.* Global and local fMRI signals driven by neurons defined optogenetically by type and wiring. *Nature.* 2010;**465**(7299):788–92.

30. Bandettini PA. Seven topics in functional magnetic resonance imaging. *J Integr Neurosci.* 2009; **8**(3):371–403.

31. Logothetis NK. What we can do and what we cannot do with fMRI. *Nature.* 2008;**453**(7197):869–78.

32. Shmuel A, Augath M, Oeltermann A, Logothetis NK. Negative functional MRI response correlates with decreases in neuronal activity in monkey visual area V1. *Nat Neurosci.* 2006;**9**(4):569–77.

33. Waldvogel D, van Gelderen P, Muellbacher W, *et al.* The relative metabolic demand of inhibition and excitation. *Nature.* 2000;**406** (6799):995–8.

34. Choi JK, Chen YI, Hamel E, Jenkins BG. Brain hemodynamic changes mediated by dopamine receptors: role of the cerebral microvasculature in dopamine-mediated neurovascular coupling. *Neuroimage.* 2006;**30**(3):700–12.

35. Nicola SM, Surmeier J, Malenka RC. Dopaminergic modulation of neuronal excitability in the striatum and nucleus accumbens. *Annu Rev Neurosci.* 2000;**23**:185–215.

36. Knutson B, Bjork JM, Fong GW, *et al.* Amphetamine modulates human incentive processing. *Neuron.* 2004;**43**(2):261–9.

37. Zink CF, Pagnoni G, Martin-Skurski ME, Chappelow JC, Berns GS. Human striatal responses to

monetary reward depend on saliency. *Neuron.* 2004;**42**(3):509–17.

38. Dubois B, Boller F, Pillon B, Agid Y. Cognitive deficits in Parkinson's disease. In: Boller F, Grafman J, editors. *Handbook of Neuropsychology.* New York: Elsevier Science; 1991. 195–240.

39. Owen AM, James M, Leigh PN, *et al.* Fronto-striatal cognitive deficits at different stages of Parkinson's disease. *Brain.* 1992;**115**(Pt 6):1727–51.

40. Monchi O, Petrides M, Petre V, Worsley K, Dagher A. Wisconsin Card Sorting revisited: distinct neural circuits participating in different stages of the task identified by event-related functional magnetic resonance imaging. *J Neurosci.* 2001;**21**(19):7733–41.

41. Dagher A, Owen AM, Boecker H, Brooks DJ. Mapping the network for planning: a correlational PET activation study with the Tower of London task. *Brain.* 1999;**122**(Pt 10):1973–87.

42. Dagher A, Owen AM, Boecker H, Brooks DJ. The role of the striatum and hippocampus in planning: a PET activation study in Parkinson's disease. *Brain.* 2001;**124**(Pt 5):1020–32.

43. Owen AM, Doyon J, Dagher A, Sadikot A, Evans AC. Abnormal basal ganglia outflow in Parkinson's disease identified with PET. Implications for higher cortical functions. *Brain.* 1998;**121**(Pt 5):949–65.

44. Bruck A, Portin R, Lindell A, *et al.* Positron emission tomography shows that impaired frontal lobe functioning in Parkinson's disease is related to dopaminergic hypofunction in the caudate nucleus. *Neurosci Lett.* 2001;**311**(2):81–4.

45. Marié RM, Barré L, Dupuy B, *et al.* Relationships between striatal dopamine denervation and frontal executive tests in

Parkinson's disease. *Neurosci Lett.* 1999;**260**(2):77–80.

46. Cools R, Stefanova E, Barker RA, Robbins TW, Owen AM. Dopaminergic modulation of high-level cognition in Parkinson's disease: the role of the prefrontal cortex revealed by PET. *Brain.* 2002;**125**(Pt 3):584–94.

47. Mattay VS, Tessitore A, Callicott JH, *et al.* Dopaminergic modulation of cortical function in patients with Parkinson's disease. *Ann Neurol.* 2002;**51**(2):156–64.

48. Sawaguchi T, Matsumura M, Kubota K. Catecholaminergic effects on neuronal activity related to a delayed response task in monkey prefrontal cortex. *J Neurophysiol.* 1990;**63**(6):1385–400.

49. Li SC, Sikstrom S. Integrative neurocomputational perspectives on cognitive aging, neuromodulation, and representation. *Neurosci Biobehav Rev.* 2002;**26**(7):795–808.

50. Mink JW. The basal ganglia: focused selection and inhibition of competing motor programs. *Prog Neurobiol.* 1996;**50**(4):381–425.

51. Hallett M. Physiology of basal ganglia disorders: an overview. *Can J Neurol Sci.* 1993;**20**(3):177–83.

52. Monchi O, Petrides M, Doyon J, *et al.* Neural bases of set-shifting deficits in Parkinson's disease. *J Neurosci.* 2004;**24**(3):702–10.

53. Monchi O, Petrides M, Mejia-Constain B, Strafella AP. Cortical activity in Parkinson's disease during executive processing depends on striatal involvement. *Brain.* 2007;**130**(Pt 1):233–44.

54. Ng B, Palmer S, Abugharbieh R, McKeown MJ. Focusing effects of L-dopa in Parkinson's disease. *Hum Brain Mapp.* 2010;**31**(1):88–97.

55. Lewis SJ, Dove A, Robbins TW, Barker RA, Owen AM. Cognitive impairments in early Parkinson's

disease are accompanied by reductions in activity in frontostriatal neural circuitry. *J Neurosci.* 2003;**23**(15):6351–6.

56. Foltynie T, Goldberg TE, Lewis SG, *et al.* Planning ability in Parkinson's disease is influenced by the COMT val158met polymorphism. *Mov Disord.* 2004;**19**(8):885–91.

57. Williams-Gray CH, Hampshire A, Robbins TW, Owen AM, Barker RA. Catechol O-methyltransferase Val158Met genotype influences frontoparietal activity during planning in patients with Parkinson's disease. *J Neurosci.* 2007;**27**(18):4832–8.

58. Williams-Gray CH, Hampshire A, Barker RA, Owen AM. Attentional control in Parkinson's disease is dependent on COMT val 158 met genotype. *Brain.* 2008;**131**(Pt 2):397–408.

59. Gotham AM, Brown RG, Marsden CD. 'Frontal' cognitive function in patients with Parkinson's disease 'on' and 'off' levodopa. *Brain.* 1988;**111**(Pt 2):299–321.

60. Kish SJ, Shannak K, Hornykiewicz O. Uneven pattern of dopamine loss in the striatum of patients with idiopathic Parkinson's disease. Pathophysiologic and clinical implications. *N Engl J Med.* 1988;**318**(14):876–80.

61. Goldman-Rakic PS, Muly IEC, Williams GV. D1 receptors in prefrontal cells and circuits. *Brain Res Rev.* 2000;**31**(2–3):295–301.

62. Cools R, Lewis SJ, Clark L, Barker RA, Robbins TW. L-DOPA disrupts activity in the nucleus accumbens during reversal learning in Parkinson's disease. *Neuropsychopharmacology.* 2007;**32**(1):180–9.

63. Weintrau, D, Koester J, Potenza MN, *et al.* Impulse control disorders in Parkinson disease: a cross-sectional study of 3090 patients. *Arch Neurol.* 2010;**67**(5):589–95.

64. Seedat S, Kesler S, Niehaus DJ, Stein DJ. Pathological gambling behaviour: emergence secondary to treatment of Parkinson's disease with dopaminergic agents. *Depress Anxiety.* 2000;**11**(4):185–6.

65. Driver-Dunckley E, Samanta J, Stacy M. Pathological gambling associated with dopamine agonist therapy in Parkinson's disease. *Neurology.* 2003;**61**(3):422–23.

66. Voon V, Fox SH. Medication-related impulse control and repetitive behaviors in Parkinson disease. *Arch Neurol.* 2007;**64**(8):1089–96.

67. Klos KJ, Bower JH, Josephs KA, Matsumoto JY, Ahlskog JE. Pathological hypersexuality predominantly linked to adjuvant dopamine agonist therapy in Parkinson's disease and multiple system atrophy. *Parkinsonism Relat Disord.* 2005;**11**(6):381–6.

68. Voon V, Pessiglione M, Brezing C, et al. Mechanisms underlying dopamine-mediated reward bias in compulsive behaviors. *Neuron.* 2010;**65**(1):135–42.

69. van Eimeren T, Ballanger B, Pellecchia G, et al. Dopamine agonists diminish value sensitivity of the orbitofrontal cortex: a trigger for pathological gambling in Parkinson's disease? *Neuropsychopharmacology.* 2009;**34**(13)2758–66.

70. Voon V, Sohr M, Lang AE, et al. Impulse control disorders in Parkinson disease: a multicenter case–control study. *Ann Neurol.* 2011;**69**(6):986–96.

71. Gallagher DA, O'Sullivan SS, Evans AH, Lees AJ, Schrag A. Pathological gambling in Parkinson's disease: risk factors and differences from dopamine dysregulation. An analysis of published case series. *Mov Disord.* 2007;**22**(12):1757–63.

72. Rao H, Mamikonyan E, Detre JA, et al. Decreased ventral striatal activity with impulse control disorders in Parkinson's disease. *Mov Disord.* 2010;**25**(11):1660–9.

73. Pessiglione M, Seymour B, Flandin G, Dolan RJ, Frith CD. Dopamine-dependent prediction errors underpin reward-seeking behaviour in humans. *Nature.* 2006;**442**(7106):1042–5.

74. Holland PC, Gallagher M. Amygdala-frontal interactions and reward expectancy. *Curr Opin Neurobiol.* 2004;**14**(2):148–55.

75. Schonberg T, O'Doherty JP, Joel D, et al. Selective impairment of prediction error signaling in human dorsolateral but not ventral striatum in Parkinson's disease patients: evidence from a model-based fMRI study. *Neuroimage.* 2010;**49**(1):772–81.

76. Goldstein RZ, Tomasi D, Alia-Klein N, et al. Subjective sensitivity to monetary gradients is associated with frontolimbic activation to reward in cocaine abusers. *Drug Alcohol Depend.* 2007;**87**(2–3):233–40.

77. Potenza MN. Review. The neurobiology of pathological gambling and drug addiction: an overview and new findings. *Philos Trans R Soc Lond B Biol Sci.* 2008;**363**(1507):3181–9.

78. Reuter J, Raedler T, Rose M, et al. Pathological gambling is linked to reduced activation of the mesolimbic reward system. *Nat Neurosci.* 2005;**8**(2):147–8.

79. Riba J, Krämer UM, Heldmann M, Richter S, Münte TF. Dopamine agonist increases risk taking but blunts reward-related brain activity. *PLoS One.* 2008;**3**(6):e2479.

80. Frank MJ. Dynamic dopamine modulation in the basal ganglia: a neurocomputational account of cognitive deficits in medicated and nonmedicated Parkinsonism. *J Cogn Neurosci.* 2005;**17**(1):51–72.

81. Frank MJ, Samanta J, Moustafa AA, Sherman SJ. Hold your horses: impulsivity, deep brain stimulation, and medication in parkinsonism. *Science.* 2007;**318**(5854):1309–12.

82. Frank MJ, Seeberger LC, O'Reilly RC. By carrot or by stick: cognitive reinforcement learning in parkinsonism. *Science.* 2004;**306**(5703):1940–3.

83. Bodi N, Kéri S, Nagy H, et al. Reward-learning and the novelty-seeking personality: a between- and within-subjects study of the effects of dopamine agonists on young Parkinson's patients. *Brain* 2009;**132**(Pt 9):2385–95.

84. Robbins TW, Everitt BJ. A role for mesencephalic dopamine in activation: commentary on Berridge (2006). *Psychopharmacology (Berl).* 2007;**191**(3):433–7.

85. Berridge KC, Robinson TE. What is the role of dopamine in reward: hedonic impact, reward learning, or incentive salience? *Brain Res Brain Res Rev.* 1998;**28**(3):309–69.

86. Robinson TE, Berridge KC. The neural basis of drug craving: an incentive-sensitization theory of addiction. *Brain Res Brain Res Rev.* 1993;**18**(3):247–91.

87. Frosini D, Pesaresi I, Cosottini M, et al. Parkinson's disease and pathological gambling: results from a functional MRI study. *Mov Dis.* 2010;**25**(14):2449–53.

88. Djamshidian A, O'Sullivan SS, Wittmann BC, Lees AJ, Averbeck BB. Novelty seeking behaviour in Parkinson's disease. *Neuropsychologia.* 2011;**49**(9):2483–88.

89. Simioni AC, Dagher A, Fellows LK. Dissecting the effects of disease and treatment on impulsivity in Parkinson's disease. *J Int Neuropsychol Soc.* 2012;**18**(06):942–51. doi: 10.1017/S135561771200094X.

90. Voon V, Gao J, Brezing C, et al. Dopamine agonists and risk: impulse control disorders in

Parkinson's disease. *Brain.* 2011;**134**(Pt 5):1438–46.

91. Moody TD, Bookheimer SY, Vanek Z, Knowlton BJ. An implicit learning task activates medial temporal lobe in patients with Parkinson's disease. *Behav Neurosci.* 2004;**118**(2):438–42.

92. Packard MG, Hirsh R, White NM. Differential effects of fornix and caudate nucleus lesions on two radial maze tasks: evidence for multiple memory systems. *J Neurosci.* 1989;**9**(5):1465–72.

93. Grossman M, Cooke A, DeVita C, *et al.* Grammatical and resource components of sentence processing in Parkinson's disease: an fMRI study. *Neurology.* 2003;**60**(5):775–81.

94. Gusnard DA, Raichle ME. Searching for a baseline: functional imaging and the resting human brain. *Nat Rev Neurosci.* 2001;**2**(10):685–94.

95. Nagano-Saito A, Leyton M, Monchi O, *et al.* Dopamine depletion impairs frontostriatal functional connectivity during a set-shifting task. *J Neurosci.* 2008;**28**(14):3697–706.

96. Tinaz S, Schendan HE, Stern CE. Fronto-striatal deficit in Parkinson's disease during semantic event sequencing. *Neurobiol Aging.* 2008;**29**(3):397–407.

97. van Eimeren T, Monchi O, Ballanger B, Strafella AP. Dysfunction of the default mode network in Parkinson disease: a functional magnetic resonance imaging study. *Arch Neurol.* 2009;**66**(7):877–83.

98. Nagano-Saito A, Liu J, Doyon J, Dagher A. Dopamine modulates default mode network deactivation in elderly individuals during the Tower of London task. *Neurosci Lett.* 2009;**458**(1):1–5.

99. Delaveau P, Salgado-Pineda P, Fossati P, *et al.* Dopaminergic modulation of the default mode network in Parkinson's disease. *Eur Neuropsychopharmacol.* 2010;**20**:784–92.

100. Argyelan M, Carbon M, Ghilardi MF, *et al.* Dopaminergic suppression of brain deactivation responses during sequence learning. *J Neurosci.* 2008;**28**(42):10687–95.

101. Scatton B, Javoy-Agid F, Rouquier L, Dubois B, Agid Y. Reduction of cortical dopamine, noradrenaline, serotonin and their metabolites in Parkinson's disease. *Brain Res.* 1983;**275**(2):321–8.

102. Asahina M, Suhara T, Shinotoh H, *et al.* Brain muscarinic receptors in progressive supranuclear palsy and Parkinson's disease: a positron emission tomographic study. *J Neurol Neurosurg Psychiatry.* 1998;**65**(2):155–63.

103. Kuhl DE, Minoshima S, Fessler JA, *et al.* In vivo mapping of cholinergic terminals in normal aging, Alzheimer's disease, and Parkinson's disease. *Ann Neurol.* 1996;**40**(3):399–410.

104. Hilker R, Thomas AV, Klein JC, *et al.* Dementia in Parkinson disease: functional imaging of cholinergic and dopaminergic pathways. *Neurology.* 2005;**65**(11):1716–22.

105. Nagano-Saito A, Washimi Y, Arahata Y, *et al.* Cerebral atrophy and its relation to cognitive impairment in Parkinson disease. *Neurology.* 2005;**64**(2):224–9.

106. Apostolova LG, Beyer M, Green AE, *et al.* Hippocampal, caudate, and ventricular changes in Parkinson's disease with and without dementia. *Mov Disord.* 2010;**25**(6):687–8.

Networks and resting state in Parkinson's disease

Nazanin Baradaran and Martin J. McKeown

Resting-state functional magnetic resonance imaging (rs-fMRI)

Introduction

Functional magnetic resonance imaging (fMRI) has profoundly affected how the brain can be non-invasively assessed in vivo. fMRI utilizing blood oxygen level-dependent (BOLD) contrast exploits the fact that oxy- and deoxyhemoglobin have different paramagnetic properties [1]. As focal blood flow is modulated by local brain metabolism, BOLD is thus an indirect marker of neural activity. The majority of fMRI studies to date have examined changes in BOLD activity as a result of performing cognitive, motor, visual, sensory, or even taste or osmic tasks. In contrast, resting-state fMRI (rs-fMRI) explores BOLD signal fluctuations generated without any obvious external stimulus or task: neuroimaging data are acquired while individuals are instructed simply to rest quietly with their eyes closed and remain awake. In this condition, spatially widespread, unprompted activity not attributable to specific external stimuli can be observed [2]. Since first investigated by Biswal *et al.* [3], the co-activation of spontaneous fMRI BOLD time series from spatially distinct brain regions (i.e., "resting-state fMRI" – rs-fMRI) has increasingly attracted attention, and reinforces the modern notion that the brain is actively engaged during its "relaxed" state. Appropriate analysis of rs-fMRI allows the description of spontaneous networks of interaction known as resting-state networks (RSNs) [4]. RSNs are generally localized to gray matter regions [5] and include spatially distinct regions that share the same function [6]. These networks may include cortico-cerebellar [7] and cortico-subcortical [8] connectivity associations.

Origin and limitation of the BOLD signal

Determining the biological significance of rs-fMRI requires knowledge of the exact origin of resting-state BOLD signals, yet this is unclear. It can be difficult to ascertain what constitutes physiological noise, such as that induced by cardiac pulsation and respiration, and what reflects neuronal activity in the BOLD signal, resulting in a vigorous debate in the literature [9, 10]. Strong support for the neuronal basis of BOLD signals is based on examining the relation between RSNs and diffusion tensor imaging (DTI) [11]. DTI is a relatively new imaging method, used to measure structural brain connectivity by measuring the diffusion profile of water molecules in the brain, allowing, under fairly strong assumptions, the reconstruction of white matter tracts [12]. A review of studies comparing resting-state functional connectivity with structural connectivity concluded that the close relationship between rs-fMRI and structural connectivity is strongly suggestive of a neuronal origin for RSNs [13]. However, co-activation of the BOLD signal between regions can potentially be strongly affected by cardiac and respiratory activity, hence pre-processing methods to reduce these influences are crucial for accurate rs-fMRI analysis [9, 10].

Anatomy of resting-state networks (RSN)

A meticulous cataloging of RSNs in healthy populations is essential to infer any potential alteration in brain synchronicity due to neurological disease. While RSNs have also been consistently identified with the electroencephalogram (EEG) [14] and $H_2^{15}O$ positron emission tomography (PET) studies [14], the majority of studies examining RSNs have employed rs-fMRI. The patterns of RSN activity in

Magnetic Resonance Imaging in Movement Disorders, ed. Paul Tuite and Alain Dagher. Published by Cambridge University Press. © Cambridge University Press 2013.

rs-fMRI demonstrate individual differences, as they may reflect a combination of conscious activity and internal neural dynamics [15], but at least six independent functional networks have been consistently found across a number of studies (summarized below). Further discrepancy in the regions constituting individual networks may be due to data acquisition and analysis technique variations [3, 5]. For instance, the frequent frontoparietal network (FPN) observed may be composed of distinct right and left lateralized networks [16].

Of particular relevance for this chapter is that a number of studies have revealed that the normally observed RSNs are frequently and significantly disrupted in neurological disorders [17–20].

- **Default mode network (DMN)**

The most consistently reported RSN with strong reproducibility across studies is the DMN [14, 21]. Raichle et al. [14] introduced the term "default mode network" to describe activity seen in $H_2^{15}O$ PET when the brain was not performing a specific task. Although it has been found that the DMN emerges predominantly under resting state, and is relatively deactivated during many different types of cognitive tasks [14], some studies have shown that its engagement is correlated with individual task performance [22].

The DMN may function as the key process of cognitive and emotional processing as well as monitoring the world around us [23] and/or may facilitate performance during active tasks, for example working memory performance [22]. The latter role was suggested based on a positive correlation between the intensity of functional connectivity and task performance [24].

The main regions contributing to the DMN include the precuneus/posterior cingulate cortex (PCC), the mesial prefrontal cortex (PFC), and the lateral parietal cortex [14, 21, 23]. The precunecus/PCC node, a region of interest (ROI) which is widely connected with other regions [25], has a major role in introspective mental activity; including the ability to think about the past, picture future events, and possess awareness [26]. The intense interconnectivity with other brain regions is consistent with its position as a key node in overall functional connectivity [27]. Some studies have suggested an anterior and posterior categorization of DMN [28] depending upon the task performed.

- **Sensorimotor network (SMN)**

The precentral gyrus, postcentral gyrus, and supplementary motor areas (SMA) [4] correspond well to sensorimotor function [3]. This network has also been observed during active tasks such as finger tapping [5].

The similarity of task-induced and spontaneous pattern of activity may represent memory of past motor performance [29].

- **Visual network (VIN)**

The VIN includes the striate, peristriate, and extrastriate visual cortex; occipital pole; and occipitotemporal regions [30]. In certain studies, separate VINs have been identified based on primary and secondary visual systems [31].

- **Auditory network (AUN)**

The AUN involves the superior and middle temporal cortices, insula, postcentral gyrus, and Heschl's gyrus [6, 32], although some discrepancies may be observed.

- **Executive control network (ECN)**

The ECN includes the medial frontal, superior frontal, and anterior cingulate cortex (ACC). This network is critical for "executive function" tasks: for example working memory or control processes [33].

- **Frontoparietal network (FPN)**

The FPN involves the inferior and medial frontal gyri and inferior parietal and angular gyri [16] and may be lateralized. It has been shown in several studies that this network contributes to different mental tasks including memory [16], language [34], attention [35], and visual [5] processes.

Methodologies

Several analysis methods have been proposed to assess functional connectivity from rs-fMRI. Assessing the functional connectivity between two brain loci can either occur at the individual voxel or the ROI level. Margulies et al. [36] reviewed six prominent categories of resting-state data analysis: seed-based functional connectivity, component-based analysis, clustering, pattern classification, graph theory, and local methods, such as the amplitude of low frequency fluctuations (ALFF) and regional homogeneity (ReHo). While discussing each of these methods is beyond the scope of this chapter, we briefly outline some of the main concepts below.

The term "functional connectivity" is sometimes used quite loosely. It may refer to different ROIs covarying over time or it may refer to direct functional connections between ROIs. As is well known in statistics, correlation does not imply causation (Figure 7.1). The terms "functional connectivity"

85

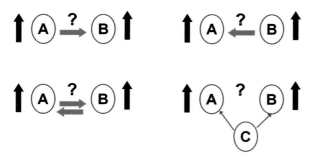

Figure 7.1 Problems associated with inferring connectivity when examining two ROIs A and B. If A and B tend to co-vary over time, is it because A is connected to B? B connected to A? Both A and B connected to each other? Or possibly a third ROI C that is connected to both A and B, and A and B are not connected at all? Causal methods attempt to distinguish between these possibilities, while direct correlative methods cannot.

and "effective connectivity" are sometimes used to try and distinguish between correlative and causative relations between regions respectively.

Seed-based method

The most straightforward method of analysis for functional connectivity is the seed-based or ROI-based method. This method starts by extracting the mean time course of the BOLD signal from a pre-defined ROI, and then this time course is correlated with all other brain regions. The outcome of such a procedure is a functional connectivity map (fcMAP) representing how much different ROIs are connected with the given region [3, 23]. The main benefit of the seed-based method is that it results in an unambiguous functional map with a straightforward interpretation, while the main disadvantage is the dependence of resulting fcMAPs on the choice of seed ROI [6, 37].

Independent component analysis (ICA)

ICA decomposes BOLD patterns into spatially independent maps and their associated time courses [38], which was a significant shift from the traditional hypothesis-based approach to fMRI analysis. If two or more voxels are part of the same independent component, then it means that at least some components of their raw time courses are co-varying. Because no time course of activation needs to be specified a priori, ICA is ideally suited to assessing rs-fMRI data [16, 39]. ICA analysis of rs-fMRI has been widely used to study clinical populations, for example Alzheimer's disease [17], depression [18], schizophrenia [40], mild

cognitive impairment [41], and non-communicative brain-damaged patients [42].

Causal methods

Assessment of a causal relationship is non-trivial, and an active area of research [43]. Most of these methods are based on conditional probability. Since, in general, $P(A|B) \neq P(B|A)$ it is possible to infer directional connectivity with these methods. As most statistical techniques require sufficient data to make reliable estimates, the situation in fMRI, where the timepoints are relatively few (~100–300) and the number of ROIs or voxels is very large, may cause problems for these methods.

The PCfdr network approach

The so-called PC (Peter Spirtes and Clark Glymore) algorithm can be used to learn which ROIs within a group of ROIs are directly functionally linked together, and not driven by another common ROI [44]. For two correlated ROIs A and B, the algorithm determines if the correlation is still present after taking into account the influence of a third region. It then proceeds to rigorous examination of all other ROIs (and combinations of ROIs) to see if the correlation between A and B can be completely explained by these external factors. If it can be explained by external influence(s), then no direct connection between ROIs A and B is inferred. The algorithm uses the false discovery rate (FDR) approach to ensure that inferred connections are established with a given level of significance [45]. This approach, while well suited to the fMRI situation with few timepoints and large numbers of ROIs, cannot determine the direction or the strength of association between each pair of ROIs.

Dynamic Bayesian networks (DBNs)

DBNs are a type of graphical model where statistical relations between variables are shown as "edges" and each ROI is considered a "node." With the DBN approach, many (e.g., thousands) candidate models are selected to see how well they describe the relationships between ROIs, and the best model, based on a criterion which determines a balance between accuracy and parsimony, is selected. This approach can be computationally expensive, but when the PCfdr method is first used to determine *what* ROIs are connected, this greatly restricts the number of candidate models that need to be tested with the DBN. The end result of a PCfdr–DBN approach is a network describing the relation between each pair of ROIs in terms of (a) whether or not a significant connection exists, (b) the direction of that connection, and (c) the strength of that connection.

Group network studies in causal networks

Assessing group network studies is difficult because of inherent inter-subject variability. Typically, one wants to answer the question, "How does the resting-state causal network differ between PD subjects and controls?" This necessitates trying to estimate a "typical" PD network and a "typical" control network. Since each subject's network can differ between subjects not only in *what* ROIs are connected, but also *how strongly* they are connected, it is desirable to determine the best way to combine individual subject models into a group model. Li *et al.* rigorously assessed this and found that for normal subjects, they were sufficiently homogeneous that it was acceptable to simply pool the data and determine a "mean" network. In contrast, in PD subjects it was more desirable to fit individual models in order to demonstrate the normalizing effect of connectivity via levodopa [46]. This research is therefore an area of ongoing study, and will be particularly important for PD research.

Graph theory analysis

Brain connectivity patterns can be represented as a graph, that is a model consisting of nodes (i.e., ROIs) and edges (i.e., the connections between the ROIs). Specifying connectivity patterns in this way facilitates the utilization of the rich theoretical framework of graph theory, allowing for the examination of the topology of complex networks. Graph theoretical measures can be used to describe the intrinsic properties of network configuration, such as the local and global organization of functional brain networks [47]. Many graphs found in nature, including the connectivity patterns in the brain, demonstrate "small-world" topology, where the typical distance between two randomly chosen nodes is proportional to the logarithm of the number of nodes in the network. Graph theoretic measures applied to graphs derived from rs-fMRI studies suggest that many brain networks are organized as efficient small-world networks with a high level of local connectedness and low mean path length [48]. Disruption of small-world topography may be seen in disease states: for instance a significant

reduction of clustering coefficient in Alzheimer's disease individuals was reported by Supekar *et al.* [49].

Advantages of rs-fMRI
Diverse patient population

Examining RSNs allows for a comprehensive picture of intrinsic neural organization without relying on active performance or engagement of the patient. It is an easy paradigm to apply, specifically for subjects who may find it difficult to perform complex motor and/or cognitive tasks. It broadens the patient population that can be recruited for rs-fMRI studies, for example infants, people with severe cognitive or physical impairment, and varying consciousness states including sleep [50], anesthesia [11], and disorders of consciousness [42].

rs-fMRI changes as a marker of dysfunction

RSNs were initially used solely as a research tool to investigate the functional architecture of the brain in healthy volunteers. In fact, functional connectedness is so important for normal brain function that alterations in RSNs can be used as a marker of network dysfunction [17], resulting in many clinical applications. In fact, a rapidly developing area in clinical neuroscience over the past decade has been an appreciation of the relation between altered neural connectivity patterns and neuropsychiatric, neurodevelopment, and also neurodegenerative disorders. This has prompted rs-fMRI studies in normal aging [28, 37], human cognition, behavior, and psychiatric, for example depression [18], and various neurological disorders [11, 18, 19, 47], and even sleep [50]. RSN patterns in patients in a minimally conscious state have suggested conscious awareness and some cognitive processing [42, 51, 52]. RSN properties may correlate with clinical measures, such as Mini-Mental State Examination (MMSE) scores [53]. In fact, there may be a link between organization of brain networks and intellectual performance [54] consistent with EEG findings, suggesting that people with higher levels of education tend to have shorter mean path lengths [55]. Nevertheless, many have observed that further technical enhancement and experimental refinement may be required to describe robustly and completely the complex architecture of different RSNs, especially in disease scenarios [18, 40].

While RSN disruption has been studied in dozens of disorders, the most consistent results have been obtained with Alzheimer's disease and schizophrenia [17, 56]. Among all RSNs, DMN activation and connectivity has been of special interest as a marker of cognitive ability [19, 56]. Hence, the strength of this network might be of diagnostic value for different clinical conditions and diseases, and this may be due to its involvement in the consolidation of episodic memory.

Another key clinical area where RSN evaluation may play an increasingly important role is that of pre-surgical assessment. Pre-surgical brain mapping based on neuroimaging data is usually required by the neurosurgical team to assess preoperative risk, predict outcome, and create patient-specific surgical strategies during surgical planning. Traditionally, such pre-surgical brain mapping requires intensive subject cooperation and depends on the selection of appropriate paradigms and tasks that reliably activate the brain areas of interest. However, slight changes in task design, task performance, or data analysis can have substantial impact on the final brain mapping results [57]. Moreover, subject cooperation may be problematic for patients, particularly those who are impaired and/or anxious and frightened by their condition, and thus rs-fMRI has been suggested for pre-surgical motor/brain mapping [58].

An interesting extension of rs-fMRI methods is to assess changes in RSNs after a therapeutic intervention, such as exercise. For example, Mayer et al. [59] examined changes in the DMN before and after exercise in concussed individuals and found reduced connectivity from the PCC with the ACC and right supramarginal gyrus. Alterations in RSNs in the sub-acute phase of injury may therefore be of use clinically in assessing the severity of injury and offering some insight into the pathophysiology of the disorder [59].

Parkinson's disease (PD)
Studies of altered functional connectivity in PD

Despite the extensive application of resting-state imaging modalities to aforementioned brain disorders, relatively fewer studies have assessed altered connectivity in Parkinson's disease (PD). PD is a common neurodegenerative disorder, clinically characterized by tremor, rigidity, and akinesia (difficulty in initiating movements). A prominent pathological feature is relentless substantia nigra *pars compacta* dopaminergic cell loss [60] in the densely connected striatum [61]. The motor physiology of PD has emphasized the classical cortico-striato-pallido-thalamo-cortical circuit model of motor pathway including, more recently, the hyperdirect pathway between the motor cortex and subthalamic nucleus (STN) [62].

Given the tight interconnectedness between the basal ganglia and cortex, disruption of functional networks in PD individuals is perhaps unsurprising, suggesting network approaches for exploring the development of novel therapeutic strategies is critical [63, 64]. Distinct patterns of functional network dysfunction in PD can be observed in the striatum, globus pallidus, thalamus, STN, substantia nigra, and cortical motor areas (primary motor cortex, SMA, premotor cortex) [65]. Altered connectivity patterns in PD related to motor task performance have been described in a number of fMRI [66–68], and electrophysiological [66, 69], studies. However, in addition to these task-related studies, the study of RSNs in PD may provide a number of advantages, including less bias during performance of a specific motor task or cognitive function. They also require a minimal degree of cooperation, which may introduce extensive variability in performance.

Resting-state studies in PD

A few studies have investigated rs-fMRI brain network characteristics in PD [70–74]. A consistent finding among all of them is increased connectivity between the basal ganglia and motor regions.

Helmich et al. [72] examined the functional connectivity of three cortico-striatal loops that included the posterior putamen, the anterior putamen, and the caudate nucleus, regions that have been deemed important in DTI [75] and rs-fMRI of normal controls [8]. They suggest that the normal cortical SMN may be conceptually partitioned into two different cortico-striatal loops, with connectivity to/from the posterior putamen or to/from the anterior putamen (with less severe dopamine depletion in PD). PD subjects demonstrated reduced functional connectivity between the posterior putamen and inferior parietal cortex, suggesting this network alteration may underlie abnormal sensorimotor integration observed in PD [72]. In contrast, connectivity between the anterior putamen and the pre-SMA, and between the caudate nucleus and the dorsal PFC, did not differ from normal controls.

Wu et al. [70] used graph theory-based connectivity analysis to study resting-state in PD and found increased overall network coupling in M1 (primary motor cortex) and cerebellum while global functional connectivity was reduced in the SMA, PFC, and putamen. Their results were consistent with ^{18}F-fluorodeoxyglucose (FDG)-PET resting state results in PD demonstrating patterns of altered cerebral metabolic activity [76]. In a more recent rs-fMRI study, Wu et al. [71] employed the seed-based method to demonstrate altered connectivity between pre-SMA (important for motor preparation and initiation [77]) and primary motor cortex (M1) (critical in motor execution) in PD subjects. The greater network connectivity changes observed in regions related to motor preparation and initiation, compared to those for motor execution (M1), may imply a lack of readiness for movement in PD. They postulate that the strengthened connectivity to/from M1 they observed may reflect compensatory functional reorganization and/or the incapacity to suppress contextually improper functional circuits [71].

None of the aforementioned studies explicitly focused on the STN, which probably plays a crucial role in normal motor functioning and also in the pathophysiology of PD. An increased synchronized link between the STN and motor cortex, which is mediated via the hyperdirect pathway, has been suggested as fundamental to the pathophysiology of PD. Therefore, Baudrexel et al. [74] set out to describe the rs-fMRI STN network differences between PD and normal controls using a seed-region approach based on the STN. They found increased rs-fMRI connectivity between the STN and cortical motor regions in PD, suggestive of an important key role for the STN in modulation of basal ganglia–cortical motor network activity in PD. Their results complement the ones from electrophysiological findings indicating excessive synchronization in basal ganglia–cortical circuitries [78].

Tremor

Baudrexel et al. [74] revealed functional connectivity differences between tremor-predominant (increased STN–primary motor cortex) and non-tremor-dominant patients (increased STN–midline cortical motor regions) based on the rs-fMRI. In another study, tremor was related to a transient increase in basal ganglia–motor cortex functional connectivity, suggesting the emergence of tremor from abnormal interactions between the basal ganglia and cerebello-thalamo-cortical circuit [72].

Akinesia and freezing of gait

Freezing of gait, which can occur during gait initiation or turning [79], is frequently associated with PD, and may be independent from akinesia [80]. Dysfunction of the SMA may be an important underlying mechanism for akinesia in PD and task-related studies have shown that increased activity in the SMA is highly correlated with clinical improvement of akinesia [81]. It is therefore expected that an rs-fMRI study found reduced functional connectivity within both ECN and VIN associated with freezing of gait in PD [82].

Effects of dopaminergic treatment

The increased cortico-striatal functional connectivity observed in PD is largely normalized by decreased connectivity strength after levodopa administration [71, 83].

A recent study compared the ALFF in BOLD signals before and after dopaminergic treatment [83]. It observed an increase in the cortico-striatal functional connectivity strength, which was down-regulated after administration of levodopa.

Cognitive assessment

rs-fMRI studies have described RSNs not only related to motor symptoms, but also to non-motor features of PD, such as cognitive dysfunction. Although cognitive impairment in PD is generally milder than that seen in Alzheimer's disease, cognitive dysfunction is frequently observed in PD, and plays a major role in clinical disability. Early studies using FDG-PET imaging demonstrated independent patterns of metabolic dysfunction related to cognitive and motor function [84].

Apathy and depression have been assessed in PD using resting state. Although both entities may occur in PD and have some overlapping features, resting-state data have shown separate underlying circuits involved in each one of the features. Apathy score is best predicted by ALFF signal in the left supplementary motor cortex, the right orbitofrontal cortex, and the right middle frontal cortex, whereas depression score is best predicted by the changes in the right putamen [85].

DMN in PD during task performance

A number of fMRI and $H_2^{15}O$ PET studies have suggested that performance of an executive or attentional task requires deactivation of the DMN [14, 21]. In general, the complexity of a task correlates with the degree of DMN deactivation, but this relationship might be lost in PD patients [86]. The normal deactivation of the DMN may also be impaired in different conditions such as normal aging, demented patients, and neuropsychiatric diseases [87].

Tinaz *et al.* [88] found that in contrast to controls, PD patients did not show decreased activation of the DMN during task performance. The same findings were found during a Montreal card sorting task [89]. Normal aging has a different pattern of DMN activation and deactivation [87].

Future potential as a biomarker

PD can be regarded as a fundamental disruption of network connectivity, and appropriate network assessments may eventually guide loci for treatments. Intrinsic connectivity network measures may prove sufficiently reliable to be used as biomarkers for disease progression and treatment responses [90]. Similar to the case for Alzheimer's disease [91], rs-fMRI has been suggested as a useful biomarker in PD-related dementia, showing inter-regional network disruption in the cortico-striatal loop [92]. Furthermore, in addition to being used as a biomarker and analytical tool for evaluation of PD, rs-fMRI could potentially be used for prediction of the development of PD [93]. From a clinical perspective, further pursuit of network-based strategies might lead to development of sensitive and specific biomarkers for diagnostic, prognostic, and disease-monitoring purposes.

Summary

In summary, rs-fMRI has the advantage of accurately assessing brain connectivity patterns without requiring subjects to engage actively in complex cognitive or motor tasks. As a number of task-related fMRI studies have suggested that a critical characteristic of PD is disruption of systems-level connectivity, rs-fMRI appears to be an ideal tool to assess various motor and non-motor alterations in PD. While some technical aspects remain, it is anticipated that rs-fMRI will continue to expand its role as a quantitative assay of brain function in PD.

References

1. Ogawa S, Lee TM, Kay AR, Tank DW. Brain magnetic-resonance-imaging with contrast dependent on blood oxygenation. *Proc Natl Acad Sci U S A*. 1990;**87**(24):9868–72.

2. Friston KJ, Frith CD, Frackowiak RSJ. Principal component analysis learning algorithms – a neurobiological analysis. *Proc Biol Sci*. 1993;**254**(1339):47–54.

3. Biswal B, Yetkin FZ, Haughton VM, Hyde JS. Functional connectivity in the motor cortex of resting human brain using echo-planar MRI. *Magn Reson Med*. 1995;**34**(4):537–41.

4. Rosazza C, Minati L. Resting-state brain networks: literature review and clinical applications. *Neurol Sci*. 2011;**32**(5):773–85.

5. De Luca M, Smith S, De Stefano N, Federico A, Matthews PM. Blood oxygenation level dependent contrast resting state networks are relevant to functional activity in the neocortical sensorimotor system. *Exp Brain Res*. 2005;**167**(4):587–94.

6. Cordes D, Haughton VM, Arfanakis K, *et al*. Mapping functionally related regions of brain with functional connectivity MR imaging. *Am J Neuroradiol*. 2000;**21**(9):1636–44.

7. Habas C, Kamdar N, Nguyen D, *et al*. Distinct cerebellar contributions to intrinsic connectivity networks. *J Neurosci*. 2009;**29**(26):8586–94.

8. Zhang DY, Snyder AZ, Fox MD, *et al*. Intrinsic functional relations between human cerebral cortex and thalamus. *J Neurophysiol*. 2008;**100**(4):1740–8.

9. Chang C, Cunningham JP, Glover GH. Influence of heart rate on the BOLD signal: the cardiac response function. *Neuroimage*. 2009;**44**(3):857–69.

10. Birn RM, Smith MA, Jones TB, Bandettini PA. The respiration response function: the temporal dynamics of fMRI signal fluctuations related to changes in respiration. *Neuroimage*. 2008;**40**(2):644–54.

11. Greicius MD, Supekar K, Menon V, Dougherty RF. Resting-state functional connectivity reflects structural connectivity in the

default mode network. *Cereb Cortex.* 2009;**19**(1):72–8.

12. Le Bihan D. Looking into the functional architecture of the brain with diffusion MRI. *Nat Rev Neurosci.* 2003;**4**(6):469–80.

13. Damoiseaux JS, Greicius MD. Greater than the sum of its parts: a review of studies combining structural connectivity and resting-state functional connectivity. *Brain Struct Funct.* 2009;**213**(6):525–33.

14. Raichle ME, MacLeod AM, Snyder AZ, *et al.* A default mode of brain function. *Proc Natl Acad Sci U S A.* 2001;**98**(2):676–82.

15. Buckner RL. Human functional connectivity: new tools, unresolved questions. *Proc Natl Acad Sci U S A.* 2010;**107** (24):10769–70.

16. Damoiseaux JS, Rombouts SARB, Barkhof F, *et al.* Consistent resting-state networks across healthy subjects. *Proc Natl Acad Sci U S A.* 2006;**103**(37):13848–53.

17. Greicius MD, Srivastava G, Reiss AL, Menon V. Default-mode network activity distinguishes Alzheimer's disease from healthy aging: evidence from functional MRI. *Proc Natl Acad Sci U S A.* 2004;**101**(13):4637–42.

18. Greicius MD, Flores BH, Menon V, *et al.* Resting-state functional connectivity in major depression: abnormally increased contributions from subgenual cingulate cortex and thalamus. *Biol Psychiatry.* 2007;**62**(5): 429–37.

19. Mohammadi B, Kollewe K, Samii A, *et al.* Changes of resting state brain networks in amyotrophic lateral sclerosis. *Exp Neurol.* 2009;**217**(1):147–53.

20. Bonavita S, Gallo A, Sacco R, *et al.* Distributed changes in default-mode resting-state connectivity in multiple sclerosis. *Mult Scler.* 2011;**17**(4):411–22.

21. Raichle ME, Snyder AZ. A default mode of brain function: a brief history of an evolving idea. *Neuroimage.* 2007;**37**(4):1083–90; discussion 1097–9.

22. Esposito F, Aragri A, Latorre V, *et al.* Does the default-mode functional connectivity of the brain correlate with working-memory performances? *Arch Ital Biol.* 2009;**147**(1–2):11–20.

23. Greicius MD, Krasnow B, Reiss AL, Menon V. Functional connectivity in the resting brain: a network analysis of the default mode hypothesis. *Proc Natl Acad Sci U S A.* 2003;**100**(1):253–8.

24. Hampson M, Driesen NR, Skudlarski P, Gore JC, Constable RT. Brain connectivity related to working memory performance. *J Neurosci.* 2006;**26**(51):13338–43.

25. Cavanna AE, Trimble MR. The precuneus: a review of its functional anatomy and behavioural correlates. *Brain.* 2006;**129**:564–83.

26. Buckner RL, Andrews-Hanna JR, Schacter DL. The brain's default network – anatomy, function, and relevance to disease. *Ann N Y Acad Sci* 2008;**1124**:1–38.

27. Fransson P, Marrelec G. The precuneus/posterior cingulate cortex plays a pivotal role in the default mode network: evidence from a partial correlation network analysis. *Neuroimage.* 2008; **42**(3):1178–84.

28. Damoiseaux JS, Beckmann CF, Arigita EJS, Barkhof F, Scheltens P, Stam CJ, *et al.* Reduced resting-state brain activity in the "default network" in normal aging. *Cereb Cortex.* 2008;**18**(8):1856–64.

29. Fox MD, Corbetta M, Snyder AZ, Vincent JL, Raichle ME. Spontaneous neuronal activity distinguishes human dorsal and ventral attention systems. *Proc Natl Acad Sci U S A.* 2006;**103**(26):10046–51.

30. Stevens WD, Buckner RL, Schacter DL. Correlated low-Frequency BOLD fluctuations in the resting human brain are modulated by recent experience in category-preferential visual regions. *Cereb Cortex.* 2010; **20**(8):1997–2006.

31. Rocca MA, Valsasina P, Pagani E, *et al.* Extra-visual functional and structural connection abnormalities in Leber's hereditary optic neuropathy. *PloS One.* 2011;**6**(2):e17081.

32. Seifritz E, Esposito F, Hennel F, *et al.* Spatiotemporal pattern of neural processing in the human auditory cortex. *Science.* 2002; **297**(5587):1706–8.

33. Seeley WW, Menon V, Schatzberg AF, *et al.* Dissociable intrinsic connectivity networks for salience processing and executive control. *J Neurosci.* 2007;**27**(9):2349–56.

34. Smith SM, Fox PT, Miller KL, *et al.* Correspondence of the brain's functional architecture during activation and rest. *Proc Natl Acad Sci U S A.* 2009; **106**(31):13040–5.

35. Dosenbach NUF, Fair DA, Miezin FM, *et al.* Distinct brain networks for adaptive and stable task control in humans. *Proc Natl Acad Sci U S A.* 2007; **104**(26):11073–8.

36. Margulies DS, Bottger J, Long XY, *et al.* Resting developments: a review of fMRI post-processing methodologies for spontaneous brain activity. *MAGMA.* 2010;**23** (5–6):289–307.

37. Andrews-Hanna JR, Snyder AZ, *et al.* Disruption of large-scale brain systems in advanced aging. *Neuron.* 2007;**56**(5):924–35.

38. McKeown MJ, Makeig S, Brown GG, *et al.* Analysis of fMRI data by blind separation into independent spatial components. *Hum Brain Mapp.* 1998;**6**(3): 160–88.

39. Esposito F, Aragri A, Pesaresi I, *et al.* Independent component model of the default-mode brain function: combining individual-level and population-level analyses in resting-state fMRI. *Magn Reson Imaging.* 2008;**26**(7):905–13.

40. Jafri MJ, Pearlson GD, Stevens M, Calhoun VD. A method for functional network connectivity among spatially independent resting-state components in schizophrenia. *Neuroimage.* 2008;**39**(4):1666–81.

41. Qi Z, Wu X, Wang Z, *et al.* Impairment and compensation coexist in amnestic MCI default mode network. *Neuroimage.* 2010;**50**(1):48–55.

42. Vanhaudenhuyse A, Noirhomme Q, Tshibanda LJF, *et al.* Default network connectivity reflects the level of consciousness in non-communicative brain-damaged patients. *Brain.* 2010;**133**:161–71.

43. Pearl J. Causal inference from indirect experiments. *Artif Intell Med.* 1995;**7**(6):561–82.

44. Li JN, Wang ZJ, McKeown MJ. Controlling the false discovery rate in modeling brain functional connectivity. 2008 *IEEE International Conference on Acoustics, Speech and Signal Processing,* Vols **1–12**; 2008: 2105–8.

45. Li JN, Wang ZJ. Controlling the false discovery rate of the association/causality structure learned with the PC algorithm. *J Mach Learn Res.* 2009;**10**: 475–514.

46. Li JN, Wang ZJ, Palmer SJ, McKeown MJ. Dynamic Bayesian network modeling of fMRI: a comparison of group-analysis methods. *Neuroimage.* 2008;**41**(2):398–407.

47. Bullmore E, Sporns O. Complex brain networks: graph theoretical analysis of structural and functional systems. *Nat Rev Neurosci.* 2009;**10**(3):186–98.

48. Watts DJ, Strogatz SH. Collective dynamics of 'small-world' networks. *Nature.* 1998;**393**(6684):440–2.

49. Supekar K, Menon V, Rubin D, Musen M, Greicius MD. Network analysis of intrinsic functional brain connectivity in Alzheimer's disease. *PloS Comput Biol.* 2008;**4**(6):e1000100.

50. Horovitz SG, Braun AR, Carr WS, *et al.* Decoupling of the brain's default mode network during deep sleep. *Proc Natl Acad Sci U S A.* 2009;**106**(27):11376–81.

51. Boly M, Garrido MI, Gosseries O, *et al.* Preserved feedforward but impaired top-down processes in the vegetative state. *Science.* 2011;**332**(6031):858–62.

52. Owen AM, Coleman MR, Boly M, *et al.* Detecting awareness in the vegetative state. *Science.* 2006;**313**(5792):1402.

53. Li SJ, Li Z, Wu GH, *et al.* Alzheimer disease: evaluation of a functional MR imaging index as a marker. *Radiology.* 2002;**225**(1):253–9.

54. van den Heuvel MP, Mandl RCW, Kahn RS, Pol HEH. Functionally linked resting-state networks reflect the underlying structural connectivity architecture of the human brain. *Hum Brain Mapp.* 2009;**30**(10):3127–41.

55. Micheloyannis S, Pachou E, Stam CJ, *et al.* Using graph theoretical analysis of multi channel EEG to evaluate the neural efficiency hypothesis. *Neurosci Lett.* 2006;**402**(3):273–7.

56. Harrison BJ, Yucel M, Pujol J, Pantelis C. Task-induced deactivation of midline cortical regions in schizophrenia assessed with fMRI. *Schizophr Res.* 2007;**91**(1–3):82–6.

57. McGonigle DJ, Howseman AM, Athwal BS, *et al.* Variability in fMRI: An examination of intersession differences. *Neuroimage.* 2000;**11**(6):708–34.

58. Liu HS, Buckner RL, Talukdar T, *et al.* Task-free presurgical mapping using functional magnetic resonance imaging intrinsic activity. *J Neurosurg.* 2009;**111**(4):746–54.

59. Mayer AR, Mannell MV, Ling J, Gasparovic C, Yeo RA. Functional connectivity in mild traumatic brain injury. *Hum Brain Mapp.* 2011;**32**(11):1825–35.

60. Hoehn MM, Yahr MD. Parkinsonism: onset, progression and mortality. *Neurology.* 1967;**17**(5):427–42.

61. Brooks DJ, Piccini P. Imaging in Parkinson's disease: the role of monoamines in behavior. *Biol Psychiatry.* 2006;**59**(10):908–18.

62. Brown P, Oliviero A, Mazzone P, *et al.* Dopamine dependency of oscillations between subthalamic nucleus and pallidum in Parkinson's disease. *J Neurosci.* 2001;**21**(3):1033–8.

63. Eckert T, Van Laere K, Tang C, *et al.* Quantification of Parkinson's disease-related network expression with ECD SPECT. *Eur J Nucl Med Mol Imaging.* 2007;**34**(4):496–501.

64. Eidelberg D. Metabolic brain networks in neurodegenerative disorders: a functional imaging approach. *Trends Neurosci.* 2009;**32**(10):548–57.

65. Alexander GE, Delong MR, Strick PL. Parallel organization of functionally segregated circuits linking basal ganglia and cortex. *Annu Rev Neurosci.* 1986; **9**:357–81.

66. Palmer SJ, Lee PWH, Wang ZJ, Au WL, McKeown MJ. Theta, beta but not alpha-band EEG connectivity has implications for dual task performance in Parkinson's disease. *Parkinsonism Relat Disord.* 2010;**16**(6):393–7.

67. Palmer SJ, Eigenraam L, Hoque T, *et al.* Levodopa-sensitive, dynamic changes in effective connectivity during simultaneous movements

in Parkinson's disease. *Neuroscience*. 2009;**158**(2):693–704.

68. Helmich RC, Aarts E, de Lange FP, Bloem BR, Toni I. Increased dependence of action selection on recent motor history in Parkinson's disease. *J Neurosci*. 2009;**29**(19):6105–13.

69. Tropini G, Chiang J, Wang ZJ, Ty E, McKeown MJ. Altered directional connectivity in Parkinson's disease during performance of a visually guided task. *Neuroimage*. 2011;**56**(4):2144–56.

70. Wu T, Wang L, Chen Y, *et al.* Changes of functional connectivity of the motor network in the resting state in Parkinson's disease. *Neurosci Lett*. 2009;**460**(1):6–10.

71. Wu T, Long X, Wang L, Hallett M, Zang Y, Li K, *et al.* Functional connectivity of cortical motor areas in the resting state in Parkinson's disease. *Hum Brain Mapp*. 2011;**32**(9):1443–57.

72. Helmich RC, Derikx LC, Bakker M, *et al.* Spatial remapping of cortico-striatal connectivity in Parkinson's disease. *Cereb Cortex*. 2010;**20**(5):1175–86.

73. Kwak Y, Peltier SJ, Bohnen NI, *et al.* L-DOPA changes spontaneous low-frequency BOLD signal oscillations in Parkinson's disease: a resting state fMRI study. *Front Syst Neurosci*. 2012;**6**:52.

74. Baudrexel S, Witte T, Seifried C, *et al.* Resting state fMRI reveals increased subthalamic nucleus-motor cortex connectivity in Parkinson's disease. *Neuroimage*. 2011;**55**(4):1728–38.

75. Lehericy S, Ducros M, Van de Moortele PF, *et al.* Diffusion tensor fiber tracking shows distinct corticostriatal circuits in humans. *Ann Neurol*. 2004;**55**(4):522–9.

76. Huang C, Tang C, Feigin A, *et al.* Changes in network activity with the progression of Parkinson's

disease. *Brain*. 2007;**130**(Pt 7):1834–46.

77. Cunnington R, Windischberger C, Deecke L, Moser E. The preparation and execution of self-initiated and externally-triggered movement: a study of event-related fMRI. *Neuroimage*. 2002;**15**(2):373–85.

78. Lalo E, Thobois S, Sharott A, *et al.* Patterns of bidirectional communication between cortex and basal ganglia during movement in patients with Parkinson disease. *J Neurosci*. 2008;**28**(12):3008–16.

79. Nutt JG, Bloem BR, Giladi N, *et al.* Freezing of gait: moving forward on a mysterious clinical phenomenon. *Lancet Neurol*. 2011;**10**(8):734–44.

80. Giladi N. Freezing of gait. Clinical overview. *Adv Neurol*. 2001;**87**:191–7.

81. Jahanshahi M, Jenkins IH, Brown RG, *et al.* Self-initiated versus externally triggered movements. I. An investigation using measurement of regional cerebral blood flow with PET and movement-related potentials in normal and Parkinson's disease subjects. *Brain*. 1995;**118** (Pt 4):913–33.

82. Tessitore A, Amboni M, Esposito F, *et al.* Resting-state brain connectivity in patients with Parkinson's disease and freezing of gait. *Parkinsonism Relat Disord*. 2012;**18**(6):781–7.

83. Kwak Y, Peltier S, Bohnen NI, *et al.* Altered resting state cortico-striatal connectivity in mild to moderate stage Parkinson's disease. *Front Syst Neurosci*. 2010;**4**:143.

84. Lozza C, Baron JC, Eidelberg D, *et al.* Executive processes in Parkinson's disease: FDG-PET and network analysis. *Hum Brain Mapp*. 2004;**22**(3):236–45.

85. Skidmore FM, Yang M, Baxter L, *et al.* Apathy, depression, and

motor symptoms have distinct and separable resting activity patterns in idiopathic Parkinson disease. *Neuroimage*. 2011; [Epub ahead of print].

86. Nagano-Saito A, Liu J, Doyon J, Dagher A. Dopamine modulates default mode network deactivation in elderly individuals during the Tower of London task. *Neurosci Lett*. 2009;**458**(1):1–5.

87. Lustig C, Snyder AZ, Bhakta M, *et al.* Functional deactivations: change with age and dementia of the Alzheimer type. *Proc Natl Acad Sci U S A*. 2003;**100**(24):14504–9.

88. Tinaz S, Schendan HE, Stern CE. Fronto-striatal deficit in Parkinson's disease during semantic event sequencing. *Neurobiol Aging*. 2008;**29**(3):397–407.

89. van Eimeren T, Monchi O, Ballanger B, Strafella AP. Dysfunction of the default mode network in Parkinson disease: a functional magnetic resonance imaging study. *Arch Neurol*. 2009;**66**(7):877–83.

90. Chou YH, Panych LP, Dickey CC, Petrella JR, Chen NK. Investigation of long-term reproducibility of intrinsic connectivity network mapping: a resting-state fMRI study. *AJNR Am J Neuroradiol*. 2012;**33**(5):833–8.

91. Fleisher AS, Sherzai A, Taylor C, *et al.* Resting-state BOLD networks versus task-associated functional MRI for distinguishing Alzheimer's disease risk groups. *Neuroimage*. 2009;**47**(4):1678–90.

92. Seibert TM, Murphy EA, Kaestner EJ, Brewer JB. Interregional correlations in Parkinson disease and Parkinson-related dementia with resting functional MR imaging. *Radiology*. 2012;**263**(1):226–34.

93. Skidmore FM, Yang M, Baxter L, *et al.* Reliability analysis of the resting state can sensitively and specifically identify the presence of Parkinson disease. *Neuroimage*. 2013;**75**:249–61.

Chapter

8

MRI for targeting in surgical treatment of movement disorders

Aviva Abosch and Noam Harel

Background

Deep brain stimulation (DBS) is approved by the US Food and Drug Administration and has *Conformité Européenne* CE Mark approval in Europe for the treatment of Parkinson's disease (PD), dystonia, and essential tremor, with additional indications currently under investigation. The success of this technique is critically dependent on the accurate placement of a DBS electrode into the appropriate target structure. Currently, DBS targets for the treatment of PD include the subthalamic nucleus (STN) or the globus pallidus internus (GPi) [1], for dystonia the target is GPi [2], and for essential tremor the target is the ventral intermediate nucleus (VIM) of the thalamus [3]. Each of these brain targets is relatively small, and the optimal location for a DBS electrode within each structure is even more restricted. The challenge is thus one of placing an electrode array many centimeters deep to the cortical surface, within the motor territory of the structure of interest, but not so close to boundaries with surrounding structures that current spread to these structures results in intolerable side effects. Compounding this challenge is the fact that the target structures can be difficult, if not impossible, to resolve and visualize on standard clinical magnetic resonance (MR) imaging. Various strategies have therefore arisen to improve the likelihood of placing the DBS electrode into the optimal location. Nonetheless, suboptimal electrode location remains a significant problem besetting DBS surgery – with an incidence of 40% in a study of etiologies underlying "failed DBS surgery" [4], in a population of patients referred to a DBS center for evaluation. There remains, therefore, room for further work on the optimization of stereotactic targeting for the DBS procedure.

Stereotactic neurosurgery refers to the use of a rigid external reference frame applied to the human skull, for the purpose of localizing brain targets. The term derives from the Greek word *stereos*, meaning solid, and the Latin word *tactis* for touch [5]. Spiegel *et al.* first described their apparatus for human stereotactic neurosurgery in 1947 [5, 6]. The early stereotactic technique made use of fixed extracranial bony landmarks to create a tri-planar coordinate system, in order to determine the location of intracranial structures by referencing historical brain atlases [7]. However, use of this technique resulted in significant inconsistencies in targeting due to variability of human cranial bony landmarks relative to intracranial structures. To overcome this variability, two techniques – X-ray imaging and skull-mounted stereotactic frames – were combined in the late 1940s, resulting in a dramatic advance in deep brain targeting. The advent of ventriculography – injection of a contrast agent into the ventricular system followed by acquisition of anteroposterior and lateral skull X-rays – enabled the visualization of the anterior commissure (AC) and posterior (PC) commissure as protrusions into the third ventricle [8]. Intracerebral coordinates could then be determined by visualization of the AC and PC, and referenced to the skull-mounted stereotactic frame. A vector could then be determined between the AC–PC coordinates and the desired target structure, using historical human brain atlases. This technique is termed *indirect* targeting, as it requires reference to a historical human brain atlas – such as the one developed by Schaltenbrand and Wahren [9], which uses histological sections in frontal, coronal, and sagittal planes, with transparent overlays delineating nuclear structures and fiber pathways. Indirect targeting is still in use today, although ventriculography has largely been supplanted by stereotactic MR, or fused stereotactic computed tomography (CT)/MR-based imaging, which can be used by the surgeon to modify the initial target and trajectory. *Direct* targeting refers to the use of a patient's own MR images, on which the desired structure can be visualized, in order to place the electrode. Regardless of which targeting technique is used, some form of intraoperative electrophysiological corroboration is typically then used to confirm the target location.

Anatomical and functional considerations of DBS targets for the treatment of movement disorders

Three specific DBS targets are currently in widespread use for the treatment of specific movement disorders. These are VIM for the treatment of tremor (parkinsonian or essential), STN for PD, and GPi for PD and for dystonia. Other targets and other indications are under investigation – such as the pedunculopontine area (PPN area) for the treatment of PD-associated postural instability [10] – and will not be reviewed here.

The subthalamic nucleus (STN)

The STN is a small midbrain nucleus, situated approximately 9 cm from the cortical surface, 12 mm lateral to midline, and measures approximately 6 mm anteroposteriorly, 4 mm mediolaterally, and 5 mm dorsoventrally [11]. Within this small area, the motor territory, which is the intended target for DBS surgery, lies in the posterolateral portion of the nucleus, whereas the limbic territory lies anteromedially [12]. The STN is bounded above by the zona incerta, posteromedially by the medial lemniscus and red nucleus, posteroventrally by the Edinger–Westphal nucleus, which sends fibers to the tract of the third cranial nerve, ventrally by the substantia nigra *pars reticulata*, and laterally and anteriorly by the internal capsule. The proximity of these surrounding structures, and of discrete motor and limbic territories within the STN, accounts for the specific stimulation-induced side effects noted when the DBS electrode is placed in a suboptimal location within the STN, or even at supra-clinical voltages of stimulation delivered through an optimally positioned DBS electrode. The STN can be delineated on MRI, using T_2-weighted sequences, and appears as a

hypointense signal bordered superiorly by the structures detailed above. The resolution of current clinical imaging, however, is usually insufficient to allow for clear visualization of the entire STN border. In particular, the distinction between the inferior border of the STN and the superior border of the substantia nigra (SN) is difficult, if not impossible, to resolve on current clinical imaging modalities [13].

Globus pallidus internus (GPi)

The GPi is situated approximately 2 cm lateral to the AC–PC line. Although not as small as the STN, the GPi is similarly divided into motor and limbic territories, and lies in close proximity to neighboring structures such as the optic tract ventrally, globus pallidus *externa* (GPe) laterally and dorsally, and the internal capsule posteromedially. GPi can be delineated on MR, using T_2-weighted or inversion recovery sequences (Figure 8.1) [14]. Within the GPi lies the *lamina partialis interna*, which separates the internal (GPi-i) and external (GPi-e) segments of the GPi [13]. It should be noted that the GPi, although a larger target than STN, is similarly bounded by structures to which current spread from a suboptimally placed electrode would cause unwanted side effects – for example, optic tract inferiorly and internal capsule posteromedially. The motor territory of the GPi is situated in the posterolateral portion of the GPi, with the associative territory situated anteromedially [15].

Ventral intermediate nucleus (VIM)

VIM (ventral intermediate nucleus or motor thalamus), which cannot be distinguished from surrounding thalamic nuclei on conventional (1.5 or 3 tesla; T) MRI scans, is a narrow, columnar structure measuring approximately 2–4 mm in anteroposterior dimension, 7–10 mm in dorsoventral extent, and 4–6 mm in mediolateral extent. The ventral caudalis (Vc) lies immediately posterior to VIM, and is the principal sensory nucleus of the thalamus; the medial lemniscus lies ventrally, the internal capsule laterally, the ventrooralis posterior (Vop) nucleus anteriorly, and the dorsal tier nuclei are situated dorsal to VIM. VIM is organized in a somatotopic fashion, with the face lying medially and leg laterally. Again, the close proximity of these surrounding structures both within and adjacent to the thalamus means that an electrode that is, for example, too close to the posterior border of

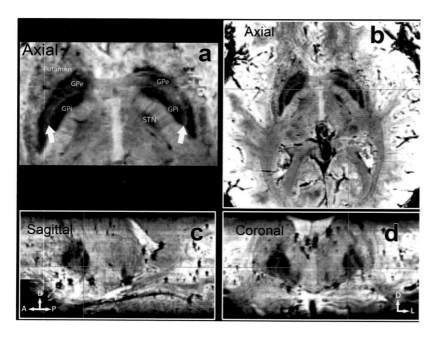

Figure 8.1 Globus pallidus interna (GPi) and globus pallidus externa (GPe) in human subjects imaged at 7T MRI. Axial, sagittal, and coronal imaging demonstrating the boundary between GPi and GPe with susceptibility-weighted imaging. GPi appears (b–d) immediately caudal to the commissural plane. (a) Arrows indicate lamina pallidi medialis, the thin layer separating GPi from GPe. (From Abosch et al., 2010 [13].)

VIM with Vc can result in stimulation-induced paresthesias that limit the therapeutic effect of an implanted DBS electrode within VIM.

Current technique for targeting in DBS surgery

All DBS surgeries currently require some form of stereotaxy, which is a means of translating information from two-dimensional (2D) brain images to the three-dimensional (3D) operative field. Two types of stereotactic approaches are available for DBS surgery. The first of these, frame-based stereotaxy, remains prevalent and provides accuracy, stability, and reproducibility. However, drawbacks to frame-based stereotaxy include patient discomfort during frame placement, and immobilization of the head and neck during surgery. So-called "frameless" stereotaxy – which involves mounting mini-frames directly on the skull surrounding the operative site – is also used, and studies have demonstrated that this technique provides comparable efficacy to traditional frame-based stereotaxy [16]. Frameless stereotaxy requires the placement of multiple skull-mounted fiducials, usually on the day prior to surgery, which are also associated with some discomfort. For the minority of patients whose head circumference is too large to fit within a standard stereotactic frame, frameless stereotaxy is a useful alternative.

Frame-based stereotaxy involves the application of a stereotactic frame to a patient's head, to which is affixed a fiducial localizer box, followed by CT and/or MR imaging. A variety of different MR-compatible stereotactic frames exist, including the Leksell, Cosman–Roberts–Wells (CRW), and Riechert–Mundinger (RM) frames, and selection of a particular frame is based on surgeon preference. Following the acquisition of stereotactic images, the patient is transported to the operating room, and the images transferred to a neuro-navigational workstation. Fiducial marks are registered on the workstation, and the location of the AC, PC, and three midline points – allowing correction for pitch, yaw, and roll of brain position in 3D space – are designated on the images.

Frame-based or frameless stereotactic preoperative imaging is used for surgical targeting. Attributes of these imaging protocols include the use of contiguous, non-overlapping, 1- to 2-mm-thick slices, 3D acquisitions that are then reformatted into axial, coronal, and sagittal planes, image matrices of 512 × 512 and a field-of-view (FOV) that encompasses the AC and PC, target region, cortical entry site and trajectory, and stereotactic frame fiducial marks.

Table 8.1. Consensus target coordinates for the STN, GPi, and VIM

STN

3–4 mm posterior to mid-AC–PC point

3–5 mm caudal to IC plane

12 mm lateral to AC–PC line

GPi

2–3 mm anterior to mid-AC–PC point

3–6 mm caudal to IC plane

20–21 mm lateral to AC–PC line

VIM

25–50% of AC–PC length from PC at IC plane

½ (third ventricular width) + 11.5 mm

IC, intercommissural plan.

Consensus target coordinates

Based on the Schaltenbrand–Wahren Atlas [9], specific indirect target coordinates have been selected as the accepted starting point for localizing deep brain structures for movement disorder surgery. These consensus target coordinates for the STN, GPi, and VIM are listed in Table 8.1.

Indirect versus direct targeting

As mentioned above, the success of DBS surgery is critically dependent on accurate localization of the target structure of interest. Two different approaches to initial target localization exist, and frequently are combined in the operating room: indirect and direct targeting. The use of consensus target coordinates, or indirect targeting, relies on the application of normalized atlas-derived diagrams. These atlas diagrams, which are composites of mapped brains of a *limited* number of subjects, use set distances from the AC–PC line (see Table 8.1). When the atlas diagrams are superimposed on a given patient's MRI scan, they yield *approximate* coordinates for target localization in that patient [9, 14]. Software programs then allow modification of these atlas diagrams, in order to approximate more closely the specific patient's scan. Although indirect targeting offers a reasonable approximation of target location, the actual axial and coronal orientation of

basal ganglia structures and thalamic nuclei in humans can vary significantly in control subjects [17, 18], without adding in the potential confounds of age and neurodegenerative processes. Furthermore, no consensus exists regarding how best to compensate for these individual variations.

In contrast, direct targeting relies on *direct* visualization of the structures in question. The small size, depth, difficulty with visualization of STN (see above), and variability in rotation of the STN – coupled with limitations in the accuracy of the stereotactic technique – can lead to targeting errors in the operating room when relying solely on indirect targeting.

Current MRI sequences for visualization of the STN, GPi, and VIM

A variety of different MR sequences have been reported for visualizing the STN and GPi, in an effort to identify reliably the anatomical borders of these structures on preoperative imaging [19]. Iron deposition in the STN has been shown to be the source of T_2-weighted hypointensity in this structure [20], and is typically exploited for the purposes of STN visualization – through the use of susceptibility-weighted imaging (SWI) or T_2^* sequences [21, 22]. Of note, internal thalamic nuclei are difficult, if not impossible, to visualize on current clinically available MRI systems [23]. Abosch and colleagues have used 7T imaging with SWI to visualize the pulvinar and Vc, with the VIM appearing as an area of signal hyperintensity immediately anterior to Vc (see Table 8.2 and Figure 8.2) [13].

Typical MR pulse sequences for stereotactic imaging of the STN and GPi have been published elsewhere [14].

Brain shift

One disadvantage of both consensus coordinate-based and direct targeting is their reliance on static preoperative imaging studies. The target coordinates are determined on brain atlases or on the individual patient's brain, which is imaged prior to surgical alteration and imaged in a different patient position than the one assumed in the operating room. Brain shift, or the alteration in brain position within the cranial vault relative to preoperative imaging data, is a known confound in all neurosurgical procedures that rely on preoperative imaging for guidance. In DBS surgical procedures, brain shift can result in deviation

Table 8.2. Magnetic resonance imaging parameters for SWI of thalamus at 7T

	FOV, mm	Matrix	Resolution, mm	Slices, n	TR/TE, ms	Flip angle, degrees	Bandwidth, Hz/pixel	PI, n	Repetitions, n	Total acquisition time, min
SWI-1	192 × 192	512 × 512	0.375 × 0.375 × 1	72	28/20	10	120	4	1	7
SWI-2	256 × 160	384 × 240	0.67 × 0.67 × 0.67	88	28/20	10	120	2	4	15

PI, parallel imaging; TE, echo time; TR, repetition time.
Abosch et al., 2010 [13].

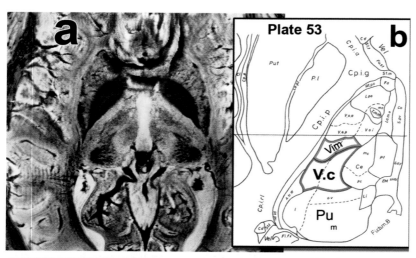

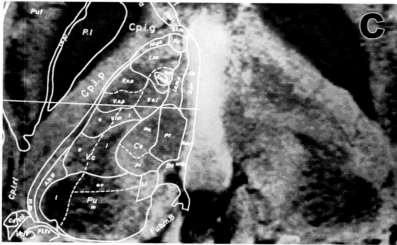

Figure 8.2 Visualization of human internal thalamic nuclei in vivo. (a) Axial SWI slice through thalamus, at the level of the AC–PC plane. (b) Corresponding histologically defined outline (plate # 53 from Schaltenbrand and Wahren Atlas), superimposed on the MRI image, in Panel (c). Note visualization of pulvinar, the arrowhead shape of Vc (red; compare with unmarked right hemisphere), and image contrast modulation within thalamus corresponding to Vim (green). (From Abosch, et al., 2010 [13].)

from the predetermined target coordinates, and may arise from a number of causes, including cerebrospinal fluid (CSF) loss and resulting pneumocephalus, the effect of patient head position on the location of intracranial structures [24], and/or brain deformation due to an advancing electrode. A few millimeters of brain displacement in the target region can adversely affect the efficacy of the surgical intervention, by resulting in the need for multiple extra passes with a recording electrode through the brain in order to achieve an optimal location, or in the suboptimal placement of electrode contacts within the desired target. For these reasons, care is taken to minimize the amount of shift that occurs [25], and efforts are underway to incorporate intraoperative imaging into the DBS surgical procedure, as described below.

Problems with current surgical targeting techniques

Microelectrode recording

As mentioned above, current clinical MR imaging cannot resolve the internal structure of the thalamus, and is insufficient to resolve consistently and accurately the entire boundary of the STN or GPi, and completely distinguish these structures from surrounding structures. Some form of intraoperative electrophysiological technique is therefore used in order to confirm or modify the initial targeting, and the majority of implanting centers use microelectrode recording for this purpose [26]. Microelectrodes are used to sample single-unit extracellular neuronal activity from brain regions en route to, and including, the intended target. Although providing extremely useful electrophysiological information about electrode location, microelectrode recording is an invasive procedure and has been linked to an increase in hemorrhage rate [27]. Additionally, patients are generally kept awake during microelectrode recording, so as not to suppress neural activity with anesthetic agents. This can contribute to patient anxiety and discomfort during the procedure.

Variability in target location

Reliance solely on indirect targeting is problematic in that significant inter-subject variability exists in the location of basal ganglia and thalamic targets. Direct visualization of nuclear boundaries is of obvious utility in allowing fine adjustments in the indirect coordinates to be made [28, 29].

Accuracy of current stereotactic systems

The mean accuracy of the Leksell and CRW stereotactic frames has been demonstrated in phantom studies to be 1.7 ± 0.1 and 1.8 ± 0.11 mm, respectively, when using CT (slice thickness of 1 mm) for fiducial

registration [30, 31]. This accuracy decreases in the clinical setting owing to some combination of the following potential factors: (1) the head frame must bear the weight of the stereotactic arc system, which causes some amount of deflection from target, (2) some degree of positional and operative brain shift occurs between preoperative stereotactic and postoperative imaging, and (3) inter-rater variation exists in the identification of the actual DBS electrode location and AC–PC coordinates on postoperative imaging. Starr and colleagues assessed the accuracy of frame-based stereotaxy in DBS procedures, and found the mean difference between predicted and actual lead coordinates to be 1.4 to 2 mm in all dimensions, despite the use of microelectrode recording, but with much higher deviations in individual cases [32]. Holloway and colleagues have reported that no significant difference exists in the accuracy of frame-based versus frameless stereotactic systems [31].

Use of intraoperative magnetic resonance imaging for DBS surgery

Because of the drawbacks to using preoperative imaging for DBS procedures highlighted above, the use of intraoperative MRI guidance for the placement of DBS electrodes is gaining considerable interest. Starr and colleagues have recently reported their experience with 53 electrodes implanted into 29 patients, using frameless stereotaxy and intraoperative 1.5T MRI guidance in patients under general endotracheal anesthesia for the procedure, and without the use of intraoperative electrophysiological techniques – such as microelectrode recording or macrostimulation – to confirm or modify ultimate electrode location (see below). Postoperative imaging disclosed acceptable anatomical accuracy of lead placement based on consensus target coordinates, and motor subscale of the Unified Parkinson Disease Rating Scale testing in those patients implanted bilaterally (n = 13) indicated an improvement of 60% at 9 months, demonstrating acceptable clinical outcome [33]. Complications included two device infections – attributed to having to shift patient location from the intraoperative MR suite to an anteroom for drilling – and suboptimal placement of both DBS electrodes in one patient due to inadequate visualization of the STN.

Currently, MRI plays a crucial role in targeting electrodes for DBS surgery. A 1.5T stereotactic MR scan is routinely used preoperatively to visualize the AC and PC for indirect targeting. With T_2-weighted imaging it is possible to visualize deep brain structures such as the STN for direct targeting. However, even with T_2-weighted 3T MRI, the border between the SN and STN is difficult to resolve, as are internal thalamic nuclei, such as VIM.

Recent work using high-field strength MRI (at 7T) combined with the contrast provided by SWI sequences has demonstrated a significant improvement in the ability to resolve these deep brain structures [13, 21, 34]. Using 7T and SWI, the border of the STN and SN can be clearly resolved, and internal thalamic nuclei can be visualized. Furthermore, the technical challenges of visualizing deep brain nuclei with functional MRI (fMRI) at 7T are being addressed, holding the promise of identifying functional territories within these small deep brain structures. As mentioned above, intraoperative MRI is being used to guide leads directly into deep brain structures, and has the advantage of accounting for brain shift following the opening of the dura and resulting CSF egress. However, currently available intraoperative MR suites use low-field MR systems – typically 1.5T – and therefore fail to resolve targets such as VIM, and routinely miss the boundary between the STN and SN. With currently available registration algorithms, however, image co-registration using different imaging modalities – such as CT and MRI – and different sequences within a given modality – such as T_1, T_2, and SWI – can be accomplished with sub-voxel accuracy [35]. This capability enables the use of preoperative high-field imaging, as will be discussed below, for intraoperative fusion to clinically available stereotactic imaging (e.g., 1.5T).

High-field MRI: the promise and the challenges

Ultra-high-field (7T and beyond) MRI systems are proving invaluable for basic science research and neuroscience applications [36–38].

fMRI studies conducted at high field, capitalizing on the enhanced sensitivity and specificity of the measured blood oxygen level-dependent (BOLD) signal, have successfully demonstrated the functional organization of neuronal architecture in the cerebral cortex, with an unprecedented level of detail [39, 40].

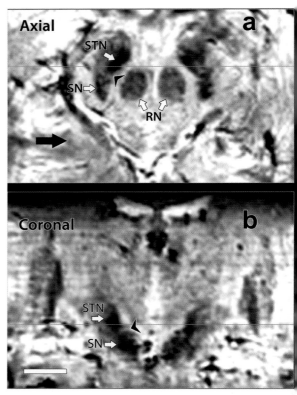

Figure 8.3 Subthalamic nucleus (STN) and substantia nigra (SN) on MRI at 7T susceptibility-weighted imaging axial (a) and coronal (b) images. A boundary between STN and SN is visible on both coronal and axial images. Examination of red nucleus (RN) reveals a complex internal structure (A). (From Abosch et al., 2010 [13].

Structural (i.e., anatomical) images of the human brain acquired at 7T exhibit rich informational content with potential utility for clinical applications [13, 22, 34, 41]. Such publications have led to the expanding interest in high-field MRI for research and clinical applications.

The use of 7T MRI with its enhanced signal-to-noise ratio (SNR), combined with MR sequences that are more advantageous at higher magnetic field, such as SWI [42–44], has yielded high-resolution images with enhanced contrast. The high spatial resolution afforded by 7T MRI enables the clear delineation of structures such as the thalamus, GPe, GPi (Figure 8.1), STN, and SN from surrounding structures (Figure 8.3) [13]. It also enables the detailed reconstruction of the white matter tracts that comprise the basal ganglia and thalamic circuitry (Figure 8.4), and a quantification of the relative strengths of these

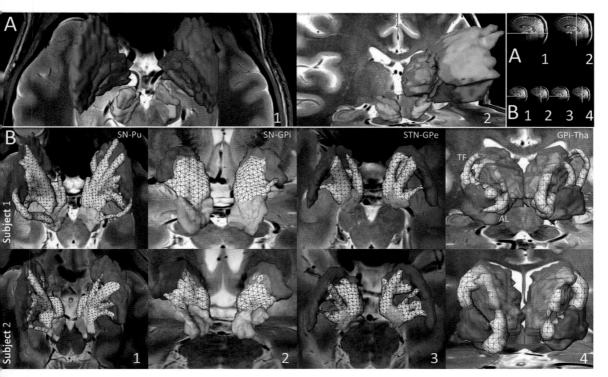

Figure 8.4 Segmentation and reconstruction of fiber pathways of basal ganglia and thalamus. (Panel A) Three-dimensional visualization of manual segmentations of basal ganglia and thalamus from high-resolution SWI, T_2-weighted images, and fractional anisotropy maps. Segmentations are superimposed on T_2-weighted images. (Panel B) White matter pathways identified using diffusion MRI probabilistic tractography. Wireframe volumes represent white matter tracts identified as pathways of interest. From left to right: (1) nigrostriatal, (2) nigropallidal, (3) subthalamopallidal, and (4) pallidothalamic pathways (AL: ansa lenticularis; TF: thalamic fasciculus). Background images are T_2-weighted 7T MR images. (Top right inset; yellow lines denote orientation and location of T_2-weighted images in each panel, with (A1) axial image through SN; (A2) coronal image through posterior Tha; (B1) Axial image through SN, caudo-rostral orientation; (B2) coronal image at the level of the anterior GPi; (B3) axial image slightly inferior to STN; (B4) coronal image through posterior Tha, rostro-caudal orientation. Caudate nucleus, CN: light blue; Putamen, Pu: red; External globus pallidus, GPe: dark blue; Internal globus pallidus, GPi: green; Substantia nigra, SN: yellow; Subthalamic nucleus, STN: magenta; Thalamus, Tha: orange. (From Lenglet et al., PLoS One., 2012 [34].)

various connections [34]. The combination of multiple imaging modalities at high field has enabled the in vivo visualization of individual human basal ganglia and thalamic nuclei (Figure 8.5), and the reconstruction of white matter pathways and their connectivity probability that previously had only been reported in animal studies, histopathologically in human cadaver studies, or in group-averaged MRI population studies [34]. High-resolution data obtained at 7T allow for the exploration of the fine spatial relationships and connectivity patterns of brain structures – details which are typically lost when MRI data are averaged across multiple subjects, due to the limited sensitivity of the acquired data. The technique of group analysis – which involves the pooling of data across subjects – arose out of a lack of

sufficient SNR to resolve structures within individual subjects. With the advent of 7T imaging, however, sufficient SNR now exists to allow for the resolving of smaller structures without the need to average across multiple subjects [34]. It should be noted, however, that the exact relationship between MRI signal and histo-architectural properties of brain tissue has yet to be fully defined [45].

Although of obvious interest, there are potential obstacles to the clinical implementation of 7T MRI. Of primary concern are the following issues at 7T: (1) increased power deposition, (2) the substantial increase in susceptibility artifact, and perhaps most important for surgical applications, (3) geometrical distortion [13, 35]. Each of these issues increases in magnitude with increasing magnetic field strength,

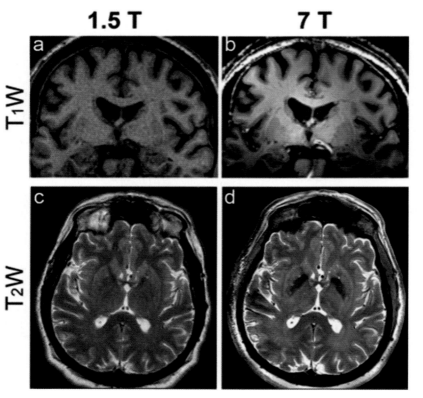

1.5 T   **7 T**

T1W — a, b

T2W — c, d

Figure 8.5 Visual demonstration of registration of 7T to 1.5T MRI. Edges of brain structures obtained from the registered 7T image (right column) are superimposed on the 1.5T image (left column). Top row: T_1W coronal images acquired at (a) 1.5T and (b) 7T. Bottom row: T_2W axial images acquired at (c) 1.5T and (d) 7T, respectively. Note the high degree of correspondence between the 7T red iso-contour edge lines superimposed on the 1.5T images, indicating minimal distortion in the 7T images compared to the clinical 1.5T images. This method follows the current standard practice used in the operating room, in which the surgeon overlays the registered image on top of the reference image and toggles between them in order to determine, visually, how well regional brain structures coincide in the different image sets. (From Duchin et al., PLoS One; 2012 [35].)

and can significantly compromise image acquisition and the interpretability of the images.

In a recent publication by Duchin and colleagues [35], the authors sought to characterize, in vivo, the amount of geometrical distortion present at 7T relative to standard clinical imaging obtained on a 1.5T scanner, in subjects undergoing preoperative evaluation for DBS surgery. These authors demonstrated that co-registration of clinical stereotactic MR images to CT images – which is routinely performed as part of the surgical procedure in order to eliminate possible geometric distortion – can also be performed using 7T images, the same as with 1.5T images, and without any significant geometrical distortion in the region of basal ganglia or thalamic DBS targets. Images acquired at 7T were found to exhibit minimal distortion in midbrain and thalamic regions compared to 1.5T images, and distortion could be corrected by regionally based linear registrations, thereby documenting the feasibility of using high-field MRI as a clinical tool [35].

Clinically available MR systems use 1.5 or 3T magnetic fields for imaging. Significant advances in

MRI technology over the past decade have led to increased field strength and improvements in the SNR, yielding enhanced resolution of the deep brain structures that are the targets of DBS. As mentioned above, frequently neither 1.5 nor 3T imaging allows clear delineation of the STN, especially the caudal boundary with the SN. Furthermore, current clinical MR imaging systems frequently do not allow for a clear delineation between the GPe and GPi, or for visualization of internal structure within the GPi. As mentioned previously, though, using particular sequences (e.g., SWI) at 7T results in significant enhancement of image contrast and resolution [13]. The use of connectivity-based probabilistic tractography enables mapping of white matter projections between structures and within structures, allowing for the identification of various known sub-territories of the basal ganglia and thalamic nuclei [34]. These advances raise the possibility that the technique of microelectrode recording might one day be replaced by a combination of high-resolution anatomical and functional imaging.

MRI compatibility

As mentioned above, intraoperative MRI is being used to assist in the placement of DBS electrodes, and advances in MR technology are yielding important information about DBS targets and their 3D surroundings. Leveraging this improved imaging technology for the benefit of the DBS patient population seems the appropriate next step, but major safety concerns remain. Implanted DBS devices are both conductive and electronically activated [46]. Subjecting an implanted DBS device to a magnetic field can cause heating, induction of currents, and subsequent magnetic interactions, with the potential to (1) create artifacts, (2) cause functional disruption of the device, and most importantly, (3) generate thermal injury to deep brain structures [47, 48]. To date, two deaths and a reversible injury have been reported in patients with implanted DBS systems who underwent MRI or diathermy, respectively [49]. It should be noted that in each of these cases, the manufacturer's guidelines and recommendations for safety in patients with implanted DBS devices were not followed [49, 50]. Furthermore, thousands of MRI scans have been performed on DBS patients without incident [51, 52]. Nonetheless, with the trend towards higher magnetic field-strength imaging systems, and the proliferation of DBS surgeries and indications for this surgery worldwide, there is an urgent need for the development of MRI-compatible devices that will eliminate this risk of thermal injury or device malfunction.

References

1. Follett KA, Weaver FM, Stern M, et al. Pallidal versus subthalamic deep-brain stimulation for Parkinson's disease. N Engl J Med. 2010;362:2077–91.

2. Kupsch A, Benecke R, Muller J, et al. Pallidal deep-brain stimulation in primary generalized or segmental dystonia. N Engl J Med. 2006;355:1978–90.

3. Rehncrona S, Johnels B, Widner H, et al. Long-term efficacy of thalamic deep brain stimulation for tremor: double-blind assessments. Mov Disord. 2003;18:163–70.

4. Okun MS, Tagliati M, Pourfar M, et al. Management of referred deep brain stimulation failures: a retrospective analysis from 2 movement disorders centers. Arch Neurol. 2005;62:1250–5.

5. Pereira EA, Green AL, Nandi D, Aziz TZ. Stereotactic neurosurgery in the United Kingdom: the hundred years from Horsley to Hariz. Neurosurgery. 2008;63:594–606; discussion 607.

6. Spiegel EA, Wycis HT, Marks M, Lee AJ. Stereotaxic apparatus for operations on the human brain. Science. 1947;106:349–50.

7. Horsley V, Clark RH. The structure and functions of the cerebellum examined by a new method. Brain. 1908;31:45–124.

8. Talairach J, Tournoux P. Co-planar Stereotaxic Atlas of the Human Brain. 3-Dimensional Proportional System: An Approach to Cerebral Imaging. Stuttgart; New York: Georg Thieme; 1988.

9. Schaltenbrand G, Wahren W. Atlas for Stereotaxy of the Human Brain. Stuttgart: Thieme; 1977.

10. Stefani A, Lozano AM, Peppe A, et al. Bilateral deep brain stimulation of the pedunculopontine and subthalamic nuclei in severe Parkinson's disease. Brain. 2007;130:1596–607.

11. Richter EO, Hoque T, Halliday W, Lozano AM, Saint-Cyr JA. Determining the position and size of the subthalamic nucleus based on magnetic resonance imaging results in patients with advanced Parkinson disease. J Neurosurg. 2004;100:541–6.

12. Mallet L, Schupbach M, N'Diaye K, et al. Stimulation of subterritories of the subthalamic nucleus reveals its role in the integration of the emotional and motor aspects of behavior. Proc Natl Acad Sci U S A. 2007;104:10661–6.

13. Abosch A, Yacoub E, Ugurbil K, Harel N. An assessment of current brain targets for deep brain stimulation surgery with susceptibility-weighted imaging at 7 tesla. Neurosurgery. 2010;67:1745–56; discussion 56.

14. Starr PA. Placement of deep brain stimulators into the subthalamic nucleus or globus pallidus internus: technical approach. Stereotact Funct Neurosurg. 2002;79:118–45.

15. Vitek JL, Bakay RA, Hashimoto T, et al. Microelectrode-guided pallidotomy: technical approach and its application in medically intractable Parkinson's disease. J Neurosurg. 1998;88:1027–43.

16. Bronte-Stewart H, Louie S, Batya S, Henderson JM. Clinical motor outcome of bilateral subthalamic nucleus deep-brain stimulation for Parkinson's disease using image-guided frameless stereotaxy. Neurosurgery. 2010;67:1088–93; discussion 1093.

17. Patel NK, Khan S, Gill SS. Comparison of atlas- and magnetic-resonance-imaging-based stereotactic targeting of the subthalamic nucleus in the surgical treatment of Parkinson's

disease. *Stereotact Funct Neurosurg.* 2008;**86**:153–61.

18. Ashkan K, Blomstedt P, Zrinzo L, *et al.* Variability of the subthalamic nucleus: the case for direct MRI guided targeting. *Br J Neurosurg.* 2007;**21**:197–200.

19. O'Gorman RL, Shmueli K, Ashkan K, *et al.* Optimal MRI methods for direct stereotactic targeting of the subthalamic nucleus and globus pallidus. *Eur Radiol.* 2011;**21**:130–6.

20. Dormont D, Ricciardi KG, Tande D, *et al.* Is the subthalamic nucleus hypointense on T2-weighted images? A correlation study using MR imaging and stereotactic atlas data. *AJNR Am J Neuroradiol.* 2004;**25**:1516–23.

21. Vertinsky AT, Coenen VA, Lang DJ, *et al.* Localization of the subthalamic nucleus: optimization with susceptibility-weighted phase MR imaging. *AJNR Am J Neuroradiol.* 2009;**30**:1717–24.

22. Cho ZH, Min HK, Oh SH, *et al.* Direct visualization of deep brain stimulation targets in Parkinson disease with the use of 7-tesla magnetic resonance imaging. *J Neurosurg.* 2010;**113**:639–47.

23. Traynor CR, Barker GJ, Crum WR, Williams SC, Richardson MP. Segmentation of the thalamus in MRI based on T1 and T2. *Neuroimage.* 2011;**56**:939–50.

24. Huston OO, Watson RE, Bernstein MA, *et al.* Intraoperative magnetic resonance imaging findings during deep brain stimulation surgery. *J Neurosurg.* 2011;**115**:852–7.

25. Petersen EA, Holl EM, Martinez-Torres I, *et al.* Minimizing brain shift in stereotactic functional neurosurgery. *Neurosurgery.* 2010;**67**:ons213–21; discussion ons221.

26. Bour LJ, Contarino MF, Foncke EM, *et al.* Long-term experience with intraoperative microrecording during DBS neurosurgery in STN and GPi. *Acta Neurochir (Wien).* 2010;**152**:2069–77.

27. Zrinzo L, Foltynie T, Limousin P, Hariz MI. Reducing hemorrhagic complications in functional neurosurgery: a large case series and systematic literature review. *J Neurosurg.* 2012; **116**:84–94.

28. Starr PA, Vitek JL, DeLong M, Bakay RA. Magnetic resonance imaging-based stereotactic localization of the globus pallidus and subthalamic nucleus. *Neurosurgery.* 1999;**44**:303–13; discussion 313–14.

29. Patel NK, Khan S, Gill SS. Comparison of atlas- and magnetic-resonance-imaging-based stereotactic targeting of the subthalamic nucleus in the surgical treatment of Parkinson's disease. *Stereotact Funct Neurosurg.* 2008;**86**:153–61.

30. Maciunas RJ, Galloway RL, Jr., Latimer JW. The application accuracy of stereotactic frames. *Neurosurgery.* 1994;**35**:682–94; discussion 694–5.

31. Holloway KL, Gaede SE, Starr PA, *et al.* Frameless stereotaxy using bone fiducial markers for deep brain stimulation. *J Neurosurg.* 2005;**103**:404–13.

32. Starr PA, Christine CW, Theodosopoulos PV, *et al.* Implantation of deep brain stimulators into the subthalamic nucleus: technical approach and magnetic resonance imaging-verified lead locations. *J Neurosurg.* 2002;**97**:370–87.

33. Starr PA, Martin AJ, Ostrem JL, *et al.* Subthalamic nucleus deep brain stimulator placement using high-field interventional magnetic resonance imaging and a skull-mounted aiming device: technique and application accuracy. *J Neurosurg.* 2010;**112**:479–90.

34. Lenglet C, Abosch A, Yacoub E, *et al.* Comprehensive in vivo mapping of the human basal ganglia and thalamic connectome in individuals using 7T MRI. *PLoS One.* 2012;**7**:e29153.

35. Duchin Y, Abosch A, Yacoub E, Sapiro G, Harel N. Feasibility of using ultra-high field (7 T) MRI for clinical surgical targeting. *PLoS One.* 2012;**7**:e37328.

36. Kerchner GA. Ultra-high field 7T MRI: a new tool for studying Alzheimer's disease. *J Alzheimer's Dis.* 2011;**26** Suppl 3:91–5.

37. Lotfipour AK, Wharton S, Schwarz ST, *et al.* High resolution magnetic susceptibility mapping of the substantia nigra in Parkinson's disease. *J Magn Reson Imaging.* 2012;**35**:48–55.

38. Metzger CD, Eckert U, Steiner J, *et al.* High field FMRI reveals thalamocortical integration of segregated cognitive and emotional processing in mediodorsal and intralaminar thalamic nuclei. *Front Neuroanat.* 2010;**4**:138.

39. Yacoub E, Harel N, Ugurbil K. High-field fMRI unveils orientation columns in humans. *Proc Natl Acad Sci U S A.* 2008;**105**:10607–12.

40. Harel N, Lin J, Moeller S, Ugurbil K, Yacoub E. Combined imaging-histological study of cortical laminar specificity of fMRI signals. *Neuroimage.* 2006;**29**:879–87.

41. Duyn JH, van Gelderen P, Li TQ, *et al.* High-field MRI of brain cortical substructure based on signal phase. *Proc Natl Acad Sci U S A.* 2007;**104**:11796–801.

42. Haddar D, Haacke E, Sehgal V, *et al.* [Susceptibility weighted imaging. Theory and applications]. *J Radiol.* 2004;**85**:1901–8.

43. Manova ES, Habib CA, Boikov AS, *et al.* Characterizing the mesencephalon using susceptibility-weighted imaging.

AJNR Am J Neuroradiol.
2009;**30**:569–74.

44. Haacke EM, Xu Y, Cheng YC,
    Reichenbach JR. Susceptibility
    weighted imaging (SWI). *Magn
    Reson Med.* 2004;**52**:612–18.

45. Yelnik J, Bardinet E, Dormont D,
    et al. A three-dimensional,
    histological and deformable atlas
    of the human basal ganglia.
    I. Atlas construction based on
    immunohistochemical and
    MRI data. *Neuroimage.*
    2007;**34**:618–38.

46. Gupte AA, Shrivastava D, Spaniol
    MA, Abosch A. MRI-related
    heating near deep brain
    stimulation electrodes: more data
    are needed. *Stereotact Funct
    Neurosurg.* 2011;**89**:131–40.

47. Rezai AR, Baker KB, Tkach JA,
    et al. Is magnetic resonance
    imaging safe for patients with
    neurostimulation systems used for
    deep brain stimulation?
    Neurosurgery. 2005;**57**:1056–62;
    discussion 1062.

48. Shrivastava D, Abosch A, Hanson T,
    et al. Effect of the extracranial
    deep brain stimulation lead on
    radiofrequency heating at
    9.4 Tesla (400.2 MHz). *J Magn
    Reson Imaging.* 2010;**32**:600–7.

49. Henderson JM, Tkach J, Phillips
    M, *et al.* Permanent neurological
    deficit related to magnetic
    resonance imaging in a patient
    with implanted deep brain
    stimulation electrodes for
    Parkinson's disease: case report.

Neurosurgery. 2005;**57**:E1063;
discussion E1063.

50. Roark C, Whicher S, Abosch A.
    Reversible neurological symptoms
    caused by diathermy in a patient
    with deep brain stimulators: case
    report. *Neurosurgery.* 2008;**62**:
    E256; discussion E256.

51. Chhabra V, Sung E, Mewes K,
    et al. Safety of magnetic resonance
    imaging of deep brain stimulator
    systems: a serial imaging and
    clinical retrospective study.
    J Neurosurg. 2010;**112**:497–502.

52. Larson PS, Richardson RM,
    Starr PA, Martin AJ. Magnetic
    resonance imaging of implanted
    deep brain stimulators: experience
    in a large series. *Stereotact Funct
    Neurosurg.* 2008;**86**:92–100.

Chapter 9

Magnetic resonance imaging and spectroscopy in Huntington's disease

Isabelle Iltis and Janet Dubinsky

Introduction

Huntington's disease (HD) is a hereditary neurodegenerative disorder that manifests with motor control, cognitive, and psychiatric symptoms. HD is caused by an expansion of CAG repeats in the huntingtin gene, leading to an abnormally long polyglutamine stretch in the N-terminal tail of the protein that interferes with its normal function, and causes the accumulation of the mutated protein [1–3]. Normal huntingtin is a large protein (350 kDa) whose structure favors protein–protein interaction, and is more specifically involved with shuttling stress-induced signal proteins from the endoplasmic reticulum in and out of the nucleus [4], and with microtubule-associated axonal vesicular and mitochondrial trafficking, thereby facilitating neurotransmission [5–10]. Both loss of its normal function and the accumulation of the abnormal protein affect neuronal function by altering cell signaling, axonal transport, mitochondrial metabolism, and neurotransmission. Histologically, the GABAergic medium spiny neurons of the striatum, projecting to the globus pallidus and the substantia nigra, are largely affected in HD. This is manifested in the brain of patients by striatal (caudate and putamenal) atrophy and consequent malfunctioning of the long loop feedback pathways involving this region. More subtle, widespread cortical defects have also recently been identified in patients at an early stage, which increase over time [11]. Reactive microglia along with activated astrocytes and oligodendrocytes are also associated with HD pathology in the striatum and cortex [3, 12–14]. Altered energy production and utilization, identified in the muscles of patients, also affect the striatal neurons, which are more sensitive to mitochondrial defects [10, 15, 16].

Because HD is an autosomal dominant transmitted disorder for which the culprit gene is identified, diagnosis is often made by genetic testing. As such, magnetic resonance (MR) techniques rarely have a significant role in clinical diagnosis. However, because MR provides a non-invasive approach, the processes involved in HD pathogenesis (structural changes of the brain, neuronal death, gliosis, energy production and utilization deficits), it is an attractive and promising tool for clinical and fundamental research. In this chapter, we will focus on the main findings and advances brought by magnetic resonance imaging (MRI) and magnetic resonance spectroscopy (MRS) to the understanding of prodromal and early-stage patients. We will also review new approaches used in animal models that will hopefully be translated in clinical studies in the near future.

Role of MR in research and multicentric studies

In HD, as in many neurodegenerative disorders, accurate markers of disease progression that reflect pathogenic mechanisms are currently lacking, and therefore are an important focus of current research. Although no cure is available at this time, development of treatments or cures is governed by the availability of reliable, sensitive biomarkers that can accurately measure treatment efficacy in the smallest number of patients possible. MR techniques are a particularly promising tool in the identification of such biomarkers.

In uncommon neurodegenerative disorders such as HD, natural history studies and clinical trials within one institution are difficult because of the small numbers of patients available to participate

Control (60 yo)   Huntington (57 yo)

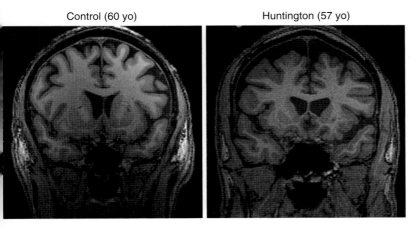

Figure 9.1 Coronal MP-RAGE (T_1-weighted) images from a 60-year-old (60 yo) healthy control and a 57-year-old (57 yo) patient with early-stage Huntington disease (stage I). The enlargement of the ventricles, the decrease in the overall brain volume, and the atrophy of the striatal structures are clearly visible on this coronal view of the brain.

within one location. Multicenter investigations are therefore required. In the effort to discover biomarkers, two major international studies were conducted: PREDICT-HD (for "neurobiological predictors of Huntington disease onset") and TRACK-HD (a multicenter, multinational prospective, observational biomarker study of premanifest and early-stage HD with no experimental treatment). Started in 2001 and still ongoing, PREDICT-HD is a longitudinal study following persons who have undergone a predictive genetic testing for the number of CAG repeats [17]. The goal of this study is to identify measurable changes years before diagnosis. TRACK-HD is a similar study (longitudinal observation of persons knowing their genetic status prior to disease onset), but designed as a potential clinical trial: volunteers are examined every year for 3 years, looking at annual measurable changes. Together, these studies have shed some light on the pathogenesis of HD [18–22]. These studies which are international multicentric in nature have employed MRI systems (including higher field 3T platforms) which are available in most hospitals and universities. Such studies, though, require coordination and calibration of the methods employed for the data to be comparable across institutions.

Main MRI findings

When examining MR data obtained in patient studies, notable and important discrepancies are seen. A large part of this heterogeneity is attributable to two factors: (1) distinctions were not always made between "prodromal," "early" stage, or later stages, in earlier studies;

and (2) the definition of the "prodromal" stage itself varies between researchers. The term "prodromal" usually defines the stage before the appearance of at least one permanent neurological dysfunction (usually, a motor symptom) needed for formal diagnosis. Even when patients are not formally diagnosed and therefore still considered in the prodromal stage, subtle alterations of the motor, cognitive, and mood performance are detectable, as recently demonstrated in the PREDICT-HD study where subjects were followed 8 years after enrollment [19]. Meanwhile, progressive atrophy has been shown during this "prodromal" phase [23]. Since subtle motor dysfunctions can be present in a prodromal patient, volunteers recruited in the prodromal phase probably are clinically heterogeneous, thereby complicating the interpretation of study results.

Volumetric analysis

Examination of anatomical brain images from patients with early-stage HD reveals a decrease in both striatal and overall volume compared to controls, as expected from the pathological hallmarks of HD (Figure 9.1) [24]. To evaluate when these changes in brain anatomy occur and to quantify their extent, three different strategies have been employed in HD: (1) measurement (or "segmentation") of the whole brain volume (Figure 9.2A) and distinct brain structures such as the caudate and putamen; (2) measurement of the cortical thickness (Figures 9.2C and 9.3) [20, 22, 25]; and (3) a voxel-based morphometry (VBM) approach, which permits additional estimation of cerebrospinal fluid (CSF), gray and white matter volumes compared to a control "template" of

107

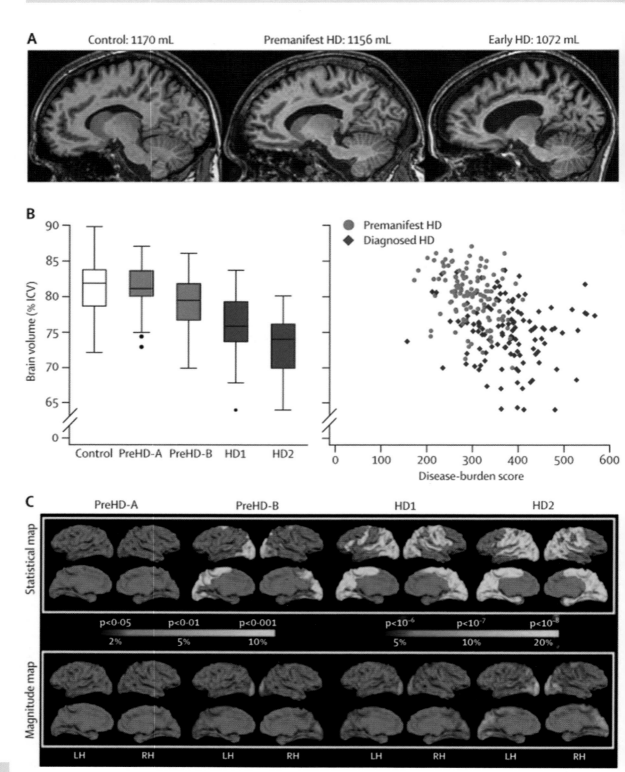

Figure 9.2 Whole brain and regional atrophy in the controls, premanifest, and early Huntington's disease groups. (A) 3T volumetric MRI scan in a 50-year-old control, a 55-year-old individual with preHD, and a 49-year-old with early Huntington's disease. Brain volumes

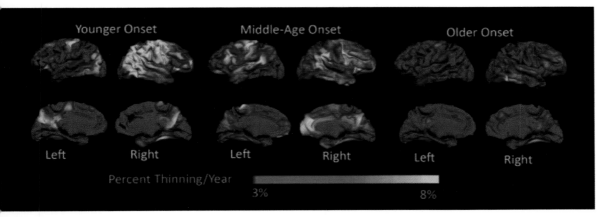

Figure 9.3 Surface-based maps of the rate of cortical thinning: young, middle aged, old. Younger patients had a much more rapid rate of thinning, especially in the sensorimotor and parietal cortical regions. The general distribution of thinning was similar, however, in the young and middle-aged groups. In older patients, the rate of thinning was much slower than either of the other groups. Maps are presented on a semi-inflated cortical surface of an average brain. The color scale at the bottom represents the yearly rate of thinning, transitioning from red (3% or greater) to yellow (8% or greater). (From Rosas *et al.*, *Mov Disord.* 2011 [25].)

the brain (by averaging anatomical images over control subjects after corrections for differences in shapes and size) (Figure 9.4) [26]. VBM is a voxel-wise statistical comparison of anatomical images between controls and patients, and as such requires extensive computational capability. The brain template must be carefully prepared specifically for each study (matching for gender and age), and a rigorous consistency in acquisition sequences, input parameters of the processing software, and statistical analysis is required, as the apparent results are highly dependent on the input parameters and statistical analysis, potentially biasing results [27–29]. The main advantages of VBM are that it is a semi-automated method (free software packages, such as FSL, http://www.fmrib.ox.ac.uk/fsl/, are available for the processing of such data) and that it can be applied to the whole brain.

Volumetric methods showed striatal atrophy which also correlated with the number of CAG repeats, disease severity, motor symptoms, and total functional capacity score [23, 30–35]. Importantly, the volumes of the caudate and putamen were decreased up to 15 years before diagnosis [36]. The rate of cortical thinning is also faster in earlier onset patients (Figure 9.3) [11, 25]. VBM analysis of early-stage and prodromal patients reveals that the atrophy of striatal gray and white matter starts in the caudate 8–10 years before predicted onset, propagates to the putamen, and finally extends to the cortical layers 1–2 years before predicted onset of symptoms (Figure 9.4) [21, 34]. Thalamic atrophy has also been observed in the prodromal period [36]. In clinically diagnosed patients who are in early stages of disease, gray matter atrophy is seen in other regions such as the globus pallidus, hippocampus, amygdala, and cerebellum, and the rate of atrophy is faster in patients with larger CAG repeats [35].

In conclusion, these anatomical measurements provided insights into the natural course of the disease in patients before and after onset of symptoms. However, when examined in large cohorts they also proved not to be sensitive enough to be used as biomarkers (note the large error bars in Figure 9.2B) [18, 21, 37]. However, more subtle functional and biochemical changes may precede the gross structural alteration that volumetric analyses measure. MR methodologies assessing such physiological characteristics have been used with the hope of unveiling additional functional biomarkers.

Caption for Figure 9.2 (*cont.*) are corrected for intracranial volume. (B) Brain volume as a percentage of intracranial volume across all groups (horizontal lines are median; boxes are upper and lower quartiles; bars are range; dots are outliers) and scatter plot of brain volume as a percentage of intracranial volume against disease burden. (C) Cortical thinning in the Huntington's disease groups compared with controls. The top panel shows statistical maps corrected with the false discovery rate; magnitude maps are shown below. All results are adjusted for age and sex. ICV = intracranial volume. LH = left hemisphere. RH = right hemisphere. (From Tabrizi *et al.*, *Lancet Neurol.* 2009 [20].)

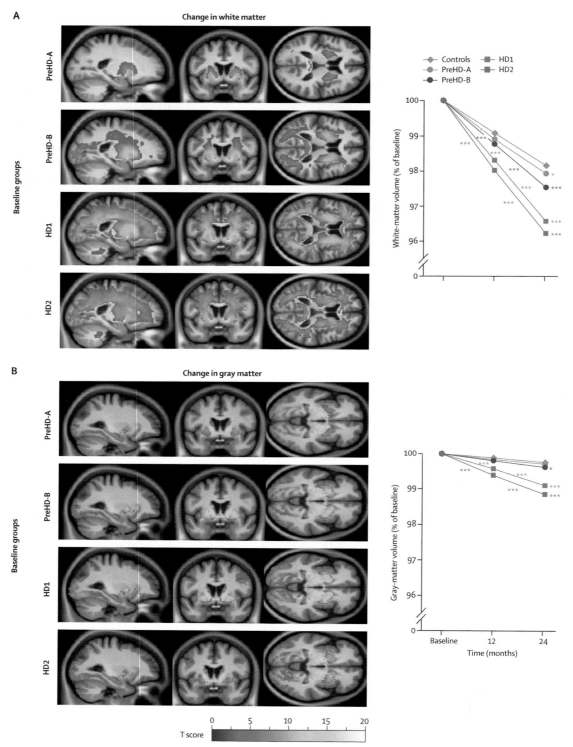

Figure 9.4 Longitudinal changes in gray and white matter. Parametric maps showing regions with statistically significant atrophy in (A) white matter and (B) gray matter over 24 months, relative to controls. Results were adjusted for age, sex, study site, and scan interval and are corrected for multiple comparisons with family-wise error at the p < 0.05 level. Corresponding longitudinal plots show mean values at baseline, 12 months, and 24 months. Significant change differences relative to controls over 0–12, 12–24, and 0–24 months are represented by *p < 0.05, **p < 0.01, and ***p < 0.001. (From Tabrizi *et al.*, *Lancet Neurol.* 2012 [21].)

Diffusion imaging

Diffusion-weighted imaging (DWI) measures the diffusivity and directionality of water molecules, by observing the water signal decaying along a field gradient (the higher the diffusion, the more the signal loss) [38, 39]. Diffusion of water depends on its physical location: water constrained in axonal fibers diffuses in a restricted, directional manner along these structures, whereas water from CSF and extracellular spaces diffuses more freely. Diffusion imaging therefore measures the disorganization of fibers, cell swelling, edema, as well as axonal and/or myelin loss (although the method still does not permit distinguishing between these two features, extensive work is ongoing to differentiate between both processes). With DWI, "apparent diffusion coefficients" (ADCs) for each pixel of the image can be derived from the MR acquisition. Alterations in ADCs (or diffusivity) can reflect a number of physiological events, among them neuronal fiber density, orientation changes, and the loss of membrane integrity. Fractional anisotropy (FA), another parameter that can be derived from diffusion images, is the ratio between the longitudinal and the radial diffusivity, hence the coherence of the axonal and myelin fibers. A loss in local axonal fiber organization translates as a lower FA value, but it does not provide information on the directionality of the fibers, nor on demyelination versus axonal loss. To estimate the directionality of the fibers, mathematical operators called "tensors" can be applied to the diffusivity (or ADC) maps. Using this technique (called diffusion tensor imaging or DTI) the most probable fiber trajectory between two predefined brain regions (or "seeds") can be estimated [38–40]. Diffusion imaging therefore provides insights into the microstructure of the brain, and how brain structures are connected to each other.

In HD, few studies have been conducted using diffusion imaging. In both prodromal and early-stage patients, increased diffusivity has been consistently found in the caudate, putamen, and overall brain compared to controls [41–44]. Interestingly, FA is also decreased in the putamen, but not the caudate, of both prodromal and early-stage patients [43]. Although not fully understood, both these results are potentially related to the microglial activation, axonal membrane degeneration, early gliotic processes, disruption in axonal transport, and loss in fiber organization (more importantly in the putamen)

reported in HD [13]. White matter also exhibits a decrease in FA in both prodromal and early-stage patients observed longitudinally, suggesting demyelination and/or axonal loss and providing evidence for white matter involvement in the pathogenesis of HD [45, 46]. In addition, the FA decrease and diffusivity increase in the occipital, frontal, parietal, and temporal white matter of symptomatic patients are correlated with clinical measures of disease severity [45]. Since both diffusivity and FA correlate with measures of disease progression, both could represent valid biomarkers of the disease [42, 43, 45].

Perfusion and functional MRI

Using MRI, cerebral blood flow (CBF) or perfusion can be quantitatively measured using a technique named arterial spin labeling (ASL). The principle of measuring perfusion with ASL is based on manipulating the magnetization of water protons so that the water signal becomes an endogenous contrast agent [47]. Using this technique, maps of CBF can be obtained, and perfusion can be measured both at rest and also during brain activity (i.e., with functional MRI or fMRI). Thus ASL permits measurement of the change in blood flow related to the activity of the brain [47, 48]. For measuring brain activity, another technique can be used, namely blood oxygen level-dependent (BOLD) imaging [49]. BOLD contrast is indirectly related to blood flow, as it relies on the difference in contrast between oxygenated and deoxygenated hemoglobin. Deoxygenated hemoglobin is paramagnetic while oxygenated hemoglobin is diamagnetic, or virtually non-magnetic.

Only one study reports data on absolute resting CBF in early-stage patients, showing that cortical and striatal regions are lower in early HD, although this decrease is not correlated with the degree of atrophy of these regions (Figure 9.5) [50]. In fMRI, different stimulation or "activation paradigms" are used, designed to elicit activity in specific regions of the brain. Tasks eliciting striatal activity result in a decrease in the striatal ASL signal in symptomatic patients [51, 52] and, more interestingly, in presymptomatic patients as well (Figure 9.6) [53–55]. In cortical regions, early-stage patients exhibit lower neuronal activation (as detected by the change in blood flow), whereas in prodromal patients, the activation is higher in these same regions, possibly due to compensatory recruitment to maintain normal

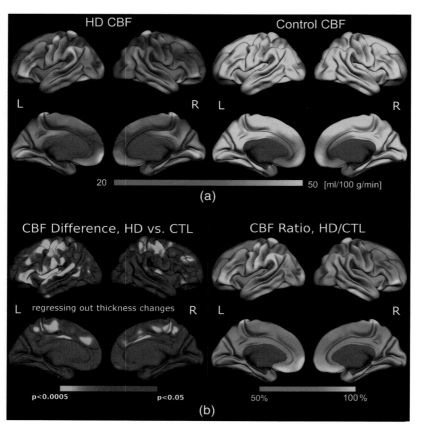

Figure 9.5 Cortical mapping of quantitative CBF for early HD patients an controls. (a) CBF in HD subjects (left) wa on the average of 48.4±12.5 ml/100 g/mi over the entire cortex, markedly lower than CBF in controls (right), averaging 62.9±9.7 ml/100 g/min. (b) Left: CBF wa significantly reduced in the HD group (shown in blue) relative to the control population (adjusted for multiple comparisons). CBF was primarily compromised in the superior frontal, insular, lateral occipital and posterior cingulate regions, with the inferior temporal and medial occipital cortical regions comparatively "spared." Right: Ratio between the mean CBF in the HD and control groups, showing regional CBF to be reduced by as much as 50% i the HD group. (From Chen *et al.*, *Neuroimage* 2012 [50].)

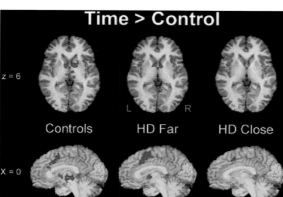

Figure 9.6 Activation foci (p < .01) derived from the T-minus-C comparison for the control, far, and close groups. *Top row*, Axial sections are 6 mm superior to the anterior commissure–posterior commissure line. *Bottom row*, Sections represent the midsagittal plane. From Paulsen *et al.*, *AJNR Am J Neuroradiol.* 2004 [53].)

performance [56]. Using a working memory task, Wolf *et al.* [57] observed a decrease in the left dorsolateral prefrontal cortex in presymptomatic patients compared to controls. However, this initial decrease did not worsen over time when the patients were reexamined after 2 years, indicating that there may not be a worsening of the prefrontal cortex activity over time. Therefore, the prefrontal cortex activation elicited with this task does not seem to be a useful measure to track the disease. In prodroma and early-stage HD, only one publication reports results in patients using BOLD fMRI [58]. The authors focused on eye movements as an activation task of subjects; utilizing that clinical feature that saccadic eye movements deteriorate in HD and therefore may represent a means to monitor disease progression. They observed a decrease in the BOLD signal of the presupplementary motor area and dorsal anterior cingulate cortex in patients in early stage, while the signal between prodromal and control subjects was comparable. Cross-sectional and prospective fMRI studies using different tasks which activate other brain regions, for example the striatum, have not yet been performed, and therefore this remains an untapped area of inquiry in biomarker development.

Magnetic resonance spectroscopy (MRS) in Huntington's disease

MRS is a technique that permits the measurement of the absolute concentration of small metabolically relevant molecules in the region observed (see Chapter 15 for more details on MRS principles). MR-observable atoms (such as ^1H) have frequencies dependent on their neighboring atoms, and the signal intensity of each frequency is directly proportional to its concentration in vivo. MRS is a particularly attractive tool to identify biochemical changes which are expected to precede neuronal loss and accompanying atrophy that is present at the time of diagnosis [59].

An advantage of MRS (as opposed to structural imaging) is that it is less dependent on data processing strategies than methods requiring extensive computation or model-based interpretation, such as VBM or DTI. It is important to note, however, that the spectral quality is of major importance in MRS for the accurate analysis of the data obtained. Several atomic nuclei with biological relevance can be observed using MRS techniques; in particular proton (^1H), carbon 13 (^{13}C), phosphorus 31 (^{31}P), and oxygen 17 (^{17}O). Because of its natural presence and abundance in the body, the most popular and least technically challenging nucleus observable in MRS is ^1H (^1H MRS). Several studies have been conducted using ^1H MRS in HD.

Quality of the ^1H MR spectrum and quantification of the metabolites

MRI is based on the detection of the proton signal within water molecules. In ^1H MRS, we observe protons that are attached to other biochemically relevant molecules present in the brain. To accomplish this, the overwhelmingly large water signal is suppressed by manipulating its frequency. In ^1H MRS the concentration of numerous neurochemicals relevant to the cellular function of both neurons and astrocytes can be detected: glutamate and glutamine (Glu and Gln, a major excitatory neurotransmitter and its metabolite), N-acetylaspartate and N-acetylaspartyl glutamate (NAA and NAAG, together also referred to as NAA + NAAG or tNAA, total NAA, markers of neurons, with NAAG likely participating in neurotransmission [60]), creatine and phosphocreatine (Cr and PCr, or tCr for total PCr + Cr content, reflecting energy metabolism), choline compounds (Cho, involved in the integrity and quantity of cellular membranes), γ-aminobutyric acid (GABA, a major inhibitory neurotransmitter), antioxidants (glutathione and ascorbate) and *myo*-inositol (*myo*-Ins or Ins, a marker of astrocytes), to name a few. These molecules can be detected on the same spectrum (Figure 9.7, top spectrum), where each peak corresponds to the spectral pattern of a specific metabolite, with the area under the peak being directly proportional to the concentration of the metabolite in the voxel. Therefore, quantitative information on the metabolism and functional integrity of the cells can be obtained within a same region of interest or voxel.

The quality of the spectrum determines the quality and reliability of the concentration measurement [61]. Spectral quality depends on a number of methodological considerations. First, for optimal data acquisition, higher-order shimming methods and efficient water suppression are necessary to achieve a high signal-to-noise ratio. Individual spectra should be acquired every 4–5 seconds, which permits corrections for phase and frequency and exclusion of spectra affected by motion. To increase the signal-to-noise ratio, the multiple spectra (usually 64 to 128) are then summed to obtain the final spectrum. Corrections for eddy currents, specific to each scanner and hardware, should be applied at that stage. In addition, using higher field strengths improves the quantification because frequencies of more metabolites are more accurately distinguished. If the original spectral quality is poor, the resulting concentrations may be inaccurate.

The quantification method must also be considered when evaluating experimental conclusions. Most studies rely on metabolite ratios, that is, normalizing concentrations of reported metabolites to the concentration of one metabolite, usually creatine, and assume no change in this reference between patients and controls. As such, any change in creatine between patients and controls will be masked, and apparent concentrations of other metabolites will be biased. A widely used quantification software named LCModel (for "linear combination of metabolite models") normalizes the concentrations to the water signal from the same voxel, thereby avoiding such bias [62]. LCModel requires the a-priori knowledge of the individual spectra of metabolites, or "models," constituting a basis set. This basis set must be accurate for the proper fitting of the experimental data.

113

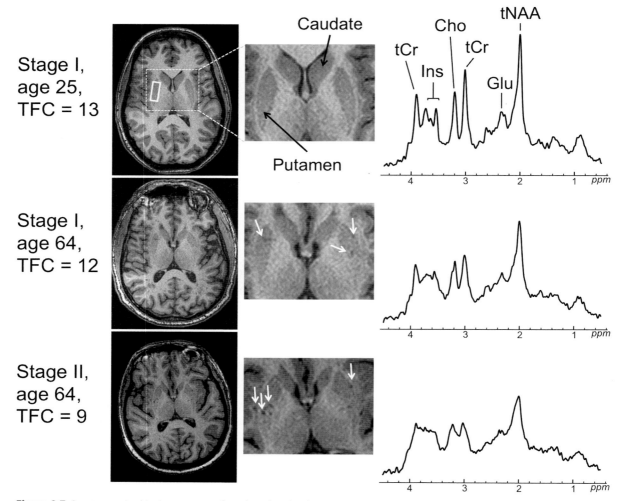

Figure 9.7 Spectra acquired in the putamen of prodromal and early-stage patients with HD. The images are axial views of the brain, and the enlargement shows the region containing the basal ganglia (caudate and putamen). The box illustrates the location of the voxel in which the spectra were acquired (stimulated echo acquisition mode [STEAM] sequence, echo time [TE] = 8 ms, transverse magnetization [TM] = 32 ms, repetition time [TR] = 4 s, voxel size = 4.1 ml). The white arrows indicate the location of microvessels, which are not detected in the prodromal patient. TFC, total functional score; tNAA, N-acetylaspartate; Glu, glutamate; Cho, choline compounds; tCr, creatine + phosphocreatine; Ins, myo-inositol.

In addition to methodological issues, the quality of a spectrum is also affected by the characteristics of the disease. In the specific case of patients with HD, movements can affect data quality. To minimize these effects, padding can be used on the side of the head, and as mentioned above, individual scans affected by a sudden movement can be discarded from the final spectrum. It is also expected that MR-compatible motion tracking devices will also be useful to correct for motion during the acquisition. Even in the absence of movements, we have also observed a broadening of the peaks as the patients show more severe symptoms of the disease (Figure 9.7). Although the causes of this increase are not fully understood, we have observed that patients at more advanced stages tend to present larger and more numerous microvessels inside the putamen (Figure 9.7). These vessels create inhomogeneity inside the structure, resulting in less resolved peaks, and affecting the overall quality of the data. This issue seems not specific to HD but to neurodegenerative disorders, as a similar broadening has also been observed in patients with Parkinson's disease (cf. Chapter 15 and [63]). In contrast, in the putamen of a prodromal patient with HD

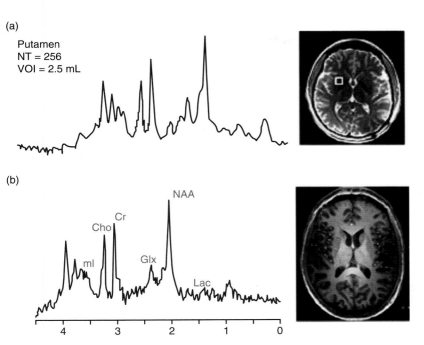

(a)

Putamen
NT = 256
VOI = 2.5 mL

(b)

NAA

Cr
Cho

ml   Glx

Lac

4   3   2   1   0

Figure 9.8 Comparison of the quality obtained in the putamen of control subjects at 7T between two studies. (A) ^{1}H MR spectrum obtained with the stimulated echo acquisition mode (STEAM) (TR = 5 s; TE = 8 ms; mixing time, 32 ms) from the putamen (voxel size = 2.5 ml). NT, number of transients. (From Emir et al., *NMR Biomed*. [68]). (B) Spectrum obtained in the same region of interest (voxel size up to 3.4 ml) with the STEAM sequence (TR = 2 s, TE = 19 ms, TM = 25 ms) (From van den Bogaard et al., *J Neurol*. 2011 [67]). The positions of the voxels (VOIs) are shown in the images. The bottom spectrum has visibly a lower signal-to-noise ratio, and the peaks are less resolved. Such differences in spectral quality can affect the accuracy of the quantification. Lac, lactate; NAA, *N*-acetylaspartate; Glx, glutamate + glutamine; Cr, creatine + phosphocreatine; Cho, choline compounds; ml, *myo*-inositol.

(unaffected by microvessel proliferation), a good quality spectrum was acquired (Figure 9.7). Peaks from metabolites are clearly distinguished and the baseline is "flat," meaning that proper water suppression and eddy currents compensation have been used. On such a spectrum, the quantification is reliable. Acquisition methods for MRS have been extensively described [64].

^{1}H MRS in Huntington's disease

HD results in the MRS literature should be carefully reviewed as the findings vary depending on the field strength used and the methodological pitfalls mentioned above. Also, the heterogeneity of the premanifest and manifest groups among studies contributes to a lack of consistency between different reports.

For example, Sanchez-Pernaute et al. [65] reported data at 1.5T, and could only detect three metabolites. At 7T, a field strength still restricted to research but permitting a greater number of detectable metabolites, Unschuld et al. recently measured accurately 11 metabolites in the posterior cingulate cortex in 12 early-stage and prodromal patients [66]. van den Bogaard et al. [67] also report data at 7T on six metabolites in prodromal and early-stage patients. However, in this study, the data quality is not consistent with previous reports at the same field

strength where 11–14 metabolites were distinguished (Figure 9.8) [63, 66, 68]. Moreover, the cohorts observed in these studies were rather small (between 12 and 14 volunteers in the patient groups), which restricts the statistical power of the analysis. Sturrock et al. [69] benefited from a larger cohort which was one of the TRACK-HD study sites (n = 25 and 30 for premanifest and manifest groups, respectively), but used a 3T system. While 3T systems are increasingly available in clinical centers and hospitals, opening the prospect of a multicenter clinical study, 7T systems benefit from a higher signal-to-noise ratio and increased precision to detect and quantify more metabolites when methodologically optimized [70].

Despite the technological shortcomings in these studies, the consistent observation among them is a decrease in putaminal tNAA in symptomatic, early-stage patients [67, 69, 71]. A decrease in tNAA in the posterior cingulate cortex, along with a decrease in glutamate, has also been reported [66]. In addition, in the putamen [65, 67, 69] and the caudate [65, 67], but not in the posterior cingulate cortex, tCr decreases in early-stage patients, indicating an impairment of energy metabolism in these structures. The decrease in tNAA correlates with clinical measures of disease severity across early-stage and prodromal patients [67, 69], and with the Montreal Cognitive Assessment

115

scale (MOCA, designed to detect mild cognitive impairment) in the posterior cingulate cortex of prodromal and early-stage patients [66]. In one study, tCr correlated with disease severity in manifest patients [67]. In the posterior cingulate cortex, glutamate concentration also correlates with cognitive impairment [66]. Glutamate also may be decreased in the putamen, although no correlation with clinical measures has been found [67, 69]. myo-Ins, indicative of gliosis, increases in symptomatic patients as well [69]. Rather disappointingly, no change in metabolite concentration has been consistently observed in the basal ganglia of presymptomatic patients [67, 69].

Overall, the information from ^{1}H MRS in patient studies is still scarce, and the cited studies attempted to capture the necessary spectra under the constraints of a clinical study and with suboptimal technical conditions. However, in animals, high quality ^{1}H MRS has proven a suitable method for identifying candidate biomarkers [72–74]. A significant effort is underway to optimize consistency among MRS software and sequences tailored for achieving high quality scans across centers and institutions (discussed during the International Society for Magnetic Resonance in Medicine 2012 meeting), along with the sharing of state-of-the-art acquisition techniques across institutions. With this and the slowly increasing availability of 7T systems, a more detailed analysis of a greater number of metabolites may be achieved, bringing the promise of pathologically based, quantitative biomarkers to HD diagnosis and progression, as already demonstrated in animal studies.

^{1}H MRS in animal models of HD

Technically precise ^{1}H MRS studies in rodent models of HD at high field strength have yielded information on up to 17 metabolites [72–74]. Studies in animal models of HD are critical for obtaining an understanding of the pathogenesis and pathophysiology, but also for preclinical testing of potential therapies. The first step for such testing is the characterization of the animal models and the evaluation of markers comparable across species, that is, between human and rodents. Initial cross-sectional studies of mouse models with advanced disease stages reported decreased tNAA, as shown in patients with HD [67, 69, 71, 75]. Recently, we have also shown that an early decrease in tNAA is detectable in the R6/2 transgenic mouse model as early as 4 weeks of age in the cortex and 8 weeks in the striatum, prior to

motor deficits, and that tNAA concentration steadily decreases up until 12 weeks of age [72, 74]. Increases in both striatal and cortical myo-Ins are also observed in 8-week-old mice; similar to findings in patients. Creatine increases in these mice, which has not been shown in patients to date. Thus, studies of additional patients are warranted to confirm this result. Remarkably, Zacharoff et al. demonstrated using sophisticated statistical methods that not a single metabolite but a group of them pooled together form excellent predictors of the disease, and as such are good candidate biomarkers [74]. Likewise, using a multimodality MRI approach combining data from various imaging methods such as MRS, DTI, etc. may have the potential to provide sensitive and accurate measures of disease progression.

^{31}P MRS

^{31}P MRS measures concentrations of phosphorylated metabolites such as PCr, ATP, and inorganic phosphate (P_i), which are important in energy metabolism (Figure 9.9). Given the negative energy balance present in early-stage and manifest HD and documented in muscle studies [76–78], ^{31}P has the potential to contribute to our understanding of altered energetics in HD. ^{31}P MRS also permits measurement of intracellular pH, using the relative chemical shift difference (i.e., the distance between the frequencies of two peaks) between PCr and P_i [79]. Although still restricted to research magnets equipped with specific hardware, there are some encouraging studies from animal models of HD and HD patients [80–82]. Because of the challenging aspects of these techniques, however, the region of the human brain evaluated has been limited to the visual cortex. At rest, no change in the concentration of PCr, ATP, or P_i was observed between patients and controls [83]. However, Mochel et al. showed that when early-stage patients receive visual stimulation, P_i/PCr did not increase as it did in the control cohort, suggesting a defect in energy metabolism in these patients. Additionally, the P_i/PCr ratio was found to correlate to disease severity assessed by the Unified Huntington Disease Rating Scale (UHDRS) in patients [81]. These findings show that brain energy metabolism is impaired in early-stage patients, which may represent a new functional measure of HD that could prove useful in monitoring treatments and disease progression (Figure 9.9). Longitudinal studies in presymptomatic and symptomatic patients will help determine the utility of the P_i/PCr ratio in HD research.

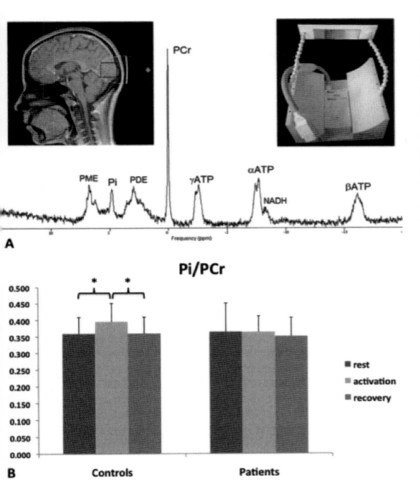

A

B

Pi/PCr

■ rest
■ activation
■ recovery

Figure 9.9 Representative ^{31}P-NMR spectrum from the occipital cortex of a control subject at 3T (pulse-acquire, 240 repetitions, TR = 2 s, 8 minutes total acquisition time). (A) A 2-Hz Lorentzian line broadening was applied. In addition, a ^{1}H image shows the position of the sphere used for reference at the center of the ^{31}P surface coil, aligned with the visual cortex (upper left). The surface coil is drawn on the image to show the size and position of the coil relative to the head. The dashed white line indicates the sensitive volume of the coil encompassing most of the visual cortex. The square on the ^{1}H image shows the region used for localized ^{1}H shimming. A picture of the ^{31}P coil also shows how the ^{31}P coil could slide inside the holder for precise position adjustment (upper right). (B) Pi/PCr ratio before, during, and after visual stimulation in 15 early HD patients and 15 age- and gender-matched controls. In controls, the Friedman test was significant for Pi/PCr (p = .006), and the Bonferroni-corrected Wilcoxon signed-rank test indicated increased Pi/PCr between rest and activation (p = .024) followed by a decrease between activation and recovery (p = .012). These changes were absent in HD patients; *p < .05. From Mochel *et al.*, *Mov Disord.* 2012 [81].

Interestingly, both in manifest patients and in the 3-nitropropionic acid (3-NP) rat model, intracellular pH is higher in the brain (likely from neuronal dysfunction or loss) [80]. Furthermore, in the rats, the authors detected a change in intracellular pH before the striatal degeneration. Although the origin of the change in intracellular pH is not yet understood, it provides insights into cellular dysfunction in HD.

Conclusion

Because of the multimodality and the non-invasiveness of MR methods, MRI and MRS have brought insights about pathogenic factors of HD. While MR techniques have a limited impact in diagnosis, they may prove useful in tracking disease progression and treatment responses in clinical trials. Structural imaging with cortical and striatal volume measurements have shown early and progressive atrophy in HD, even prior to clinical diagnosis; but these techniques do not provide insights into the pathogenic mechanisms of disease. Meanwhile, imaging modalities such as diffusion, perfusion, and fMRI offer insights into the microstructure of the brain and its function in HD pathology, but are not yet proven sensitive enough to be useful in clinical trials [19, 21]. Because of its ability to demonstrate aspects related to cellular function, MRS may offer insights into pathogenic mechanisms of disease; which may precede or coincide with volumetric changes. Nonetheless, prospective multicenter patient studies will be needed to determine the validity of these various methods. In addition to human studies, validation of MR techniques in rodent models of HD will facilitate comparisons and smoother translation of these methods in order to guide their use in human clinical trials.

References

1. DiFiglia M, Sapp E, Chase KO, *et al*. Aggregation of huntingtin in neuronal intranuclear inclusions and dystrophic neurites in brain. *Science*. 1997;**277**(5334):1990–3.

2. Hatters DM. Protein misfolding inside cells: the case of huntingtin and Huntington's disease. *IUBMB Life*. 2008;**60**(11):724–8.

3. Schulte J, Littleton JT. The biological function of the Huntingtin protein and its relevance to Huntington's Disease pathology. *Curr Trends Neurol*. 2011;**5**:65–78.

4. Atwal RS, Xia J, Pinchev D, *et al*. Huntingtin has a membrane association signal that can modulate huntingtin aggregation, nuclear entry and toxicity. *Hum Mol Genet*. 2007;**16**(21):2600–15.

5. Stefani IC, Wright D, Polizzi KM, Kontoravdi C. The role of ER stress-induced apoptosis in neurodegeneration. *Curr Alzheimer Res*. 2012;**9**(3):373–87.

6. Vidal R, Caballero B, Couve A, Hetz C. Converging pathways in the occurrence of endoplasmic reticulum (ER) stress in Huntington's disease. *Curr Mol Med*. 2011;**11**(1):1–12.

7. Correia SC, Santos RX, Perry G, *et al*. Mitochondrial importance in Alzheimer's, Huntington's and Parkinson's diseases. *Adv Exp Med Biol*. 2012;**724**:205–21.

8. Block-Galarza J, Chase KO, Sapp E, *et al*. Fast transport and retrograde movement of huntingtin and HAP 1 in axons. *Neuroreport*. 1997;**8**(9–10):2247–51.

9. Bossy-Wetzel E, Petrilli A, Knott AB. Mutant huntingtin and mitochondrial dysfunction. *Trends Neurosci*. 2008;**31**(12):609–16.

10. Oliveira JM. Nature and cause of mitochondrial dysfunction in Huntington's disease: focusing on huntingtin and the striatum. *J Neurochem*. 2010;**114**(1):1–12.

11. Rosas HD, Liu AK, Hersch S, *et al*. Regional and progressive thinning of the cortical ribbon in Huntington's disease. *Neurology*. 2002;**58**(5):695–701.

12. Myers RH, Vonsattel JP, Paskevich PA, *et al*. Decreased neuronal and increased oligodendroglial densities in Huntington's disease caudate nucleus. *J Neuropathol Exp Neurol*. 1991;**50**(6):729–42.

13. Sapp E, Kegel KB, Aronin N, *et al*. Early and progressive accumulation of reactive microglia in the Huntington disease brain. *J Neuropathol Exp Neurol*. 2001;**60**(2):161–72.

14. Vonsattel JP, Myers RH, Stevens TJ, *et al*. Neuropathological classification of Huntington's disease. *J Neuropathol Exp Neurol*. 1985;**44**(6):559–77.

15. Oliveira JM. Mitochondrial bioenergetics and dynamics in Huntington's disease: tripartite synapses and selective striatal degeneration. *J Bioenerg Biomembr*. 2010;**42**(3):227–34.

16. Reis SA, Thompson MN, Lee JM, *et al*. Striatal neurons expressing full-length mutant huntingtin exhibit decreased N-cadherin and altered neuritogenesis. *Hum Mol Genet*. 2011;**20**(12):2344–55.

17. Paulsen JS, Hayden M, Stout JC, *et al*. Preparing for preventive clinical trials: the Predict-HD study. *Arch Neurol*. 2006;**63**(6):883–90.

18. Paulsen JS, Nopoulos PC, Aylward E, *et al*. Striatal and white matter predictors of estimated diagnosis for Huntington disease. *Brain Res Bull*. 2010;**82**(3–4):201–7.

19. Paulsen JS, Wang C, Duff K, *et al*. Challenges assessing clinical endpoints in early Huntington disease. *Mov Disord*. 2010;**25**(15):2595–603.

20. Tabrizi SJ, Langbehn DR, Leavitt BR, *et al*. Biological and clinical manifestations of Huntington's disease in the longitudinal TRACK-HD study: cross-sectional analysis of baseline data. *Lancet Neurol*. 2009;**8**(9):791–801.

21. Tabrizi SJ, Reilmann R, Roos RA, *et al*. Potential endpoints for clinical trials in premanifest and early Huntington's disease in the TRACK-HD study: analysis of 24 month observational data. *Lancet Neurol*. 2012;**11**(1):42–53.

22. Tabrizi SJ, Scahill RI, Durr A, *et al*. Biological and clinical changes in premanifest and early stage Huntington's disease in the TRACK-HD study: the 12-month longitudinal analysis. *Lancet Neurol*. 2011;**10**(1):31–42.

23. Aylward E, Mills J, Liu D, *et al*. Association between age and striatal volume stratified by CAG repeat length in prodromal Huntington disease. *PLoS Curr*. 2011;**3**:RRN1235.

24. Graveland GA, Williams RS, DiFiglia M. Evidence for degenerative and regenerative changes in neostriatal spiny neurons in Huntington's disease. *Science*. 1985;**227**(4688):770–3.

25. Rosas HD, Reuter M, Doros G, *et al*. A tale of two factors: what determines the rate of progression in Huntington's disease? A longitudinal MRI study. *Mov Disord*. 2011;**26**(9):1691–7.

26. Ashburner J, Friston KJ. Voxel-based morphometry – the methods. *Neuroimage*. 2000;**11**(6 Pt 1):805–21.

27. Ridgway GR, Henley SM, Rohrer JD, *et al*. Ten simple rules for reporting voxel-based morphometry studies. *Neuroimage*. 2008;**40**(4):1429–35.

28. Henley SM, Ridgway GR, Scahill RI, *et al*. Pitfalls in the use of voxel-based morphometry as a biomarker: examples from Huntington disease. *AJNR Am J Neuroradiol*. 2010;**31**(4):711–19.

29. Senjem ML, Gunter JL, Shiung MM, Petersen RC, Jack CR, Jr. Comparison of different methodological implementations of voxel-based morphometry in neurodegenerative disease. *Neuroimage*. 2005;**26**(2):600–8.

30. Aylward EH, Codori AM, Rosenblatt A, *et al.* Rate of caudate atrophy in presymptomatic and symptomatic stages of Huntington's disease. *Mov Disord*. 2000;**15**(3):552–60.

31. Aylward EH, Li Q, Stine OC, *et al.* Longitudinal change in basal ganglia volume in patients with Huntington's disease. *Neurology*. 1997;**48**(2):394–9.

32. Aylward EH, Liu D, Nopoulos PC, *et al.* Striatal volume contributes to the prediction of onset of Huntington disease in incident cases. *Biol Psychiatry*. 2012;**71**(9):822–8.

33. Aylward EH, Nopoulos PC, Ross CA, *et al.* Longitudinal change in regional brain volumes in prodromal Huntington disease. *J Neurol Neurosurg Psychiatry*. 2011;**82**(4):405–10.

34. Henley SM, Wild EJ, Hobbs NZ, *et al.* Relationship between CAG repeat length and brain volume in premanifest and early Huntington's disease. *J Neurol*. 2009;**256**(2):203–12.

35. Ruocco HH, Bonilha L, Li LM, Lopes-Cendes I, Cendes F. Longitudinal analysis of regional grey matter loss in Huntington disease: effects of the length of the expanded CAG repeat. *J Neurol Neurosurg Psychiatry*. 2008;**79**(2):130–5.

36. Paulsen JS, Magnotta VA, Mikos AE, *et al.* Brain structure in preclinical Huntington's disease. *Biol Psychiatry*. 2006;**59**(1):57–63.

37. Paulsen JS. Cognitive impairment in Huntington disease: diagnosis and treatment. *Curr Neurol Neurosci Rep*. 2011;**11**(5):474–83.

38. Mukherjee P, Berman JI, Chung SW, Hess CP, Henry RG. Diffusion tensor MR imaging and fiber tractography: theoretic underpinnings. *AJNR Am J Neuroradiol*. 2008;**29**(4):632–41.

39. Mukherjee P, Chung SW, Berman JI, Hess CP, Henry RG. Diffusion tensor MR imaging and fiber tractography: technical considerations. *AJNR Am J Neuroradiol*. 2008;**29**(5):843–52.

40. Mori S, Zhang J. Principles of diffusion tensor imaging and its applications to basic neuroscience research. *Neuron*. 2006;**51**(5):527–39.

41. Seppi K, Schocke MF, Mair KJ, *et al.* Diffusion-weighted imaging in Huntington's disease. *Mov Disord*. 2006;**21**(7):1043–7.

42. Mascalchi M, Lolli F, Della Nave R, *et al.* Huntington disease: volumetric, diffusion-weighted, and magnetization transfer MR imaging of brain. *Radiology*. 2004;**232**(3):867–73.

43. Rosas HD, Tuch DS, Hevelone ND, *et al.* Diffusion tensor imaging in presymptomatic and early Huntington's disease: selective white matter pathology and its relationship to clinical measures. *Mov Disord*. 2006;**21**(9):1317–25.

44. Dumas EM, van den Bogaard SJ, Ruber ME, *et al.* Early changes in white matter pathways of the sensorimotor cortex in premanifest Huntington's disease. *Hum Brain Mapp*. 2012;**33**(1):203–12.

45. Delmaire C, Dumas EM, Sharman MA, *et al.* The structural correlates of functional deficits in early huntington's disease. *Hum Brain Mapp*. 2012; [Epub ahead of print].

46. Weaver KE, Richards TL, Liang O, *et al.* Longitudinal diffusion tensor imaging in Huntington's disease. *Exp Neurol*. 2009;**216**(2):525–9.

47. Detre JA, Alsop DC. Perfusion magnetic resonance imaging with continuous arterial spin labeling: methods and clinical applications in the central nervous system. *Eur J Radiol*. 1999;**30**(2):115–24.

48. Alsop DC, Dai W, Grossman M, Detre JA. Arterial spin labeling blood flow MRI: its role in the early characterization of Alzheimer's disease. *J Alzheimers Dis*. 2010;**20**(3):871–80.

49. Ogawa S, Lee TM, Kay AR, Tank DW. Brain magnetic resonance imaging with contrast dependent on blood oxygenation. *Proc Natl Acad Sci U S A*. 1990;**87**(24):9868–72.

50. Chen JJ, Salat DH, Rosas HD. Complex relationships between cerebral blood flow and brain atrophy in early Huntington's disease. *Neuroimage*. 2012;**59**(2):1043–51.

51. Clark VP, Lai S, Deckel AW. Altered functional MRI responses in Huntington's disease. *Neuroreport*. 2002;**13**(5):703–6.

52. Kim JS, Reading SA, Brashers-Krug T, *et al.* Functional MRI study of a serial reaction time task in Huntington's disease. *Psychiatry Res*. 2004;**131**(1):23–30.

53. Paulsen JS, Zimbelman JL, Hinton SC, *et al.* fMRI biomarker of early neuronal dysfunction in presymptomatic Huntington's disease. *AJNR Am J Neuroradiol*. 2004;**25**(10):1715–21.

54. Wolf RC, Vasic N, Schonfeldt-Lecuona C, Landwehrmeyer GB, Ecker D. Dorsolateral prefrontal cortex dysfunction in presymptomatic Huntington's disease: evidence from event-related fMRI. *Brain*. 2007;**130**(Pt 11):2845–57.

55. Zimbelman JL, Paulsen JS, Mikos A, *et al.* fMRI detection of early neural dysfunction in preclinical Huntington's disease. *J Int Neuropsychol Soc*. 2007;**13**(5):758–69.

56. Wolf RC, Gron G, Sambataro F, *et al.* Magnetic resonance perfusion imaging of resting-state cerebral blood flow in preclinical Huntington's disease. *J Cereb*

Blood Flow Metab. 2011;**31**(9):1908–18.

57. Wolf RC, Sambataro F, Vasic N, *et al.* Longitudinal functional magnetic resonance imaging of cognition in preclinical Huntington's disease. *Exp Neurol.* 2011;**231**(2):214–22.

58. Rupp J, Dzemidzic M, Blekher T, *et al.* Abnormal error-related antisaccade activation in premanifest and early manifest Huntington disease. *Neuropsychology.* 2011;**25**(3):306–18.

59. Aylward EH, Sparks BF, Field KM, *et al.* Onset and rate of striatal atrophy in preclinical Huntington disease. *Neurology.* 2004;**63**(1):66–72.

60. Bergeron R, Coyle JT. NAAG, NMDA receptor and psychosis. *Curr Med Chem.* 2012;**19**(9):1360–4.

61. Tkáč I, Gruetter R. Methodology of ¹H NMR spectroscopy of the human brain at very high magnetic fields. *Appl Magn Reson.* 2005;**29**:139–57.

62. Provencher SW. Automatic quantitation of localized *in vivo* ¹H spectra with LCModel. *NMR Biomed.* 2001;**14**(4):260–4.

63. Emir UE, Tuite PJ, Oz G. Elevated pontine and putamenal GABA levels in mild-moderate parkinson disease detected by 7 Tesla proton MRS. *PLoS One.* 2012;**7**(1):e30918.

64. de Graaf RAD. *In Vivo NMR Spectroscopy: Principles and Techniques.* New York: John Wiley & Sons; 2002.

65. Sanchez-Pernaute R, Garcia-Segura JM, del Barrio Alba A, Viano J, de Yebenes JG. Clinical correlation of striatal 1H MRS changes in Huntington's disease. *Neurology.* 1999;**53**(4):806–12.

66. Unschuld PG, Edden RA, Carass A, *et al.* Brain metabolite alterations and cognitive dysfunction in early Huntington's disease. *Mov Disord.* 2012;**27**(7):895–902.

67. van den Bogaard SJ, Dumas EM, Teeuwisse WM, *et al.* Exploratory 7-Tesla magnetic resonance spectroscopy in Huntington's disease provides in vivo evidence for impaired energy metabolism. *J Neurol.* 2011;**258**(12):2230–9.

68. Emir UE, Auerbach EJ, Van De Moortele PF, *et al.* Regional neurochemical profiles in the human brain measured by (1)H MRS at 7 T using local B shimming. *NMR Biomed.* 2012;**25**(1):152–60.

69. Sturrock A, Laule C, Decolongon J, *et al.* Magnetic resonance spectroscopy biomarkers in premanifest and early Huntington disease. *Neurology.* 2010;**75**(19):1702–10.

70. Tkáč I, Öz G, Adriany G, Uğurbil K, Gruetter R. In vivo ¹H NMR spectroscopy of the human brain at high magnetic fields: metabolite quantification at 4T vs. 7T. *Magn Reson Med.* 2009;**62**(4):868–79.

71. Jenkins BG, Koroshetz WJ, Beal MF, Rosen BR. Evidence for impairment of energy metabolism in vivo in Huntington's disease using localized 1H NMR spectroscopy. *Neurology.* 1993;**43**(12):2689–95.

72. Tkac I, Dubinsky JM, Keene CD, Gruetter R, Low WC. Neurochemical changes in Huntington R6/2 mouse striatum detected by in vivo 1H NMR spectroscopy. *J Neurochem.* 2007;**100**(5):1397–406.

73. Tkac I, Keene CD, Pfeuffer J, Low WC, Gruetter R. Metabolic changes in quinolinic acid-lesioned rat striatum detected non-invasively by in vivo (1)H NMR spectroscopy. *J Neurosci Res.* 2001;**66**(5):891–8.

74. Zacharoff L, Tkac I, Song Q, *et al.* Cortical metabolites as biomarkers in the R6/2 model of Huntington's disease. *J Cereb Blood Flow Metab.* 2012;**32**(3):502–14.

75. Jenkins BG, Andreassen OA, Dedeoglu A, *et al.* Effects of CAG repeat length, HTT protein length and protein context on cerebral metabolism measured using magnetic resonance spectroscopy in transgenic mouse models of Huntington's disease. *J Neurochem.* 2005;**95**(2):553–62.

76. Lodi R, Schapira AH, Manners D, *et al.* Abnormal in vivo skeletal muscle energy metabolism in Huntington's disease and dentatorubropallidoluysian atrophy. *Ann Neurol.* 2000;**48**(1):72–6.

77. Saft C, Zange J, Andrich J, *et al.* Mitochondrial impairment in patients and asymptomatic mutation carriers of Huntington's disease. *Mov Disord.* 2005;**20**(6):674–9.

78. Schapira A, Lodi R. Assessment of in vitro and in vivo mitochondrial function in Friedreich's ataxia and Huntington's disease. *Methods Mol Biol.* 2004;**277**:293–307.

79. Moon RB, Richards JH. Determination of intracellular pH by 31P magnetic resonance. *J Biol Chem.* 1973;**248**(20):7276–8.

80. Chaumeil MM, Valette J, Baligand C, *et al.* pH as a biomarker of neurodegeneration in Huntington's disease: a translational rodent-human MRS study. *J Cereb Blood Flow Metab.* 2012;**32**(5):771–9.

81. Mochel F, N'Guyen TM, Deelchand D, *et al.* Abnormal response to cortical activation in early stages of Huntington disease. *Mov Disord.* 2012;**27**(7):907–10.

82. Tkac I, Henry PG, Zacharoff L, *et al.* Homeostatic adaptations in brain energy metabolism in mouse models of Huntington disease. *J Cereb Blood Flow Metab.* 2012;**32**(11):1977–88.

83. Hoang TQ, Bluml S, Dubowitz DJ, *et al.* Quantitative proton-decoupled 31P MRS and 1H MRS in the evaluation of Huntington's and Parkinson's diseases. *Neurology.* 1998;**50**(4):1033–40.

Chapter 10

Neuroimaging of Gilles de la Tourette syndrome

Yulia Worbe and Andreas Hartmann

Introduction

In his most famous article, published in 1885, Georges Gilles de la Tourette described a strange neurological condition that he referred to as "maladie des tics." The cases presented in this article were based on the observation of nine individuals with a condition that consistently showed a number of features, including onset in childhood, heritability, waxing and waning of motor and phonic symptoms, stereotyped movements, premonitory sensation, echolalia, and coprolalia (defined below).

Over the following 125 years, Gilles de la Tourette syndrome (GTS) has been recognized as an early onset, neurodevelopmental disorder. Practically, this means that – in contrast to adult neurodegenerative diseases – access to postmortem samples is extremely difficult and therefore elucidating the precise etiology and underlying pathophysiological mechanisms remains incomplete. Consequently, the advent of modern neuroimaging techniques has provided a unique tool to investigate the pathophysiology of GTS in humans.

The goals of this chapter are to describe briefly the clinical phenomenology and pathophysiology of GTS and to review current structural and functional neuroimaging data of this fascinating neuropsychiatric condition.

Clinical aspects

GTS is a childhood onset disorder characterized by the presence of hyperkinetic movements called tics. A diagnosis of GTS is made when multiple motor tics and at least one vocal tic are present (not necessarily concurrently), develop before the age of 18 years, and last for more than 1 year from their onset, although the intensity and frequency of tics usually waxes and wanes during this period [1].

GTS was initially thought to be a very rare disorder. However, epidemiological studies suggest that the overall prevalence of this disorder in most countries could be as high as 1% in children [2].

The expression of tics ranges from brief, recurrent, and non-rhythmic motor or vocal actions (simple tics) to complex motor or vocal sequences (complex tics) such as touching behavior or repetitive word pronunciation [3]. Motor tics generally precede the development of vocal tics, and onset of simple tics often predates that of complex tics. Simple and complex tics thus differ by their phenomenological expression and are thought to represent biologically relevant symptom sub-classes [4–6].

There are various differential diagnoses for tics, which include stereotypies, myoclonus, dystonia, chorea, and epilepsy. In contrast to these disorders, however, tics are characterized by (1) premonitory sensations (also called "urge-to-do" or "urge-to-move") and (2) their possible voluntary suppression (albeit only for limited periods). Also, patients with tics often experience a sense of relief after performing the tic, which is probably explained by the release of tension caused by the "urge-to-do." Moreover, after voluntary suppression of tics one can often (but not always) observe a so-called rebound phenomenon where the patient appears to need to externalize all the tics he or she has suppressed.

Tics tend to diminish significantly with age. It is estimated that 75% of patients with a childhood diagnosis of chronic tics or GTS "lose" their tics once they reach adulthood. Of note, however, subtle tics actually persist even during adulthood in the great majority of these patients. However, they cause much less distress

Magnetic Resonance Imaging in Movement Disorders, ed. Paul Tuite and Alain Dagher. Published by Cambridge University Press. © Cambridge University Press 2013.

than during childhood and adolescence and remain often unnoticed by the patients themselves [7]. The possible cause for this spontaneous improvement is explained below [8]. Unfortunately, there are no objective criteria or predictive factors available to estimate individually long-term prognosis.

GTS patients also often develop varying degrees of one or more psychiatric and/or behavioral disorders. The most frequent of these co-morbidities are attention-deficit hyperactivity disorder (ADHD) and obsessive–compulsive disorder (OCD), but general anxiety disorder, depression, personality disorders, learning disability, reduced executive function, impulse control disorders, and other behavioral problems can also occur in conjunction with tics [9]. Therefore, the phenotypic expression of GTS is varied, ranging from simple tics to a more complex association of tics and psychiatric co-morbidities.

Pathophysiology

Many studies have shown that GTS has a strong genetic component [10, 11]. Monozygotic twins are highly concordant (60–90%); multiple affected subjects or family members with milder tics can be observed in the family in ~10% of cases; a 10- to 100-fold relative risk has been estimated for first-degree relatives; an imbalanced sex ratio is apparent with three affected males to one affected female [12, 13].

Genetic transmission models have been suggested from family studies, including single major locus models or complex inheritance models. Autosomal dominant inheritance with incomplete penetrance and intermediate patterns of inheritance, called "semi-dominant–semi-recessive" models, have been suggested. In spite of several studies using classical positional cloning, very few loci (2p, 3q, 5p, 9q, 11q, and 13q) have been described and no gene has been identified to date. In particular, since the dopamine neurotransmitter system has been suggested to be involved in GTS, genes related to dopaminergic metabolism have been at the center of genetic association studies. Rare positive associations have been reported between GTS and dopamine-related genes, including DRD4 and DRD2, encoding the dopamine receptors 4 and 2 on chromosome 11p and 11q, respectively; monoamine oxidase subtype A (MAOA) gene, encoding for the dopamine metabolic MAOA enzyme on chromosome X; and SCL6A3/dopamine transporter (DAT) gene on chromosome 5p. Finally,

a genome-wide association study has identified several susceptibility loci at 2p11, 8q22, and 11q23–24 [14]. However, these results still remain to be replicated in other studies. Chromosomal abnormalities detected by standard cytogenetic methods were identified in several patients with GTS alone or with additional clinical features. Altogether, these studies have pointed towards potential candidate regions such as 7q, 8q, and 18q, which were found to be rearranged in more than one patient. The discovery of a 13q31–q33 inversion in one GTS patient has led to the identification of two variants in the nearby SLITRK1 gene: one truncating mutation in one patient and one variant in the 3′ untranslated region (UTR) altering a binding site for micro-RNA in two patients [15–17].

Overall, these studies strongly suggest that the genetic component in GTS is heterogeneous, that is, not related to a single gene, but to many different genes, with at-risk alleles in these genes possibly transmitted according to different modes. In addition, GTS is probably polygenic in many cases, that is, is the result of the combination of several genetic variants – which alone are insufficient to produce a pathological phenotype – with environmental factors (complex inheritance). The identification of these genes would give key clues on the potential mechanisms and biological pathways altered in this disorder.

The pathophysiological origin of GTS clinical heterogeneity is far from being fully understood. Inferences from various approaches support the hypothesis that GTS is a neurodevelopmental disorder associated with dysfunction of cortico-striato-thalamo-cortical loops [18, 19]. Cortical projections to the basal ganglia are functionally and topographically organized, leading to the concept of functional divisions of cortico-striato-thalamo-cortical loops into sensorimotor, associative, and limbic circuits that are implicated in motor, cognitive, and motivational aspects of behavior, respectively (Figure 10.1) [20].

Specifically, it has been hypothesized that an aberrant focus of striatal neurons becomes inappropriately active, causing unwanted inhibition of a group of basal ganglia output neurons (especially the internal segment of the globus pallidus), which in turn disinhibit a particular movement program, leading to an involuntary movement. Repetitive overactivity of a given specific set of striatal neurons could result in involuntary and stereotyped movements such as tics [18].

Distinct cortico-basal ganglia circuits

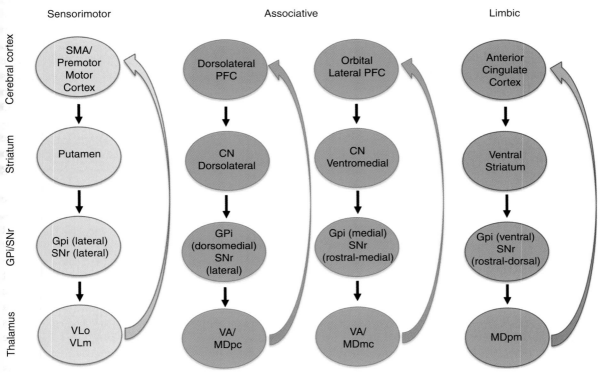

Figure 10.1 General anatomical organization of cortico-striato-thalamo-cortical networks. Abbreviations: CN, caudate nucleus; GPi, internal segment of the globus pallidus; mc, magnacellularis; MD, mediodorsal nucleus; pc, parvocellularis; PFC, prefrontal cortex; pm, posterior medial; SMA, supplementary motor area; SNr, substantia nigra pars reticulata; VA, ventral anterior nucleus; VLo, ventrolateral oral nucleus; VLm, ventrolateral medial nucleus. (Adapted from Alexander *et al.* [20].)

Although the neural circuit hypothesis for tic production was developed specifically for the motor circuits of the cortico-striato-thalamo-cortical loops, it is likely that the fundamental principles of function in the limbic and cognitive basal ganglia circuits are similar. So far, dysfunctions in these networks could lead to the emergence of various behavioral problems occurring in GTS. This hypothesis is supported by experimental data. In primate models, experiments inducing local inhibition of GABAergic transmission showed that dysfunction of the premotor and sensorimotor circuits produced abnormal movements resembling simple motor tics [21, 22], whereas dysfunction of the associative and limbic circuits resulted in behavioral disorders resembling complex tics and compulsions, respectively [22, 23].

What causes aberrant neuronal activity in GTS? Although there are several potential factors, decreased inhibitory function and/or abnormal dopamine neurotransmission probably play a major role. Neuropathological studies in GTS showed both decreased number and deviant distribution of striatal GABAergic and cholinergic interneurons [24, 25] and abnormalities in pallidal projection neurons [26]. These findings could be explained by a migration defect involving inhibitory interneurons originating in the ganglionic eminence. As cortical and basal ganglia interneurons originate from the same structures during brain development [27], reduced numbers of inhibitory interneurons may also be present in the cortex, leading to both structural changes and functional cortical abnormalities. This suggestion is in line with neurophysiological data [28, 29] showing diminished intracortical inhibition and hyperactivity of the premotor and sensorimotor cortices in GTS.

Other lines of evidence suggest that GTS is related to abnormal dopaminergic transmission [30–32]. Notably, symptoms are markedly improved by classical antipsychotics (dopamine receptor antagonists), which remain the drugs of choice for the treatment of tics. Postmortem studies have also found increased concentration of dopamine receptors and transporters in the frontal cortex and basal ganglia of GTS patients. Thus dopamine-mediated reinforcement of activity in cortico-striato-thalamo-cortical loops may explain the development and manifestation of tics and their characteristic stereotypical nature [33]. This mechanism normally occurs following unexpected reward receipt, which has been reported to elicit phasic dopamine release in both monkeys and humans. It has also been shown that phasic dopamine release is sufficient to condition behavior, possibly via modulating the efficacy of cortico-striatal synapses. Thus, following unexpected rewards, phasic dopamine may reinforce the active basal ganglia circuits such that the same action would be facilitated in the future. Antipsychotic medications would interfere with this mechanism and hence reduce reinforcement learning abilities.

These could result both in structural changes and functional abnormalities in cortico-basal ganglia networks in imaging studies, which are presented in the following parts of this chapter.

Mapping brain abnormalities in Gilles de la Tourette syndrome with structural neuroimaging

Based on our current knowledge of GTS pathophysiology, several brain regions have attracted interest. Most notably, numerous studies have reported dysfunction of cortico-striato-thalamo-cortical circuits at different levels (Table 10.1 summarizes findings from structural and diffusion studies in GTS) (Figure 10.2).

Significant neuroimaging evidence exists for a primary cortical dysfunction in GTS. In the cortex, structural changes were observed in frontal, anterior cingulate, insular, parietal, and temporal regions, using voxel-based techniques [34], region of interest [8], and cortical thickness measurements [35, 36].

The pattern of cortical thinning differs among clinical subgroups of patients [37]. In patients with simple tics, cortical thinning was mostly found in primary motor regions. In patients with simple and complex tics, thinning extended into larger premotor, prefrontal, and parietal regions. In patients with associated behavioral problems such as OCD, there was a trend for reduced cortical thickness in the anterior cingulate cortex (Figure 10.3).

Structural changes were also reported in the basal ganglia, including both the striatum and the globus pallidus. In a large cohort of both pediatric and adult GTS patients, Peterson et al. [38] identified a decrease in basal ganglia volume. In GTS children, the reduction of volume was most apparent in the caudate nucleus, whereas adult GTS patients showed volume reductions across all basal ganglia regions. A longitudinal as well as a twin study support these findings as more severely affected siblings were shown to have a smaller caudate nucleus volume [39]. Moreover, a smaller volume of the caudate nucleus head was predictive for persistence of tics in adulthood [40]. Asymmetry of the putamen, as a part of the striatum, was also reported in several studies on pediatric GTS patients [41, 42].

Besides the basal ganglia, structural changes were also described in the thalamus, midbrain [43], and cerebellum [44] in adult GTS patients.

When correlating function with structural changes, analysis showed that tic severity (measured by the Yale Global Tics Severity Scale – YGTSS) can be correlated with cortical thinning in the sensorimotor cortex and surrounding frontal and parietal areas [35, 36], gray matter increase in the ventral putamen using voxel-based techniques [45], and diffusion orientation in the thalamus [46].

In contrast, the presence of psychiatric comorbidities, such as OCD and ADHD, correlated with volume reduction in the anterior caudate nucleus [38, 40] and volume increase in the amygdala [47]. Hippocampal volume correlated both with tic severity [45] and the presence of OCD and ADHD [47].

Finally, diffusion tensor imaging (DTI), which allows evaluation of white matter integrity, has pointed to the microstructural abnormalities in white matter in GTS patients, including the corpus callosum and anterior and posterior limb of the internal capsule [48, 49] (see also Table 10.1).

Mapping brain abnormalities in Gilles de la Tourette syndrome with functional neuroimaging

Despite the numerous and extensive studies on structural abnormalities in GTS cited in the previous paragraphs, it is not always obvious how these structural

Table 10.1. Structural change in Gilles de la Tourette syndrome patients

Study	Number of subjects	Age range (years)	Findings
		Cortical thickness measurements	
Fahim et al., 2010 [36]	34	10–25	**Group comparisons:** Reduced cortical thickness in sensorimotor (L), parietal, orbitofrontal (R) areas in GTS **YGTSS was negatively correlated with cortical thinning** in orbitofrontal (R) and precentral (L) cortices and in GTS boys more than GTS girls **Gender**: prefrontal, orbitofrontal, and parietal cortices thinner in GTS boys
Sowell et al., 2008 [35]	25	7–18	**Group comparison:** Reduced cortical thickness in sensorimotor and parietal areas in GTS **YGTSS** inversely correlated with dorsal frontal, parietal (L), medial frontal (L), pre- and postcentral and occipital cortices (L)
		Volumes, regions of interest measurements, and voxel-based morphometry	
Wittforth et al., 2012 [64]	29	18–49	**Group comparison** of GTS patients with tics, associated ADHD and OCD and healthy controls **Decreased gray matter volume** was found in the left inferior frontal gyrus (IFG) in the GTS patients without ADHD In patients with associated ADHD, increased amygdalar volume (L)
Draganski et al., 2010 [65] Tobe et al., 2010 [44]	40 163	17–66 6–60	**Gray matter volume reduction** in orbitofrontal, anterior cingulate, and ventrolateral prefrontal cortices bilaterally in GTS patients **Tic severity** correlated negatively with prefrontal cortical thickness, **volume increase** in primary **somatosensory cortex** depended on the intensity of premonitory sensations. **White matter changes** were found within anterior parts of the corpus callosum **Reduced volumes of the cerebellum** bilaterally **Tic severity** and performance in a **finger tapping** test correlated with volume reduction **Gender:** males had greater volume reduction compared with females **OCD** was associated with relative enlargement of these regions in proportion to the increasing severity of OCD symptoms. No effect of ADHD. No medication effect
Muller-Vahl et al., 2009 [34]	19	17–60	**Gray matter decrease** in the anterior cingulate gyrus, sensorimotor areas, caudate nucleus (L) and postcentral gyrus (L). **White matter decrease** in inferior frontal gyrus (R), superior frontal gyrus (L), anterior corpus callosum; **white matter increase** in middle frontal gyrus (L), sensorimotor areas (L). **Tic severity** was negatively correlated with orbitofrontal structures, cingulate gyrus (R), parieto-temporo-occipital cortex
Peterson et al., 2007 [47]	154	6–63	**Larger hippocampus** and **amygdala** volumes in GTS. Regions **larger in children** than adults as compared with controls **Tic severity, OCD, and ADHD** correlated inversely with volumes in these subregions in GTS children and adults

Table 10.1. (cont.)

Study	Number of subjects	Age range (years)	Findings
Bloch *et al.,* 2005 [40]	43	9–23	Longitudinal study with first MRI at age of 9–14 years and second MRI at age 16–23 years **In GTS children**, no correlation between striatal volume and tic severity. **In GTS adults,** decreased caudate volume and putame (R) predicted the tic severity. Decreased caudate volume correlated significantly and inversely with the severity of **OCD**
Peterson, 2001 [8]	155	6–63	**Children GTS: boys** – larger dorsal prefrontal, parieto-occipital, and inferior occipital volumes; smaller premotor, orbitofrontal, and subgenial volumes; **girls** – larger dorsal prefrontal and inferior occipital volumes **Adults GTS: men** – larger premotor and parieto-occipital volumes; **women** – smaller dorso-prefrontal and parieto-occipita volumes **Tic severity** correlated with orbitofrontal and parieto-occipital volumes
Ludolph *et al.,* 2006 [45]	14	mean 12.5	**Gray matter increase** in ventral putamen bilaterally and **decrease** in the hippocampal gyrus (L) **YGTSS** correlated with gray matter changes
Garraux *et al.,* 2006 [43]	31	17–49	**Increased gray matter** in the midbrain (L)
Diffusion tensor imaging			
Govindan *et al.,* 2010 [66]	15	7–17	**White matter**: diffusion value increased in cortico-striatal pathways including external capsule (L) and subcallosal fasciculus. **Gray matter:** increased diffusion value in orbitofrontal and insular (L) cortices, putamen (L) **Tic severity** negatively associated with diffusion values in external capsule (L)
Neuner *et al.,* 2010 [48]	28	18–55	**Decreased FA and increased radial diffusivity** in the corticospinal tract and the internal capsule **Decreased FA** in the corpus callosum
Baumer *et al.,* 2010 [49]	14	Mean 35.5	Combined transcranial magnetic stimulation–DTI study Abnormal functional inter-hemispheric connectivity in GTS. No difference in FA in motor regions of the corpus callosum between the GTS and healthy volunteers, but **absence of interaction** between FA and inter-hemispheric connectivity in GTS group
Makki *et al.,* 2009 [67]	18	7–17	**Lower probability of connection** between caudate nucleus and anterior-dorsolateral-frontal region (L). **OCD** was negatively associated with connectivity score of the caudate (L) and anterior dorsolateral frontal cortex; positively associated with the subcallosal gyrus and for the lentiform nucleus
Thomalla *et al.,* 2009 [68]	15	23–45	**Increased FA** in white matter underlying the post- and precentral gyrus, supplementary motor area (L), and the ventral posterolateral part of the thalamus (R). **Tic severity** was inversely and linearly related with FA

Table 10.1. (cont.)

Study	Number of subjects	Age range (years)	Findings
Makki et al., 2008 [46]	23	5–17	Lower caudate volume (L). **Increased axial and mean diffusivity** in the putamen, **increased radial diffusivity** in thalamus (R), and a **reversed asymmetry** of FA in the thalamus **Tic severity** positively correlated with radial diffusivity in thalamus (R)

YGTSS, Yale Global Tics Severity Scale.

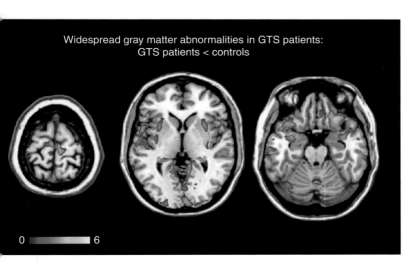

Figure 10.2 Widespread gray matter abnormalities in GTS patients compared to controls. Voxel-based morphometry of 60 GTS patients compared to 30 age- and gender matched controls showed decreased gray matter volume in the orbitofrontal, prefrontal, and ventral premotor cortex, parietal, occipital, and anterior temporal cortices in GTS. These results corroborate previous research findings obtained using structural neuroimaging methods described in this chapter.

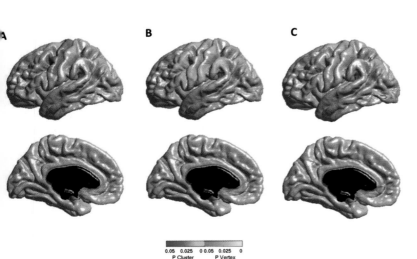

Figure 10.3 Areas of diminished cortical thickness in GTS patients compared to controls. (A) GTS patients with motor tics only had diminished cortical thickness in motor areas. (B) widespread changes in cortical thickness were noted in patients with simple and complex motor and vocal tics. The areas of diminished cortical thickness included sensorimotor, parietal and prefrontal cortices. (C) decreased ventromedial prefrontal cortical thickness was noted in GTS patients with associated obsessive–compulsive disorders. (Adapted from Worbe et al. [37].)

changes alter the functional activity of the brain and lead to heterogeneous clinical expressions of the syndrome. Several studies addressed the question of functional capacity of the brain in GTS patients using both task-specific and resting-state functional neuroimaging.

Indeed, paradigms such as suppression and imitations of tics during scanning showed activation of the sensorimotor cortico-striato-thalamo-cortical network [50, 51] with a greater BOLD activity in sensorimotor regions during expression of tics (e.g., primary motor cortex, premotor cortex, putamen). Compared to voluntary tic imitation, spontaneous expression of tics was also associated with increase activity in the amygdala/hippocampus complex [51].

In the same study, Wang et al. [51] also investigated effective connectivity among the regions of sensorimotor networks using Granger causality and found stronger connectivity within the sensorimotor pathway in the GTS group during spontaneous tics compared to the control group, which expressed voluntary tics. Interestingly, connectivity from the primary somatosensory cortex to the primary motor cortex was stronger in the GTS group. This coincides with the expected temporal relationship between premonitory sensory urges and tics. Consequently, it can be suggested from these results that greater activity within specific portions of sensorimotor pathways leads to the premonitory urges, which drive tics from another part of the same network. Despite the limitations such as a small sample size, and inclusion of medicated patients and patients with different comorbid conditions, the results of this study are of great interest as they suggest that increased activity in the primary somatosensory cortex, putamen, and amygdala/hippocampus may represent activity associated with the premonitory urge and act as a trigger for tics. They also indicate that the primary sensory cortex exerts a causal influence on the putamen that is greater in the GTS patients during spontaneous tics, confirming that a stronger generation of tics may be caused by a greater interaction between the motor cortices and striatum.

A number of studies of tic suppression also pointed to the robust activity of the frontal cortex, which was suggested to be related to a compensatory hypertrophy of the frontal cortices that helps regulate activity within the motor circuit and consequently reduces tic symptoms [52].

To date, in children suffering from GTS, only one study has combined functional and diffusion tensor imaging and demonstrated that enhanced control of motor output was predicted by the structural change in white matter within the prefrontal cortex [53]. Using a manual task-switching paradigm, the author showed that children suffering from GTS compared to controls had a significantly greater BOLD response in the right prefrontal cortex which was linearly related to behavioral (reaction time) performance in the task. An interesting dichotomy was also shown in the white matter with its relationship to the task performance: task performance in controls but not GTS patients was predicted by white matter microstructure of the corpus callosum, whereas task performance of GTS patients but not controls was significantly predicted by white matter microstructure of the frontal regions. The correlation between white matter microstructure and the severity of tics suggested that these changes might be due to neuroplastic functional adaptation rather than being a core component of the GTS. Taken together, these data provide strong evidence in support of the hypothesis that enhanced cognitive control of motor output in GTS is accompanied by adaptive functional and structural changes in the prefrontal cortex. Specifically, GTS patients who develop neuroplastic hypertrophy of the frontal cortex may remit during adolescence whereas those that do not will probably continue to have tics during adulthood.

The presence of psychiatric co-morbidities might differently contribute to the functional abnormalities found in GTS patients. Thus, functional MRI (fMRI) paradigms of reinforcement learning [54] showed different functional abnormalities in GTS patients who expressed the tics only and GTS patients who also had associated OCD.

While GTS patients with motor tics only successfully learned the stimulus–outcome association and showed abnormal activation in the motor network, GTS patients who also had OCD failed to learn from the task and showed blunted blood oxygenation level-dependent (BOLD) signal in the reward processing network, mostly in the ventromedial prefrontal cortex. These results suggest that dysfunction of reward processing in GTS patients could be linked to the presence of OCD. Moreover, as the reduction of reward sensitivity was correlated with the severity of compulsions in these patients, it could be suggested that a deficit in reinforcement learning leads to the maintenance of maladaptive behaviors such as compulsions in OCD patients with and without tics.

A small number of studies have also tried to address the question of what pathophysiological mechanisms could lead to dysfunction of functional brain networks in GTS. Using resting-state fMRI (rs-fMRI), Church et al. [55] showed decreased maturity of frontoparietal and cingulo-opercular cortical networks, both implicated in top-down cognitive control, due to abnormal patterns of connections between functional nodes in pediatric GTS patients. In adult GTS patients compared with controls, using rs-fMRI and a graph theory approach, a stronger global integration and a functional disorganization of cortico-basal ganglia circuits was demonstrated [56]. The patterns of functional changes in cortico-basal ganglia circuits in GTS, characterized by more and stronger connections between the cortex and basal ganglia, also suggest a defect in brain maturation.

In summary, defects in brain maturation could be one of the pathophysiological mechanisms that lead to emergence of the GTS symptoms in childhood and their persistence into adulthood.

Neurotransmission abnormalities in Gilles de la Tourette syndrome

Evidence from pharmacological trials, especially the fact that dopamine receptor blockers are the most effective treatment for tics to date, and postmortem analyses suggested that abnormalities of dopaminergic neurotransmission play a key role in the pathogenesis of GTS. However, most of the early analyses of striatal dopaminergic function in GTS using conventional positron emission tomography (PET) and single-photon emission computerized tomography ligands have generated equivocal or contradictory results, indicating both increased and decreased dopaminergic function in GTS.

Interestingly, a more recent study, using baseline measures and amphetamine challenge of dopaminergic function, allowed the opportunity to evaluate the specific affinity of subtypes of dopamine receptor in GTS patients [57]. The results showed that patients with GTS compared to control subjects had decreased binding potentials to D2/D3 receptors at baseline and increased dopaminergic release after amphetamine challenge in the caudate and in

many cortical regions, including the anterior cingulate, dorsolateral prefrontal, supplementary motor, premotor, and primary motor cortices as well as the superior temporal gyrus. All these regions, as already mentioned, have been postulated to play a primary role in the generation of tics. These findings could reflect both decreased receptor affinity and a primary reduction in D2/D3 receptor density. Also, reduced binding of ligands could be secondary to competition from increased release of endogenous dopamine at baseline. The increased release of - dopamine after amphetamine challenge could indicate altered function of the dopamine transporters or increased density of dopaminergic nerve terminals.

Apart from dopamine, several other neurotransmission systems have been found to be abnormal in GTS. One study has analyzed the relationship between serotonin synthesis and microstructural changes in the caudate nucleus, lentiform nucleus, and thalamus using α-[^{11}C]methyl-L-tryptophan PET scanning in GTS children. Asymmetric immature microstructure in the caudate nucleus was associated with abnormally increased serotonin synthesis [58], which corroborated a previous study on serotonin neurotransmission in GTS [59]. Interestingly, the concomitant OCD symptoms in GTS were associated with decreased serotonergic neurotransmission [60].

Finally, a recent PET neuroimaging study with a ligand for GABA$_A$ receptors, [^{11}C]-flumazenil, pointed to decreased GABAergic binding in GTS patients bilaterally in the ventral striatum, globus pallidus, thalamus, amygdala, and right insula and increased binding in the bilateral substantia nigra, left periaqueductal gray, right posterior cingulate cortex, and bilateral cerebellum [61]. These results are in agreement with neuropathological data that showed diminished number and aberrant distribution of GABAergic interneurons and support the hypothesis of cortico-striato-thalamo-cortical network hyperactivity in GTS.

Conclusions and further directions

Despite more than a century of clinical history, GTS remains an enigmatic disorder. In the past two decades, magnetic resonance and nuclear imaging techniques together with neuropathological data have enhanced our understanding of the neuroanatomical

129

and neurochemical basis of GTS. Insights on brain neuroplastic reorganization and abnormalities of brain development in GTS have emerged from these studies, using both structural and functional neuroimaging techniques.

Development of new neuroimaging techniques, namely real-time fMRI with biofeedback, suggests that neuroimaging could be useful not only for the understanding of GTS pathophysiology, but also as a treatment approach for this disorder. Thus, several recent studies have reported that biofeedback of real-time fMRI data can enable people to gain control of activity in specific parts of their brain and can alter functional connectivity between brain areas. One study, using this technique in GTS patients, showed that GTS patients were able to exert significant control over the supplementary motor area during biofeedback sessions [62]. Moreover, comparison of functional connectivity to the supplementary motor area before and after biofeedback showed that the strength of its functional connectivity with subcortical regions was reduced after biofeedback. These results suggest that biofeedback may allow GTS patients to develop greater conscious control over activity in the supplementary motor area and potentially facilitate the control over tics.

Another important area of investigation concerns endophenotypes. Endophenotypes are defined as an internal process that can be objectively measured, ideally in a robust and reliable fashion. Gottesman and Gould [63] postulated that an endophenotype should be (1) heritable, (2) co-segregate with a (neuropsychiatric) illness, (3) yet be present even when the disease is not, and (4) be found in non-affected family members at a higher rate than in the general population (which may be important for prognosis in children). To our knowledge, no endophenotypic approaches have been attempted in GTS yet. However, this is unsurprising given the clinical heterogeneity and complexity of the disease and the fact that genetic studies have been unable to identify "culprit" genes except for very rare mutations in the *SLITRK1* and *HDC* genes [10]. Nonetheless, further advances in neuroimaging and the complex genetics of GTS will lead to exciting new avenues to understand brain development and function, predict disease evolution, and tailor individual treatment approaches.

References

1. *Diagnostic and Statistical Manual of Mental Disorders*, 4th edn., text revised. Washington, DC: American Psychiatric Association; 2000.

2. Robertson MM. The prevalence and epidemiology of Gilles de la Tourette syndrome. Part 1: the epidemiological and prevalence studies. *J Psychosom Res.* 2008;**65**(5):461–72.

3. Jankovic J, Fahn S. The phenomenology of tics. *Mov Disord.* 1986;**1**(1):17–26.

4. Mathews CA, Jang KL, Herrera LD, *et al.* Tic symptom profiles in subjects with Tourette syndrome from two genetically isolated populations. *Biol Psychiatry.* 2007;**61**(3):292–300.

5. Robertson MM, Eapen V, Cavanna AE. The international prevalence, epidemiology, and clinical phenomenology of Tourette syndrome: a cross-cultural perspective. *J Psychosom Res.* 2009;**67**(6):475–83.

6. Robertson MM, Althoff RR, Hafez A, Pauls DL. Principal components analysis of a large cohort with Tourette syndrome. *Br J Psychiatry.* 2008;**193**(1):31–6.

7. Pappert EJ, Goetz CG, Louis ED, Blasucci L, Leurgans S. Objective assessments of longitudinal outcome in Gilles de la Tourette's syndrome. *Neurology.* 2003;**61**(7):936–40.

8. Peterson BS. Neuroimaging studies of Tourette syndrome: a decade of progress. *Adv Neurol.* 2001;**85**:179–96.

9. Cavanna AE, Eddy C, Rickards HE. Cognitive functioning in Tourette syndrome. *Discov Med.* 2009;**8**(43):191–5.

10. State MW. The genetics of child psychiatric disorders: focus on autism and Tourette syndrome. *Neuron.* 2010;**68**(2):254–69.

11. Deng H, Gao K, Jankovic J. The genetics of Tourette syndrome. *Nat Rev Neurol.* 2012;**8**(4):203–13.

12. Wolf SS, Jones DW, Knable MB, *et al.* Tourette syndrome: prediction of phenotypic variation in monozygotic twins by caudate nucleus D2 receptor binding. *Science.* 1996;**273**(5279):1225–7.

13. Randolph C, Hyde TM, Gold JM, Goldberg TE, Weinberger DR. Tourette's syndrome in monozygotic twins. Relationship of tic severity to neuropsychological function. *Arch Neurol.* 1993;**50**(7):725–8.

14. Simonic I, Nyholt DR, Gericke GS, *et al.* Further evidence for linkage of Gilles de la Tourette syndrome (GTS) susceptibility loci on

chromosomes 2p11, 8q22 and 11q23–24 in South African Afrikaners. *Am J Med Genet.* 2001;**105**(2):163–7.

15. O'Roak BJ, Morgan TM, Fishman DO, *et al.* Additional support for the association of SLITRK1 var321 and Tourette syndrome. *Mol Psychiatry.* 2010;**15**(5):447–50.

16. Zimprich A, Hatala K, Riederer F, *et al.* Sequence analysis of the complete SLITRK1 gene in Austrian patients with Tourette's disorder. *Psychiatr Genet.* 2008;**18**(6):308–9.

17. Abelson JF, Kwan KY, O'Roak BJ, *et al.* Sequence variants in SLITRK1 are associated with Tourette's syndrome. *Science.* 2005;**310**(5746):317–20.

18. Mink JW. The basal ganglia and involuntary movements: impaired inhibition of competing motor patterns. *Arch Neurol.* 2003;**60**(10):1365–8.

19. Albin RL. Neurobiology of basal ganglia and Tourette syndrome: striatal and dopamine function. *Adv Neurol.* 2006;**99**:99–106.

20. Alexander GE, DeLong MR, Strick PL. Parallel organization of functionally segregated circuits linking basal ganglia and cortex. *Annu Rev Neurosci.* 1986;**9**:357–81.

21. McCairn KW, Bronfeld M, Belelovsky K, Bar-Gad I. The neurophysiological correlates of motor tics following focal striatal disinhibition. *Brain.* 2009;**132**(Pt 8):2125–38.

22. Worbe Y, Baup N, Grabli D, *et al.* Behavioral and movement disorders induced by local inhibitory dysfunction in primate striatum. *Cereb Cortex.* 2009;**19**(8):1844–56.

23. Grabli D, McCairn K, Hirsch EC, *et al.* Behavioural disorders induced by external globus pallidus dysfunction in primates:

I. Behavioural study. *Brain.* 2004;**127**(Pt 9):2039–54.

24. Kalanithi PS, Zheng W, Kataoka Y, *et al.* Altered parvalbumin-positive neuron distribution in basal ganglia of individuals with Tourette syndrome. *Proc Natl Acad Sci U S A.* 2005;**102**(37):13307–12.

25. Kataoka Y, Kalanithi PS, Grantz H, *et al.* Decreased number of parvalbumin and cholinergic interneurons in the striatum of individuals with Tourette syndrome. *J Comp Neurol.* 2010;**518**(3):277–91.

26. Haber SN, Kowall NW, Vonsattel JP, Bird ED, Richardson EP, Jr. Gilles de la Tourette's syndrome. A postmortem neuropathological and immunohistochemical study. *J Neurol Sci.* 1986;**75**(2):225–41.

27. Wonders CP, Anderson SA. The origin and specification of cortical interneurons. *Nat Rev Neurosci.* 2006;**7**(9):687–96.

28. Orth M, Rothwell JC. Motor cortex excitability and comorbidity in Gilles de la Tourette syndrome. *J Neurol Neurosurg Psychiatry.* 2009;**80**(1):29–34.

29. Heise KF, Steven B, Liuzzi G, *et al.* Altered modulation of intracortical excitability during movement preparation in Gilles de la Tourette syndrome. *Brain.* 2010;**133**(Pt 2):580–90.

30. Gunther J, Tian Y, Stamova B, *et al.* Catecholamine-related gene expression in blood correlates with tic severity in Tourette syndrome. *Psychiatry Res.* 2012;**200**(2–3):593–601.

31. Herzberg I, Valencia-Duarte AV, Kay VA, *et al.* Association of DRD2 variants and Gilles de la Tourette syndrome in a family-based sample from a South American population isolate.

Psychiatr Genet. 2010;**20**(4):179–83.

32. Ferrari M, Termine C, Franciotta D, *et al.* Dopaminergic receptor D5 mRNA expression is increased in circulating lymphocytes of Tourette syndrome patients. *J Psychiatr Res.* 2008;**43**(1):24–9.

33. Groenewegen HJ, van den Heuvel OA, Cath DC, Voorn P, Veltman DJ. Does an imbalance between the dorsal and ventral striatopallidal systems play a role in Tourette's syndrome? A neuronal circuit approach. *Brain Dev.* 2003;**25** Suppl 1:S3–S14.

34. Muller-Vahl KR, Kaufmann J, Grosskreutz J, *et al.* Prefrontal and anterior cingulate cortex abnormalities in Tourette syndrome: evidence from voxel-based morphometry and magnetization transfer imaging. *BMC Neurosci.* 2009;**10**:47.

35. Sowell ER, Kan E, Yoshii J, *et al.* Thinning of sensorimotor cortices in children with Tourette syndrome. *Nat Neurosci.* 2008;**11**(6):637–9.

36. Fahim C, Yoon U, Das S, *et al.* Somatosensory-motor bodily representation cortical thinning in Tourette: effects of tic severity, age and gender. *Cortex.* 2010;**46**(6):750–60.

37. Worbe Y, Gerardin E, Hartmann A, *et al.* Distinct structural changes underpin clinical phenotypes in patients with Gilles de la Tourette syndrome. *Brain.* 2010;**133**(Pt 12):3649–60.

38. Peterson BS, Thomas P, Kane MJ, *et al.* Basal ganglia volumes in patients with Gilles de la Tourette syndrome. *Arch Gen Psychiatry.* 2003;**60**(4):415–24.

39. Hyde TM, Stacey ME, Coppola R, *et al.* Cerebral morphometric abnormalities in Tourette's syndrome: a quantitative MRI

study of monozygotic twins. *Neurology.* 1995;**45**(6): 1176–82.

40. Bloch MH, Leckman JF, Zhu H, Peterson BS. Caudate volumes in childhood predict symptom severity in adults with Tourette syndrome. *Neurology.* 2005;**65**(8):1253–8.

41. Singer HS, Reiss AL, Brown JE, *et al.* Volumetric MRI changes in basal ganglia of children with Tourette's syndrome. *Neurology.* 1993;**43**(5):950–6.

42. Zimmerman AM, Abrams MT, Giuliano JD, Denckla MB, Singer HS. Subcortical volumes in girls with Tourette syndrome: support for a gender effect. *Neurology.* 2000;**54**(12):2224–9.

43. Garraux G, Goldfine A, Bohlhalter S, *et al.* Increased midbrain gray matter in Tourette's syndrome. *Ann Neurol.* 2006;**59**(2): 381–5.

44. Tobe RH, Bansal R, Xu D, *et al.* Cerebellar morphology in Tourette syndrome and obsessive-compulsive disorder. *Ann Neurol.* 2010;**67**(4):479–87.

45. Ludolph AG, Juengling FD, Libal G, *et al.* Grey-matter abnormalities in boys with Tourette syndrome: magnetic resonance imaging study using optimised voxel-based morphometry. *Br J Psychiatry.* 2006;**188**:484–5.

46. Makki MI, Behen M, Bhatt A, Wilson B, Chugani HT. Microstructural abnormalities of striatum and thalamus in children with Tourette syndrome. *Mov Disord.* 2008;**23**(16): 2349–56.

47. Peterson BS, Choi HA, Hao X, *et al.* Morphologic features of the amygdala and hippocampus in children and adults with Tourette syndrome. *Arch Gen Psychiatry.* 2007;**64**(11):1281–91.

48. Neuner I, Kupriyanova Y, Stocker T, *et al.* White-matter abnormalities in Tourette

syndrome extend beyond motor pathways. *Neuroimage.* 2010;**51**(3):1184–93.

49. Baumer T, Thomalla G, Kroeger J, *et al.* Interhemispheric motor networks are abnormal in patients with Gilles de la Tourette syndrome. *Mov Disord.* 2010;**25**(16):2828–37.

50. Bohlhalter S, Goldfine A, Matteson S, *et al.* Neural correlates of tic generation in Tourette syndrome: an event-related functional MRI study. *Brain.* 2006;**129**(Pt 8): 2029–37.

51. Wang Z, Maia TV, Marsh R, *et al.* The neural circuits that generate tics in Tourette's syndrome. *Am J Psychiatry.* 2011;**168**(12):1326–37.

52. Mazzone L, Yu S, Blair C, *et al.* An FMRI study of frontostriatal circuits during the inhibition of eye blinking in persons with Tourette syndrome. *Am J Psychiatry.* 2010;**167**(3): 341–9.

53. Jackson SR, Parkinson A, Jung J, *et al.* Compensatory neural reorganization in Tourette syndrome. *Curr Biol.* 2011;**21**(7):580–5.

54. Worbe Y, Palminteri S, Hartmann A, *et al.* Reinforcement learning and Gilles de la Tourette syndrome: dissociation of clinical phenotypes and pharmacological treatments. *Arch Gen Psychiatry.* 2011;**68**(12):1257–66.

55. Church JA, Fair DA, Dosenbach NU, *et al.* Control networks in paediatric Tourette syndrome show immature and anomalous patterns of functional connectivity. *Brain.* 2009;**132**(Pt 1):225–38.

56. Worbe Y, Malherbe C, Hartmann A, *et al.* Functional immaturity of cortico-basal ganglia networks in Gilles de la Tourette syndrome. *Brain.* 2012;**135**(Pt 6): 1937–46.

57. Steeves TD, Ko JH, Kideckel DM, *et al.* Extrastriatal dopaminergic dysfunction in Tourette syndrome. *Ann Neurol.* 2010;**67**(2):170–81.

58. Saporta AS, Chugani HT, Juhasz C, *et al.* Multimodality neuroimaging in Tourette syndrome: alpha-[11C] methyl-L-tryptophan positron emission tomography and diffusion tensor imaging studies. *J Child Neurol.* 2010;**25**(3):336–42.

59. Behen M, Chugani HT, Juhasz C *et al.* Abnormal brain tryptophan metabolism and clinical correlate in Tourette syndrome. *Mov Disord.* 2007;**22**(15):2256–62.

60. Wong DF, Brasic JR, Singer HS, *et al.* Mechanisms of dopaminergic and serotonergic neurotransmission in Tourette syndrome: clues from an in vivo neurochemistry study with PET. *Neuropsychopharmacology.* 2008;**33**(6):1239–51.

61. Lerner A, Bagic A, Simmons JM, *et al.* Widespread abnormality of the gamma-aminobutyric acid-ergic system in Tourette syndrome. *Brain.* 2012;**135**(Pt 6):1926–36.

62. Hampson M, Scheinost D, Qiu M, *et al.* Biofeedback of real-time functional magnetic resonance imaging data from the supplementary motor area reduces functional connectivity to subcortical regions. *Brain Connect.* 2011;**1**(1):91–8.

63. Gottesman, II, Gould TD. The endophenotype concept in psychiatry: etymology and strategic intentions. *Am J Psychiatry.* 2003;**160**(4):636–45.

64. Wittforth M, Bornmann S, Peschel T, *et al.* Lateral frontal cortex volume reduction in Tourette syndrome revealed by VBM. *BMC Neurosci.* 2012;**13**:17. PMID: 22333536.

65. Draganski B, Martino D, Cavanna AE, *et al.* Multispectral brain morphometry in Tourette

syndrome persisting into adulthood. *Brain*. 2010;**133** (Pt 12):3661–75. PMID: 21071387.

66. Govindan RM, Makki MI, Wilson BJ, Behen ME, Chugani HT. Abnormal water diffusivity in corticostriatal projections in children with Tourette syndrome. *Hum Brain Mapp*.

2010;**31**(11):1665–74. PMID: 20162597.

67. Makki MI, Govindan RM, Wilson BJ, Behen ME, Chugani HT. Altered fronto-striato-thalamic connectivity in children with Tourette syndrome associated with diffusion tensor MRI and probabilistic fiber tracking. *J Child*

Neurol. 2009;**24**(6):669–78. PMID: 19491113.

68. Thomalla G, Siebner HR, Jonas M, *et al*. Structural changes in the somatosensory system correlate with tic severity in Gilles de la Tourette syndrome. *Brain*. 2009;**132**(Pt 3):765–77. PMID: 19136548.

Dystonia

Bernhard Haslinger

Introduction

Dystonias are central movement disorders that are characterized by sustained involuntary muscle contractions that lead to abnormal postures or repetitive movements. Usually different types of dystonia are categorized according to their etiology (primary, that is, without any known cause, or secondary, that is, due to another etiological factor such as neuropsychiatric drugs, cerebral ischemia, and others) and according to the clinical distribution of symptoms. Focal dystonias affect only parts of the body, such as the neck in cervical dystonia (CD), the orofacial muscles in blepharospasm/oromandibular dystonia (Meige's syndrome), or the larynx in laryngeal dystonia (LD). In action-induced dystonia, patients only become symptomatic during a specific, usually highly automated or over-learnt task like writing (focal hand dystonia = writer's cramp or WC), speaking (LD) or playing a musical instrument (musician's dystonia), such as winding in professional brass players ("embouchure" dystonia).

Dystonia is considered to represent a disorder of the basal ganglia combined with a cortical sensorimotor dysfunction [1]. Considering functional imaging and electrophysiological findings (see below), there appears to be a defective inhibitory control from the basal ganglia to cortical structures in focal dystonia. Deficient inhibitory control could lead to a failure in focusing motor output (deficient "center–surround" inhibition) and predispose to the development of abnormal cortical plasticity, resulting in altered cortical maps or increased cortical excitability [2–4]. An injury or the intensive use of the affected limb together with maladaptive sensorimotor reorganization could lead to the clinical manifestation of dystonia.

Several methodological considerations are important when talking about magnetic resonance imaging (MRI) studies in patients with dystonia. Studies in clinically symptomatic patients with generalized dystonia are nearly impossible due to the severe character of the disease, with massive involuntary hyperkinesia even at rest. This review will therefore focus mainly on MRI studies in focal dystonias. Nevertheless, involuntary movements and altered voluntary motor performance have also to be taken into account as confounding factors when interpreting functional MRI (fMRI) studies during motor tasks or even at rest in these patients with focal types of dystonia. Several studies have therefore applied sparse sampling fMRI designs with performance of the motor task during scanning pauses. Others have investigated motor or sensory stimulation tasks that do not induce the clinical appearance of dystonia or that investigate clinically asymptomatic body parts. Performing MRI at rest (resting-state MRI) in patients with action-induced dystonia (i.e., without any signs of dystonia when not performing a specific task) represents another interesting possibility to study primary pathophysiological traits of the disorder. Finally, studying the influence of peripheral muscle denervation with botulinum toxin (BTX), which represents the therapy of choice in most patients with focal dystonia, on altered sensorimotor activation patterns offers another interesting access to a better understanding of the pathophysiology of this disorder. Again, activation changes that are not reversed despite clinical improvement of symptoms following BTX therapy point to a primary trait of the disorder.

Motor activation studies in dystonia

The majority of functional imaging studies have been performed in patients with focal dystonia of the hand, especially action-induced dystonia during writing, that is, WC. Based on the intensively studied physiology of hand motor function, WC serves as a model for many other types of dystonia.

Various motor tasks have been applied to study cerebral activation when moving the clinically affected hand. Some of these investigations found overactivity whilst others described a reduced activation level of cortical sensorimotor areas in WC patients.

Previous functional imaging studies using positron emission tomography (PET) had shown reduced activation within primary motor, lateral premotor, and mesial premotor (caudal supplementary motor area [SMA]) cortices during hand movements in patients with WC [5, 6]. Oga and coworkers applied event-related fMRI in patients with WC during a task which involved active muscle contraction or relaxation of the hand. In good agreement with the earlier PET findings, they showed a reduced activation of the contralateral sensorimotor cortex and mesial premotor cortex/SMA in WC [7]. Interestingly, a similar primary motor/premotor underactivity has also been described when WC patients move their contralateral, that is, clinically unaffected hand [8].

In contrast to these findings, increased sensorimotor activation levels have been described by other studies, especially when investigating tasks explicitly provoking the manifestation of dystonic symptoms. Pujol and coworkers investigated dystonic movements on an MR-suitable guitar in musicians with task-induced hand dystonia and found a (spatially) increased activation of the primary sensorimotor cortex and reduced premotor activation (Figure 11.1) [9]. Comparable findings of an increased extent of sensorimotor activation have been reported in patients with WC when provoking dystonic symptoms by a writing task [10]. Kadota et al. described increased premotor activation in musicians with hand dystonia during a tapping task [11]. In mutation carriers for myoclonus–dystonia, activation of premotor, somatosensory, parietal, and cerebellar areas was found to be increased during a hand motor task, partly correlating to clinical penetrance of symptoms [12].

As mentioned above, differences in motor activation between patients with dystonia and healthy controls during a motor task can be confounded by unequal motor performance or superimposed dystonic symptoms. To study whether differences of sensorimotor activation as described above for hand motor tasks are primary pathophysiological traits of

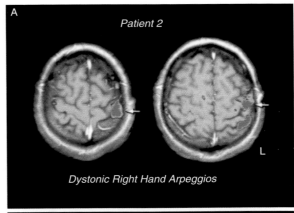

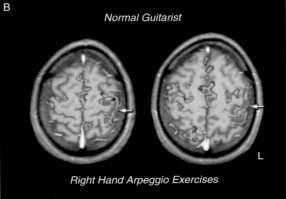

Figure 11.1 fMRI study showing spatially increased contralateral primary sensorimotor cortex activation and reduced premotor activation in a musician with action induced hand dystonia (note arrows in A) in contrast to a healthy musician during performance of right hand arpeggios (note arrows in B). (From Pujol *et al.* [9] by permission of Elsevier.)

the disorder independent of clinical motor output, we recently investigated imagination of hand writing during fMRI in patients with WC [13]. And indeed, patients with WC showed reduced activation of the premotor cortices, basal ganglia, and thalamus during motor imagination (Figure 11.2). Likewise, lateral premotor and bilateral parietal underactivity had previously been revealed in patients with CD during imagination of hand movements [14]. These results during motor imagery suggest that internal movement selection and planning during movement imagination seems to be disturbed in dystonia. This seems to be a primary pathophysiological characteristic in patients with dystonia possibly due to faulty selection and filtering of motor programs at the level of the basal ganglia.

135

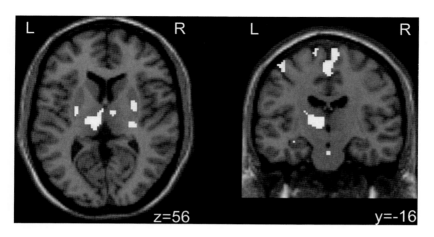

Figure 11.2 fMRI study demonstrating reduced activation of the left primary sensorimotor cortex, mesial and left dorsal premotor cortex, bilateral putamen, and bilateral thalamus in patients with writer's cramp during kinesthetic motor imagery of right hand drawing movements. (Modified from Castrop *et al.* [13].)

Although the majority of functional imaging studies have been performed in patients with action-induced focal hand dystonia, dystonias affecting craniocervical muscles are by far the most frequent clinical manifestations of adult primary dystonia. These include CD, blepharospasm, and combined blepharospasm and oromandibular dystonia (Meige's syndrome). Less frequent are action-induced dystonia of the larynx during vocalization (LD) or of the oromandibular muscles in musicians playing wind instruments ("embouchure" dystonia). Studying these subtypes of dystonia affecting the head and neck with fMRI is especially challenging due to involuntary craniocervical movements and performance monitoring in the scanner setting.

Concerning activation of the basal ganglia, an fMRI study described that involuntary eyelid spasms in patients with blepharospasm are associated with significant activation of the putamen [15]. Obermann and coworkers showed an increased activation level of the basal ganglia during a motor task involving the clinically unaffected hand in patients with blepharospasm and CD [16].

We applied special sparse sampling fMRI designs to study cerebral activation in patients with orofacial dystonia. We studied patients with blepharospasm and Meige's syndrome with a simple but well-controlled orofacial motor task (whistling) [17]. In contrast to patients with isolated blepharospasm we found deficient activation of the primary motor and ventral premotor cortices within the mouth representation area during whistling in patients with Meige's syndrome. It therefore appears that this primary motor/premotor

underactivity during the orofacial motor task is specific for the clinically affected oromandibular motor system in Meige patients (Figure 11.3). On the other hand we found increased activation of bilateral somatosensory areas and the caudal SMA in both groups of orofacial dystonia. This overactivity was partly reduced in Meige patients following BTX treatment, while the reduced motor activation that we described above was not reversed despite significant improvement of clinical symptoms.

In patients with LD, that is an action-induced dystonia of the laryngeal muscles that leads to a strained/strangled, hoarse, effortful voice, we investigated the neural correlate of dystonic speech production again with a sparse sampling fMRI paradigm (so called "silent event-related" fMRI) [18]. We found that compared to healthy controls patients with LD showed a significantly reduced activation of the primary sensorimotor, premotor, and sensory association cortices during dystonic vocalization (Figure 11.4). Interestingly, this pattern of sensorimotor underactivity was revealed in part also when investigating a neutral task where subjects were instructed to whisper and which did not lead to the clinical manifestation of dystonic symptoms in patients. As in our study in blepharospasm and Meige's syndrome, reduced sensorimotor activation could not be normalized in spite of a significant improvement of dystonic symptoms following injection of BTX into the vocal folds. Differing from these results, another fMRI study in patients with spasmodic dysphonia demonstrated that these patients

A) CONTR > Meige pre-BTX

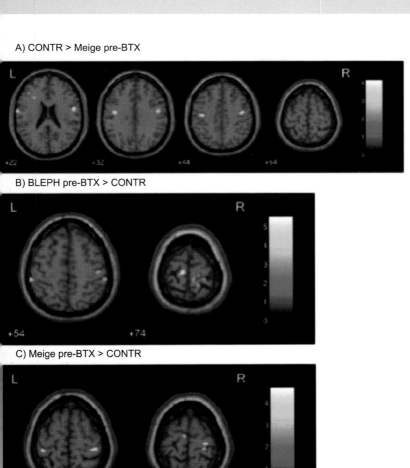

B) BLEPH pre-BTX > CONTR

C) Meige pre-BTX > CONTR

Figure 11.3 fMRI activation differences between patients with orofacial dystonia (blepharospasm, BLEPH, and Meige's syndrome) and healthy controls during an orofacial motor task. (A) Reduced primary motor and ventral premotor activation bilaterally in patients with Meige's syndrome before treatment with botulinum toxin (BTX) compared to controls. Overactivity of the primary somatosensory cortex and the caudal SMA in patients with blepharospasm (B) and patients with Meige's syndrome before BTX treatment (C). (From Dresel et al. [17] by permission of Oxford University Press).

showed a spatially increased activation of the primary sensorimotor cortex, insula, and superior temporal gyrus during symptomatic and asymptomatic tasks. On the other hand the extent of activation was decreased in the basal ganglia, thalamus, and cerebellum during the clinically asymptomatic task. The intensity of activation was higher in patients with LD in the primary somatosensory cortex during dystonic vocalization. Correlation analyses revealed a decreased correlation of activations between the primary motor and sensory cortices and stronger correlations of activations between the basal ganglia, thalamus, and cerebellum in dystonia patients [19].

We recently studied the pathophysiological basis of dystonic orofacial movements in professional brass players with a so-called "embouchure dystonia" [20].

Embouchure dystonia (ED) is a rare focal task-specific dystonia that affects wind players and manifests as playing-related involuntary movements of the orofacial muscles that control the airflow into the mouthpiece. In these patients we studied two orofacial motor tasks: again one that induces the manifestation of dystonic symptoms and a neutral task without clinical dystonia. Applying MR-suitable acrylic glass mouthpieces and a tube, the "dystonia-specific" task involved buzzing at the instrument-specific, fully functional mouthpiece; the "neutral" task involved simply blowing into a tube. Patients with ED showed a significant overactivity of the premotor, primary motor, as well as primary and secondary somatosensory cortices during both, that is the dystonia-specific as well as the clinically

137

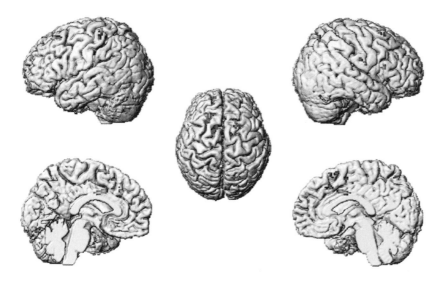

Figure 11.4 fMRI activation is significantly reduced in cortical areas in patients with laryngeal dystonia compared to healthy controls during simple vocalization. (Modified from Haslinger et al. [18].)

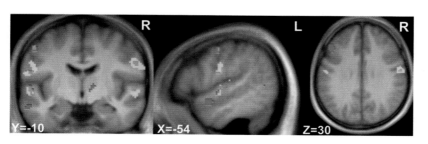

Figure 11.5 fMRI study shows areas with significantly increased activation in musicians with embouchure dystonia compared to healthy musicians. The figure shows an overactivity in dystonia patients during both the dystonia-inducing task, i.e. buzzing at a mouthpiece (yellow), as well as during a neutral task that did not induce dystonia (red). (Modified from Haslinger et al. [20].)

asymptomatic task (Figure 11.5). We hypothesize that in musicians with a potential susceptibility originally beneficial brain plasticity in response to years of intensive and repetitive motor training can go too far and shift to a maladaptation that may lead to abnormal sensorimotor processing.

Functional MRI during sensory stimulation in dystonia

Given that dystonia – on first sight – mainly manifests as a movement disorder, up to now the majority of imaging studies have investigated cerebral activation during different motor tasks as described above. Nevertheless, an important role of a dysfunction of somatosensory processing has been more and more recognized over the past years and has become one of the main focuses of research in dystonia. This is also supported clinically by sensory phenomena such as

ocular sensory discomfort in blepharospasm or hoarseness of the voice in LD. Moreover, a significant number of patients with craniocervical dystonia use a sensory trick, a so-called "geste antagonistique" such as touching or stroking the face, to alleviate their symptoms

Alterations of activity within cortical somatosensory areas have already been shown in various studies that investigated motor tasks as described above. As an example we have shown an increased activation of the primary somatosensory cortex in patients with blepharospasm and Meige's syndrome during an orofacial motor task (whispering) [17]. Obermann and coworkers reported that the primary somatosensory cortex is overactive in patients with CD during passive movement of the clinically unaffected hand [21]. The latter finding as well as our results of somatosensory overactivity in patients with isolated blepharospasm during an oral motor task, that is, a task that activates clinically unaffected

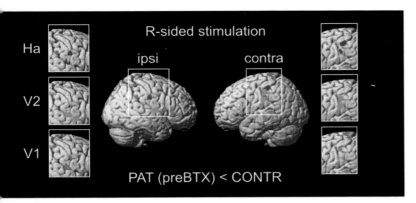

Figure 11.6 Reduced activation in patients (PAT) with orofacial dystonia (blepharospasm and Meige's syndrome) prior to botulinum toxin injection (preBTX) during right sided tactile stimulation of the right forehead (V1), right upper lip (V2), and right hand (Ha) as compared to control subjects (CONTR) projected onto a normalized rendered brain. The panels on both sides show the activation differences in the ipsilateral (ipsi) and contralateral (contra) hemisphere color-coded for each stimulation condition separately. (From Dresel *et al.* [23] by permission of Wiley and Sons.)

muscles, already might hint to a general somatosensory disinhibition in patients with dystonia. This might predispose some of them to a spread of dystonic symptoms onto neighboring muscle groups as we often see in clinical practice.

One important issue when investigating the somatosensory system with fMRI is the standardization of sensory stimuli. We therefore developed a fully automated MR-compatible device for standardized application of sensory stimuli during fMRI [22]. We applied this device for studying the cerebral activation in patients with Meige's syndrome during tactile stimulation of different regions of the face as well as of the clinically unaffected hand [23]. Our results show a significantly reduced activation of the bilateral primary somatosensory cortex as well as the right secondary somatosensory cortex in patients with Meige's syndrome during tactile stimulation in clinically affected facial areas (forehead and upper lip) but also during stimulation of a clinically unaffected hand (Figure 11.6). Reduced somatosensory activation during tactile stimulation of the hand could reflect a predisposition in some of these patients to show a segmental spread of dystonic symptoms such as the development of hand dystonia. We also studied these patients 4 weeks after treatment with BTX. Despite clinical improvement this did not lead to a reversal of cortical sensory underactivity. On the other hand we found a reduction of basal ganglia and thalamic activation during somatosensory stimulation of the forehead. A previous fMRI study showed an overactivity of the basal ganglia in patients with WC during a tactile discrimination task. This was interpreted in the context of faulty filtering of sensory signals at

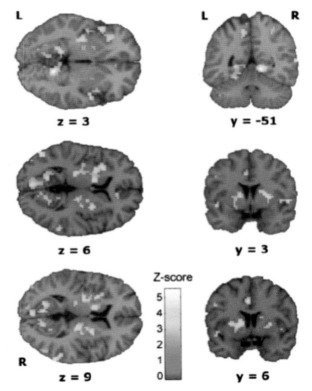

Figure 11.7 Relative overactivity of the basal ganglia and thalamus during a tactile discrimination task in patients with writer's cramp compared to healthy controls. (From Peller *et al.* [24] by permission of Oxford University Press.)

the level of the basal ganglia, possibly based on a deficient center–surround inhibition of afferent input (Figure 11.7) [24]. We hypothesize that the reduction of basal ganglia activity in patients with Meige's syndrome by BTX treatment [23] might reflect a

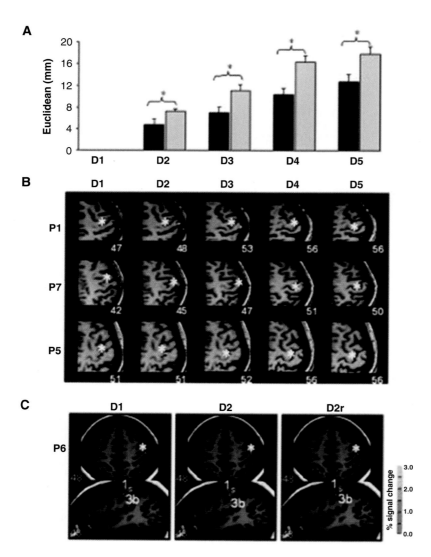

Figure 11.8 Finger representations in primary somatosensory cortex (BA3b) during vibrotactile stimulation in patients with writer's cramp and healthy controls. The mean distance (in mm) between the representation of the thumb (D1) and each of the sequential digits (D2–D5) is reduced in patients with writer's cramp (black bars) compared to healthy controls (gray bars). * = $p < 0.0125$. (From Nelson et al. [26] by permission of Wiley and Sons.)

more efficient filtering following modulation of somatosensory input.

Electrophysiological studies have shown a de-differentiation of cortical somatotopic somatosensory representations in focal dystonias. This could result from deficient subcortical filtering of somatosensory input and could contribute to the manifestation of undifferentiated motor programs in clinical dystonia. Such a rearrangement could be demonstrated with fMRI for somatotopic sensory finger representations when applying vibrotactile stimuli to the fingers of the clinically affected hand in patients with WC [25, 26]. Especially, the study by Nelson and coworkers combined high-resolution fMRI with a methodologically sophisticated design and analyses for showing that the primary somatosensory representations are spatially less separated, partially overlapping or shifted especially for digits I–III, which are the crucial digits for handwriting (Figure 11.8). In line with such a rearrangement of cortical sensory representations an earlier fMRI study showed that simultaneously applied sensory stimuli are abnormally processed in patients with WC with a non-linear interaction between individual finger stimulation and cortical sensory hemodynamic response [27].

In parallel to these findings of a somatotopic dedifferentiation at the cortical level, Delmaire and coworkers also reported a subcortical rearrangement of somatotopic representations within the basal ganglia [28]. In patients with hand dystonia, they showed that during movements of the hand, toes or lips, the normal segregation of hand and lip representations within the putamen is altered. This finding correlated to disease severity. This dedifferentiation of sensorimotor maps at the subcortical and cortical level may contribute to the clinical loss of selectivity of motor programs in patients with dystonia.

Resting-state MRI in dystonia

As mentioned above, some of the activation studies have investigated neutral tasks or tasks involving body parts not affected by dystonia. Besides that, resting-state fMRI studies of patients with action-induced dystonia can further add to our understanding of the disorder. They can determine whether abnormal activity levels within cortical and subcortical sensorimotor networks are primary pathophysiological traits of the disorder or "only" secondary due to dystonic motor performance, compensation, or alterations in sensory input during tasks applied in activation studies. Previous PET studies had already investigated resting-state activity of subcortical–cortical networks in those with dystonia gene mutations – both clinically symptomatic as well as non-manifesting carriers. They showed overactivity of a network including the basal ganglia and premotor cortices [29, 30].

Results from a previous fMRI activation study hinted towards abnormal activation levels at rest in patients with task-induced hand dystonia. Blood and coworkers showed that in these patients the activation levels of the basal ganglia remain elevated at rest after performance of a motor task with the clinically affected as well as the contralateral asymptomatic hand [31]. A recent resting-state MRI study investigated patients with WC and applied independent component analyses (ICA) to study functional connectivity of different functional networks at rest [32]. The authors reported an increased connectivity of the left putamen within the so-called default mode network. On the other hand, within the sensorimotor

network, functional connectivity of the left primary somatosensory and parietal cortices was reduced. We also recently investigated resting-state activity in patients with WC. Differing from the study of Mohammadi we performed analyses of functional connectivity within an a-priori defined network of sensorimotor regions of interest (ROIs) (C. Dresel, Y. Li, F. Castrop, C. Zimmer, B. Haslinger, unpublished data, 2012). Our results revealed a reduced functional connectivity of different subcortical and cortical areas (premotor cortex, thalamus, pallidum) to the hand area of the primary motor cortex. On the other hand, the primary motor cortex showed reduced functional connectivity at rest with premotor, prefrontal, and secondary somatosensory cortices (Figure 11.9). As patients with WC show no clinical signs of dystonia at rest, the results of these resting-state MRI studies suggest that alterations of functional connectivity within subcortical–cortical networks are a pathophysiological predisposition for the development of clinical dystonia symptoms when interacting with a dystonia-specific task.

Structural MRI in dystonia: VBM and DTI

Conventional structural imaging in primary dystonia usually shows no macroscopically detectable abnormalities. On the miscrostructural level, voxel-based morphometry (VBM) and diffusion-based MRI have been applied to investigate changes in gray matter density or fiber integrity. Several VBM studies investigated changes of brain anatomy in different forms of focal dystonia. They showed abnormalities of gray matter density in some parts of the network that has been shown to be abnormally activated in fMRI studies as reported above. One group showed that patients with WC have an increase in gray matter density within the primary somatosensory cortex [33]. Nevertheless, others have shown inconsistent or contradictory findings. Patients with CD showed an increase in gray matter density bilaterally in the motor cortex and in the cerebellar flocculus and unilaterally in the right globus pallidus internus. In addition, a decrease in gray matter density was observed in the right caudal SMA as well as in the right dorsolateral prefrontal and visual cortex [34]. Another study in patients with CD found increased gray matter density in the thalamus, caudate head bilaterally, superior

141

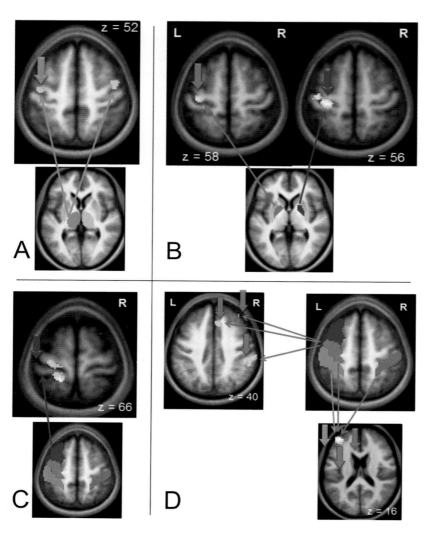

Figure 11.9 Reduced resting-state functional connectivity (FC) in patients with writer's cramp (WC) compared to healthy controls. The figure shows a reduced connectivity of the (A) left thalamus, (B) bilateral pallidum, and (C) left lateral premotor cortex to the hand area of the primary sensorimotor cortex. (D) The FC of the left primary motor cortex to the right pre-SMA, bilateral prefrontal areas, and right somatosensory cortex was impaired in writer's cramp patients. FC maps and ROIs are superimposed onto axial slices of the averaged structural image of all subjects (Montreal Neurological Institute [MNI] z-coordinate in mm) (C. Dresel, Y. Li, F. Castrop, C. Zimmer, B. Haslinger, unpublished data, 2012).

temporal lobe, and left cerebellum, while gray matter was decreased in the putamen bilaterally. In the same study, patients with blepharospasm had increased gray matter in the caudate head and cerebellum bilaterally as well as decreased in the putamen and thalamus bilaterally [35], whereas another study found gray matter increases in the bilateral putamina and decreases in the left inferior parietal lobe [36]. Common increases of gray matter density in patients with idiopathic generalized dystonia, CD, and WC were demonstrated in the globus pallidus internus, nucleus accumbens, prefrontal cortex, as well as unilaterally in the left inferior parietal lobe [37].

Besides these VBM studies of gray matter density, a number of diffusion MRI studies investigated the integrity of gray matter and white matter fiber tracts in patients with dystonia. Most of the studies employed measurements of fractional anisotropy (FA) and mean diffusivity (MD) to show differences in white matter fiber architecture related to dystonia. Carbon and coworkers performed diffusion MRI in clinically asymptomatic as well as symptomatic gene mutation carriers for generalized dystonia [38–40]. In their first study they showed significant reductions of FA in the subgyral white matter of the primary sensorimotor cortex. This finding was more pronounced in manifesting compared to non-manifesting mutation carriers [39]. They interpreted their findings as a sign of disturbed microstructural white matter integrity in afferent or efferent pathways to or from the primary sensorimotor cortex in patients with generalized dystonia. In a second study they showed that in manifesting gene mutation carriers, in addition to this subgyral primary sensorimotor white matter region, FA was reduced in the dorsal pontine brainstem at the base of the left superior cerebellar peduncle [40]. They concluded that this finding reflects either a microstructural alteration of white matter pathways to or from the pedunculopontine nucleus in manifesting mutation carriers, such as those projecting to this region from the internal globus pallidus, those projecting from this region to the thalamus, or both. Alternatively, they discussed that a pathology of white matter integrity close to the superior cerebellar peduncle reflects a role of functional/microstructural disturbances within the cerebello-thalamo-cortical loop in the pathophysiology of dystonia [40]. In a more recent study the same group applied probabilistic fiber tracking using images with high resolution of diffusion orientation to differentiate further these earlier findings of FA abnormalities. They revealed abnormalities in cerebello-thalamic and thalamo-cortical pathways in manifesting and non-manifesting dystonia mutation carriers [41]. In both groups they showed reduced fiber tract integrity in the cerebello-thalamic outflow tract (Figure 11.10). Additionally they performed $H_2^{15}O$ PET scans in a subgroup of these patients to verify if cerebellar connectivity correlates to rCBF as a correlate of brain activity during a motor task and a resting condition. Indeed their results show a positive correlation of cerebellar connectivity with motor activation in the same cerebellar region and resting activity in the thalamus. On the other hand, cerebellar connectivity was negatively correlated to motor activation within primary sensorimotor and supplementary motor areas. This puts reduced cerebello-thalamic connectivity in the context of PET resting-state overactivity as a sign for reduced cortical inhibition in basal ganglia–premotor networks in patients with generalized dystonia that were reported above [29, 30]. On the other hand, additionally reduced connectivity of thalamic projections to the sensorimotor cortex differentiated non-manifesting from clinically manifesting mutation carriers. This was suggested to "protect" the former from the effect of disrupted cerebello-thalamic

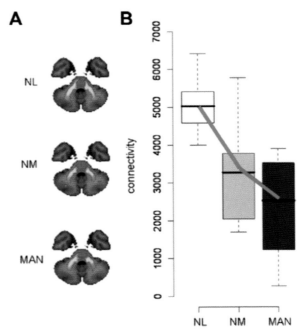

Figure 11.10 Probabilistic fiber tracking showed reduced fiber tract integrity, i.e., reduced connectivity, in the cerebello-thalamic outflow tract in nonmanifesting (NM) and manifesting (MAN) dystonia gene carriers compared to healthy "normal" (NL) controls. (From Argyelan *et al.* [41] by permission of the Society for Neuroscience.)

connectivity on cortical hyperexcitability as it was observed in manifesting mutation carriers.

In patients with idiopathic CD, Bonilha and coworkers showed reduced FA as a measure of axonal fiber integrity in the gray matter and in the white matter in the vicinity of the right thalamus and underlying the right middle frontal gyrus. MD was significantly increased in CD patients in ROIs encompassing the basal ganglia and the adjacent white matter, such as the right and left pallidum, right and left putamen, and left caudate nucleus [42]. This possibly reflects reduced cellular integrity. Applying probabilistic tractography, the same authors demonstrated a disruption of bilateral fiber tracts from the thalamus to the prefrontal cortex, suggesting that structurally abnormal thalamo-prefrontal connectivity plays an important role in the generation of dystonic movements [43]. In contrast to the results of Bonilha and coworkers [42] another diffusion MRI study in patients with CD revealed higher FA and lower MD values in the gray matter of various basal ganglia nuclei (pallidum, putamen, caudate nuclei) [44]. These authors concluded "an increased cellular density with increased fiber coherence in the basal ganglia of patients with CD compared with healthy controls." The same group later confirmed their results in CD patients by showing increased FA in the bilateral putamen compared to decreased MD in the right caudate nucleus and left putamen [45]. Additionally they showed reduced FA in the corpus callosum and increased MD in the bilateral prefrontal cortex and SMA. They concluded that these observations reflect increased cell numbers in the basal ganglia but also suggest reduced cell numbers in the prefrontal cortical areas and SMA.

In patients with WC, Delmaire and coworkers reported increased FA values in the white matter of the posterior limb of the internal capsule, in the adjacent thalamus, and in the white matter of the left posterior centrum semiovale [46]. Fiber tracking showed that especially tracts connecting subcortical (brainstem) with primary motor and sensory cortices near the hand area pass through these areas of increased FA. These tracts include the corticospinal tract, as well as thalamo-cortical and cortico-striatal fibers. Previously, abnormal hemispheric asymmetry in diffusion was observed in a group of patients with CD and hand dystonia in a region presumed to convey pallido-thalamic projections and this finding disappeared after administration of BTX [47].

A sophisticated study examined diffusion characteristics in a group of patients with LD and correlated these changes to postmortem studies of histopathological changes in a small subset of patients [48]. This study demonstrated a decrease of FA in the genu of the right-sided internal capsule and an increased diffusibility in the lentiform nucleus, ventral thalamus, and cerebellar white and gray matter in patients with LD. Reduced FA in the internal capsule was paralleled histopathologically by a loss of axonal density and myelin content in one patient. Furthermore, the authors reported "mineral accumulations in the parenchyma and vessel walls in the internal capsule, putamen, globus pallidus, and cerebellum." They conclude that white matter changes of the corticospinal and corticobulbar tract and within cerebral areas connected with/by these tracts contribute to the pathophysiology of LD.

Taken together, these voxel-based or diffusion-based imaging studies in different forms of focal dystonia show structural changes of gray matter density/integrity, white matter axonal integrity/density, or white matter cellular integrity within essential parts of the subcortical–cortical sensorimotor network. Besides the functional changes within this network as reported in various fMRI studies, this underlines an important role of altered microstructural connectivity in the pathophysiology of focal dystonias.

Summary

Taken together various fMRI, VBM, and DTI studies in patients with (focal) dystonia have shown functional and structural changes within subcortical–cortical sensorimotor networks. These findings have substantially enriched our understanding of the pathophysiology underlying dystonic symptoms.

Some of the changes have been equally detected in different forms of focal dystonias. This suggests a common pathophysiological trait independent of clinical phenotype. Especially when considering the activation level of the primary sensorimotor cortex, results in fMRI studies are inconsistent, with some showing overactivity and others reduced activation levels. This could in part be attributed to methodological differences such as the question to which extent the studied task induces dystonia with consecutive changes in somatosensory feedback or motor output.

On the other hand, functional changes have also been shown during clinically asymptomatic tasks, when examining clinically not affected body parts, despite a clinical improvement following BTX treatment, and recently at rest. Together with the reported microstructural changes, this suggests that many of these findings possibly reflect intrinsic characteristics in patients with dystonia. This could lead to the clinical presentation of dystonia in predisposed individuals. In some patients such a predisposition could contribute to a spread of dystonic symptoms to previously unaffected body parts (for example development of a contralateral WC when switching handwriting to the contralateral hand, development of Meige's syndrome in patients with initially isolated blepharospasm).

Based on possible genetic predisposition these functional and structural changes could lead to the clinical presentation of dedifferentiated motor programs in dystonia. Combining the continuously increasing knowledge about genetic factors with fMRI could further add to our knowledge. Furthermore, a multimodal combination of the above presented MR technologies that up to now have been separately applied in patients with dystonia will give further insights into dystonia pathophysiology.

References

1. Berardelli A, Rothwell JC, Hallett M, et al. The pathophysiology of primary dystonia. *Brain.* 1998;**121**(Pt 7):1195–212.

2. Siebner HR, Tormos JM, Ceballos-Baumann AO, et al. Low-frequency repetitive transcranial magnetic stimulation of the motor cortex in writer's cramp. *Neurology.* 1999;**52**(3):529–37.

3. Byl NN, Merzenich MM, Jenkins WM. A primate genesis model of focal dystonia and repetitive strain injury: I. Learning-induced dedifferentiation of the representation of the hand in the primary somatosensory cortex in adult monkeys. *Neurology.* 1996;**47**(2):508–20.

4. Meunier S, Garnero L, Ducorps A, et al. Human brain mapping in dystonia reveals both endophenotypic traits and adaptive reorganization. *Ann Neurol.* 2001;**50**(4):521–7.

5. Ceballos-Baumann AO, Sheean G, Passingham RE, Marsden CD, Brooks DJ. Botulinum toxin does not reverse the cortical dysfunction associated with writer's cramp. A PET study. *Brain.* 1997;**120**(Pt 4):571–82.

6. Ibanez V, Sadato N, Karp B, Deiber MP, Hallett M. Deficient activation of the motor cortical network in patients with writer's cramp. *Neurology.* 1999;**53**(1):96–105.

7. Oga T, Honda M, Toma K, et al. Abnormal cortical mechanisms of voluntary muscle relaxation in patients with writer's cramp: an fMRI study. *Brain.* 2002;**125**(Pt 4):895–903.

8. Islam T, Kupsch A, Bruhn H, et al. Decreased bilateral cortical representation patterns in writer's cramp: a functional magnetic resonance imaging study at 3.0 T. *Neurol Sci.* 2009;**30**(3):219–26.

9. Pujol J, Roset-Llobet J, Rosines-Cubells D, et al. Brain cortical activation during guitar-induced hand dystonia studied by functional MRI. *Neuroimage.* 2000;**12**(3):257–67.

10. Preibisch C, Berg D, Hofmann E, Solymosi L, Naumann M. Cerebral activation patterns in patients with writer's cramp: a functional magnetic resonance imaging study. *J Neurol.* 2001;**248**(1):10–17.

11. Kadota H, Nakajima Y, Miyazaki M, et al. An fMRI study of musicians with focal dystonia during tapping tasks. *J Neurol.* 2010;**257**(7):1092–8.

12. Beukers RJ, Foncke EM, van der Meer JN, et al. Disorganized sensorimotor integration in mutation-positive myoclonus-dystonia: a functional magnetic resonance imaging study. *Arch Neurol.* 2010;**67**(4):469–74.

13. Castrop F, Dresel C, Hennenlotter A, Zimmer C, Haslinger B. Basal ganglia-premotor dysfunction during movement imagination in writer's cramp. *Mov Disord.* 2012;**27**(11):1432–9.

14. de Vries PM, Johnson KA, de Jong BM, et al. Changed patterns of cerebral activation related to clinically normal hand movement in cervical dystonia. *Clin Neurol Neurosurg.* 2008;**110**(2):120–8.

15. Schmidt KE, Linden DE, Goebel R, et al. Striatal activation during blepharospasm revealed by fMRI. *Neurology.* 2003;**60**(11):1738–43.

16. Obermann M, Yaldizli O, de Greiff A, et al. Increased basal-ganglia activation performing a non-dystonia-related task in focal dystonia. *Eur J Neurol.* 2008;**15**(8):831–8.

17. Dresel C, Haslinger B, Castrop F, Wohlschlaeger AM, Ceballos-Baumann AO. Silent event-related fMRI reveals deficient motor and enhanced somatosensory activation in orofacial dystonia. *Brain.* 2006;**129**(Pt 1):36–46.

18. Haslinger B, Erhard P, Dresel C, et al. "Silent event-related" fMRI reveals reduced sensorimotor activation in laryngeal dystonia. *Neurology.* 2005;**65**(10):1562–9.

19. Simonyan K, Ludlow CL. Abnormal activation of the primary somatosensory cortex in spasmodic dysphonia: an fMRI study. *Cereb Cortex.* 2010;**20**(11):2749–59.

20. Haslinger B, Altenmuller E, Castrop F, Zimmer C, Dresel C. Sensorimotor overactivity as a pathophysiologic trait of embouchure dystonia. *Neurology.* 2010;**74**(22):1790–7.

21. Obermann M, Vollrath C, de Greiff A, et al. Sensory disinhibition on passive movement in cervical dystonia. *Mov Disord.* 2010;**25**(15):2627–33.

22. Dresel C, Parzinger A, Rimpau C, et al. A new device for tactile stimulation during fMRI. *Neuroimage.* 2008;**39**(3):1094–103.

23. Dresel C, Bayer F, Castrop F, et al. Botulinum toxin modulates basal ganglia but not deficient somatosensory activation in orofacial dystonia. *Mov Disord.* 2011;**26**(8):1496–502.

24. Peller M, Zeuner KE, Munchau A, et al. The basal ganglia are hyperactive during the discrimination of tactile stimuli in writer's cramp. *Brain.* 2006;**129**(Pt 10):2697–708.

25. Butterworth S, Francis S, Kelly E, et al. Abnormal cortical sensory activation in dystonia: an fMRI study. *Mov Disord.* 2003;**18**(6):673–82.

26. Nelson AJ, Blake DT, Chen R. Digit-specific aberrations in the primary somatosensory cortex in writer's cramp. *Ann Neurol.* 2009;**66**(2):146–54.

27. Sanger TD, Pascual-Leone A, Tarsy D, Schlaug G. Nonlinear

sensory cortex response to simultaneous tactile stimuli in writer's cramp. *Mov Disord.* 2002;**17**(1):105–11.

28. Delmaire C, Krainik A, Tezenas du Montcel S, *et al.* Disorganized somatotopy in the putamen of patients with focal hand dystonia. *Neurology.* 2005;**64**(8):1391–6.

29. Eidelberg D, Moeller JR, Ishikawa T, *et al.* The metabolic topography of idiopathic torsion dystonia. *Brain.* 1995;**118**(Pt 6):1473–84.

30. Trost M, Carbon M, Edwards C, *et al.* Primary dystonia: is abnormal functional brain architecture linked to genotype? *Ann Neurol.* 2002;**52**(6): 853–6.

31. Blood AJ, Flaherty AW, Choi JK, *et al.* Basal ganglia activity remains elevated after movement in focal hand dystonia. *Ann Neurol.* 2004;**55**(5):744–8.

32. Mohammadi B, Kollewe K, Samii A, *et al.* Changes in resting-state brain networks in writer's cramp. *Hum Brain Mapp.* 2012;**33**(4):840–8.

33. Garraux G, Bauer A, Hanakawa T, *et al.* Changes in brain anatomy in focal hand dystonia. *Ann Neurol.* 2004;**55**(5):736–9.

34. Draganski B, Thun-Hohenstein C, Bogdahn U, Winkler J, May A. "Motor circuit" gray matter changes in idiopathic cervical dystonia. *Neurology.* 2003;**61**(9):1228–31.

35. Obermann M, Yaldizli O, De Greiff A, *et al.* Morphometric changes of sensorimotor structures in focal dystonia. *Mov Disord.* 2007;**22**(8):1117–23.

36. Etgen T, Draganski B, Ilg C, *et al.* Bilateral thalamic gray matter changes in patients with restless legs syndrome. *Neuroimage.* 2005;**24**(4):1242–7.

37. Egger K, Mueller J, Schocke M, *et al.* Voxel based morphometry reveals specific gray matter changes in primary dystonia. *Mov Disord.* 2007;**22**(11):1538–42.

38. Carbon M, Argyelan M, Eidelberg D. Functional imaging in hereditary dystonia. *Eur J Neurol.* 2010;**17** Suppl 1:58–64.

39. Carbon M, Kingsley PB, Su S, *et al.* Microstructural white matter changes in carriers of the DYT1 gene mutation. *Ann Neurol.* 2004;**56**(2):283–6.

40. Carbon M, Kingsley PB, Tang C, Bressman S, Eidelberg D. Microstructural white matter changes in primary torsion dystonia. *Mov Disord.* 2008;**23**(2):234–9.

41. Argyelan M, Carbon M, Niethammer M, *et al.* Cerebellothalamocortical connectivity regulates penetrance in dystonia. *J Neurosci.* 2009;**29**(31):9740–7.

42. Bonilha L, de Vries PM, Vincent DJ, *et al.* Structural white matter abnormalities in patients with idiopathic dystonia. *Mov Disord.* 2007;**22**(8):1110–16.

43. Bonilha L, de Vries PM, Hurd MW, *et al.* Disrupted thalamic prefrontal pathways in patients with idiopathic dystonia. *Parkinsonism Relat Disord.* 2009;**15**(1):64–7.

44. Colosimo C, Pantano P, Calistri V, *et al.* Diffusion tensor imaging in primary cervical dystonia. *J Neurol Neurosurg Psychiatry.* 2005;**76**(11): 1591–3.

45. Fabbrini G, Pantano P, Totaro P, *et al.* Diffusion tensor imaging in patients with primary cervical dystonia and in patients with blepharospasm. *Eur J Neurol.* 2008;**15**(2):185–9.

46. Delmaire C, Vidailhet M, Wassermann D, *et al.* Diffusion abnormalities in the primary sensorimotor pathways in writer's cramp. *Arch Neurol.* 2009;**66**(4):502–8.

47. Blood AJ, Tuch DS, Makris N, *et al.* White matter abnormalities in dystonia normalize after botulinum toxin treatment. *Neuroreport.* 2006;**17**(12): 1251–5.

48. Simonyan K, Tovar-Moll F, Ostuni J, *et al.* Focal white matter changes in spasmodic dysphonia: a combined diffusion tensor imaging and neuropathological study. *Brain.* 2008;**131**(Pt 2):447–59.

Chapter 12

Tauopathies

Jennifer L. Whitwell and Keith A. Josephs

Introduction

Tauopathies

The term "tauopathy" defines a group of heterogeneous pathological disorders that are defined by the deposition of the microtubule-associated protein tau. A number of specific tauopathies have been described, which differ from one another by the distribution and morphological appearance of the protein-containing inclusions [1]. The most common tauopathies include progressive supranuclear palsy (PSP), corticobasal degeneration (CBD), Pick's disease (PiD), and those cases where tau deposition is associated with mutations in the microtubule-associated protein tau (MAPT) gene on chromosome 17. Over 44 different pathogenic mutations in the tau gene have been identified in over 100 families, and include missense mutations, silent mutations, single codon deletions, and intronic mutations. Rarer tauopathies include argyrophilic grain disease, globular glial tauopathy, Niemann–Pick type C, postencephalitic parkinsonism (PEP), subacute sclerosing panencephalitis (SSPE), and tangle-dominant dementia.

Clinical syndromes associated with tauopathies

It was traditionally thought that each tauopathy was associated with a specific clinical syndrome, although recent clinicopathological studies have demonstrated that this is not the case, and that, in fact, the clinical syndromes associated with these pathologically defined disorders are heterogeneous [2]. The tauopathies that are typically associated with motor syndromes, and hence will be the focus of this chapter,

are PSP, CBD, and MAPT mutations (see Table 12.1 for pathological characteristics).

The majority of PSP and CBD cases present as one of two atypical parkinsonian syndromes. The first, which has been referred to as the progressive supranuclear palsy syndrome (PSPS), or Richardson's syndrome, is characterized by postural instability, vertical supranuclear gaze palsy, and falls early in the disease course. The second is an asymmetric syndrome characterized by myoclonus, ideomotor apraxia, and extrapyramidal features, such as rigidity and dystonia, and is referred to as the corticobasal syndrome (CBS). The terms PSPS and CBS will therefore be used to refer to these clinical syndromes, while the terms PSP and CBD will only be used in reference to the pathology [2, 3]. The majority of imaging studies have assessed cohorts defined clinically, rather than pathologically. These clinical and pathological diagnoses are not, however, always the same [4–7]. Cases of PSP most commonly present with PSPS, accounting for approximately 60% of cases, although the CBS is also often observed. In contrast, CBS is more common than PSPS in CBD. Another clinical syndrome that can result from either PSP or CBD is primary progressive apraxia of speech (PPAOS) [8]. This is a motor speech syndrome that is characterized by slow speaking rate, articulatory distortions, distorted sound substitutions, and segmentation of syllables in multisyllabic words or across words. There is a suggestion that the most common pathology to underlie PPAOS is PSP, although CBD can also be observed, especially if patients also develop agrammatism. In addition to these motor-predominant syndromes, CBD also often presents with dementia and cognitive impairment, with patients diagnosed clinically with dementia of the

Table 12.1. Pathological characteristics of the four most common tauopathies

Tauopathy	Tau species	Inclusions	Typical distribution of pathology
PSP	4R	Globose neurofibrillary tangles, tufted astrocytes	Basal ganglia, subthalamic nucleus, substantia nigra, cerebellum, with relative sparing of the cortex
CBD	4R	Neuronal and glial inclusions, including astrocytic plaques, thread-like inclusions, ballooned neurons	Cortex, basal ganglia, thalamus, and brainstem
MAPT	3R, 3 + 4R or 4R	Neuronal and glial cytoplasmic inclusions in oligodendrocytes	Hippocampus, temporal and frontal lobes, subcortical nuclei, and sometimes brainstem and cerebellum
PiD	3R	Argyrophilic rounded intraneuronal inclusions (classic Pick bodies) and ballooned neurons (Pick cell)	Hippocampus, temporal lobe, frontal lobe, subcortical nuclei

PSP, progressive supranuclear palsy; CBD, corticobasal degeneration; MAPT, microtubule-associated protein tau; PiD, Pick's disease; R, repeats (i.e., number of binding domains in the carboxyl terminus of the protein).

Alzheimer's type (DAT), frontotemporal dementia (FTD), or posterior cortical atrophy (PCA).

The clinical symptoms associated with mutations in the *MAPT* gene can be heterogeneous, although patients typically present with the behavioral variant of FTD (bvFTD), characterized by changes in behavior and personality, with additional word finding and comprehension deficits often observed [9]. Parkinsonism can also be the dominant clinical presentation or can occur in addition to the behavioral syndrome, and is usually characterized by gait impairment, rigidity, bradykinesia, postural instability, and resting tremor. Clinical variability tends to occur across specific mutations, with some more associated with the dementia phenotype and others more associated with a parkinsonian syndrome. The pallidopontonigral degeneration (PPND) variant is an example of a parkinsonism-predominant syndrome that is associated with the N279K missense mutation in exon 10 of the tau gene [10]. These patients exhibit rapidly progressive parkinsonism characterized by bradykinesia, tremor, postural instability, and rigidity, and also develop pyramidal signs and eye movement abnormalities. Patients with *MAPT* mutations presenting with PSPS, CBS, or DAT have also been observed. In contrast to CBD and PSP, which are typically sporadic, mutations in the *MAPT* gene are inherited with an autosomal dominant penetrance and hence patients usually present with a family history. This disorder is often therefore referred to as familial FTD dementia and parkinsonism linked to chromosome 17 (FTDP-17). Since this is a genetic disorder, cohorts of patients for imaging studies can be identified using genetic testing, without requiring further pathological confirmation.

Patients with PiD usually present with behavioral and personality changes, and are diagnosed with bvFTD. However, word finding and comprehension deficits, or agrammatism, can also be observed as the prominent abnormality or develop later in the disease course. Parkinsonism is not usually a presenting feature, but can develop later in the disease course. A diagnosis of PiD can only be made with confidence at autopsy [1].

Role of neuroimaging in tauopathies

The most important role of neuroimaging is first, and foremost, to identify potentially treatable causes of cognitive and motor impairment, for example brain tumors, strokes, hydrocephalus, and subdural hematomas. Both computed tomography (CT) and magnetic resonance imaging (MRI) scanning will detect most of these pathologies. However, neuroimaging is also an invaluable tool to help characterize changes in brain structure and function in neurodegenerative disorders and potentially aid in clinical diagnosis.

A number of different MRI techniques are now available that allow the interrogation of different structural and functional properties of the brain:

1. **Structural MRI:** This is one of the most widely used imaging techniques and allows the

assessment of focal atrophy of the gray and white matter (typically using T_1-weighted sequences), as well as signal changes within brain tissue (typically using T_2-weighted sequences or fluid-attenuated inversion recovery, FLAIR, sequences). Detailed manual measurements can be performed on specific brain structures and sophisticated software, such as voxel-based morphometry and FreeSurfer, allows automated assessment of atrophy.

2. **Diffusion tensor imaging (DTI)**: Assesses the diffusion of water molecules through brain tissue in multiple different directions allowing the visualization of specific white matter tracts and the detection of tract degeneration.

3. **Proton magnetic resonance spectroscopy (MRS)**: Measures signals from several different metabolites within brain tissue. Each metabolite is sensitive to a different aspect of in vivo pathological processes at the molecular or cellular level, for example N-acetylaspartate (NAA), which is located in neuron bodies, axons, and dendrites and is a sensitive marker for neuronal integrity; choline (Cho), which is a potential marker of phospholipid membrane breakdown; and *myo*-inositol (*myo*-Ins), which is present in glial cells, with increased levels being associated with gliosis. The metabolite creatine (Cr) is relatively stable in neurodegenerative disease and is often used as a reference metabolite.

4. **Resting-state functional MRI (fMRI)**: Measures changes in brain functional connectivity while the patient is at rest in the scanner. Spontaneous neural activity occurs in the brain during rest and is organized into specific functional networks in which the low frequency changes in fMRI signal

intensity are highly correlated or in-phase. These networks appear to relate to structurally connected neuroanatomical systems, such as the visual, executive and memory networks, and can each be measured using resting-state fMRI. Functional connectivity between specific regions of the brain can also be measured.

Nuclear medicine techniques are also available which allow the assessment of different aspects of brain metabolism. The most commonly utilized methods are ^{18}F-fluorodeoxyglucose positron emission tomography (FDG-PET), which assesses glucose uptake, and Tc99m Neurolite or technetium-hexamethylpropyleneamine oxime (HMPAO) single-photon emission computed tomography (SPECT) imaging, which measures cerebral blood flow. The integrity of the dopaminergic system can also be assessed using presynaptic dopamine transporter ligands or postsynaptic dopamine D2 receptor ligands and either PET or SPECT imaging. These later techniques demonstrate abnormalities in the striatum and have been shown to be particularly sensitive to parkinsonian syndromes. They can be useful to differentiate these syndromes from syndromes without a dopamine deficit, such as dystonic and severe essential tremors and drug-induced Parkinsonism.

Imaging in CBD and PSP

The structural and functional neuroimaging features of the clinical syndromes known to be associated with PSP and CBD, such as PSPS, CBS, and PPAOS, have been well characterized (Table 12.2). A high proportion of patients with these syndromes will have an underlying tauopathy; although, as discussed in the section on clinical syndromes associated with

Table 12.2. Distribution of atrophy in the clinical syndromes commonly associated with CBD and PSP pathology

	Cortex				Striatum	Brainstem
	Prefrontal	**Premotor**	**Parietal**	**Temporal**		
PSPS	−	+	−	−	+	++
CBS	+	++	+	−	++	−
Hybrid syndrome*	++	++	+		++	++
PPAOS	−	+	−	−	−	−

− = typically normal, + = mild, ++ = moderate to severe.
* Patients with the hybrid syndrome display clinical features of both PSPS and the CBS.
PSPS, progressive supranuclear palsy syndrome; CBS, corticobasal syndrome; PPAOS, primary progressive apraxia of speech.

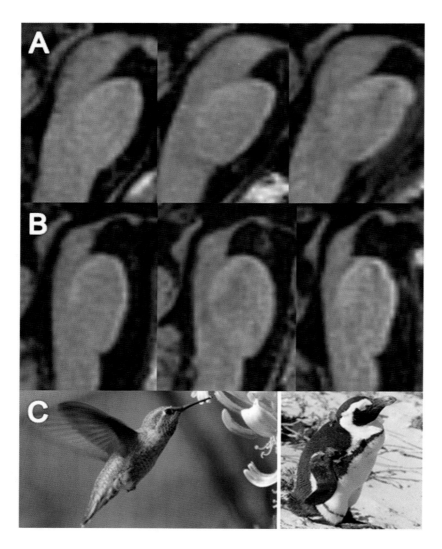

Figure 12.1 Sagittal volumetric MRI of the brainstem from three normal subjects (A) and three patients with PSPS (B). The characteristic pattern of midbrain atrophy with sparing of the pons in PSPS has been referred to as the "hummingbird" or "penguin" sign (C).

tauopathies, the pathological diagnosis could be either PSP or CBD. The imaging features associated with these syndromes are therefore not necessarily attributable to a specific pathology. Less work has focused on characterizing pathologically confirmed PSP and CBD due to difficulty obtaining cohorts of patients with pathological confirmation and standardized neuroimaging in these relatively rare disorders [11].

Progressive supranuclear palsy syndrome
Structural MRI

Atrophy of the midbrain is the most striking, and diagnostically useful, feature observed on MRI in patients with PSPS. Relative sparing of the pons,

in comparison to severe atrophy of the midbrain, produces a classic "hummingbird" or "penguin" sign (Figure 12.1). The area of the midbrain is often reduced by as much as 50% compared to a normal subject (Figure 12.2). In fact, a simple ratio of midbrain to pons area can help distinguish PSPS from other parkinsonian disorders, such as Parkinson's disease (PD) [12], and the parkinsonian form of multiple system atrophy (MSA) [13] which are not associated with atrophy of the midbrain. There is also some evidence to suggest that patients with a small midbrain are likely to progress faster clinically [14].

The superior cerebellar peduncles are also strikingly atrophic in PSPS (Figure 12.3) [15], which contrasts to a relative sparing of the middle cerebellar

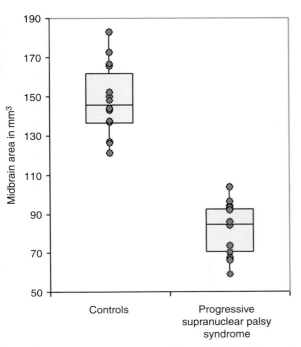

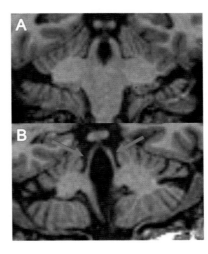

Figure 12.3 Coronal volumetric MRI from a normal subject (A) and a subject with PSPS (B) demonstrating atrophy of the superior cerebellar peduncles (red arrows).

Figure 12.2 Box-plot showing area of the midbrain for 14 normal controls and 14 patients with PSPS. No overlap is observed between groups. Each box indicates the lower quartile (25th percentile), the median, and the upper quartile (75th percentile) of the distribution. All subjects are individually indicated.

peduncles. An MRI parkinsonism index, which considers measurements of these structures along with the midbrain to pons ratio ([pons/midbrain] × [middle cerebellar peduncle/superior cerebellar peduncle]) [16], has been proposed as a useful diagnostic marker for PSPS, although it does not appear to add much diagnostic utility over and above the simple midbrain to pons ratio. Measurements of the cerebellar peduncles are difficult to perform and, due to the small size, require high-resolution MRI.

Mild cortical atrophy is observed in patients with PSPS, usually restricted to the frontal lobes. The focus of atrophy appears to be the premotor cortex, including both lateral and medial (supplementary motor area) regions, but atrophy also spreads forward into the prefrontal cortex (Figure 12.4) [17]. Cortical patterns of atrophy can be variable across patients, although premotor findings are relatively consistent. Involvement of the prefrontal cortex is typically observed in patients that develop behavioral abnormalities and executive dysfunction [18].

Striatal atrophy, particularly involving the caudate nucleus, has also been implicated in PSPS, and

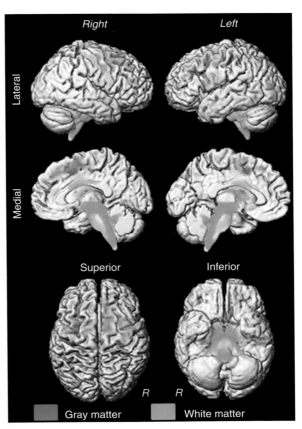

Figure 12.4 Three-dimensional renderings of the brain showing patterns of gray and white matter atrophy in a group of patients with PSPS compared to a group of normal subjects. Gray matter atrophy is observed in the medial and lateral posterior superior frontal lobe and caudate nucleus. White matter atrophy is observed in the brainstem, body of the corpus callosum, and underlying premotor cortex. Analysis was performed using voxel-based morphometry and SPM5 software (http://www.fil.ion.ucl.ac.uk/spm).

151

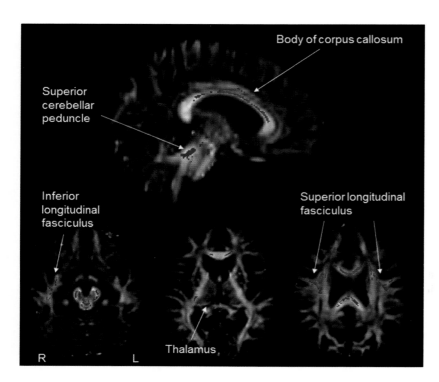

Superior
cerebellar
peduncle

Body of corpus callosum

Inferior
longitudinal
fasciculus

Superior longitudinal
fasciculus

Thalamus

R   L

Figure 12.5 Regions of white matter tract degeneration (shown in red) observed in a cohort of patients with PSPS. White matter tract degeneration is observed in the superior cerebellar peduncle, body of the corpus callosum, superior longitudinal fasciculus, inferior longitudinal fasciculus, and in the white matter laminae of the thalamus. Analysis was performed using tract-based spatial statistics and FSL software (http://www.fmrib.ox.ac.uk/fsl).

may also contribute to behavioral dysfunction [18]. Careful manual measurements of striatal structures show reductions of approximately 17% in caudate volume and 10% in putamen volume in PSPS compared to controls, with shape changes also observed in the caudate nucleus [19]. Regions of the caudate nucleus that are particularly atrophic tend to be regions associated with frontostriatal and corticostriatal circuits.

Both brainstem and cortical atrophy is progressive in nature, with decline in volume observed over time. Whole brain volumes decline at approximately 1.2% per year, with midbrain area changing at an impressive rate of 10% per year. Rates of midbrain atrophy in PSPS are significantly higher than those observed in normal subjects and patients with PD, suggesting some potential diagnostic utility. In addition, the use of a rate of midbrain atrophy as an outcome measure in a clinical trial would reduce the number of patients required to detect a treatment effect, compared to the use of whole brain atrophy or a clinical measure of disease severity. This is particularly important with the advent of potential treatments for tauopathies, since PSPS patients are a likely target.

Diffusion tensor imaging

Widespread white matter tract degeneration is observed in PSPS using diffusion tensor imaging (DTI). Consistent with structural MRI data, the superior cerebellar peduncles are particularly severely affected [20], with degeneration also observed in the cerebellar white matter tracts and the white matter laminae of the thalamus (Figure 12.5) [17]. This demonstrates involvement along the entire extent of the dentatorubrothalamic tract which runs from the cerebellum, through the superior cerebellar peduncles, synapsing in the ventrolateral thalamus. Diffusion in the superior cerebellar peduncles correlates well with clinical disease severity [21], suggesting that degeneration of these structures is central to the development of the clinical syndrome.

The body of the corpus callosum is heavily affected, with a relative sparing of the genu and splenium. This likely reflects degeneration of the commissural fibers connecting adjacent regions of the posterior frontal and premotor cortices that are commonly atrophic in PSPS. Association fibers that run through the premotor cortex and frontal lobes, particularly the superior longitudinal fasciculus, are also abnormal in PSPS. Intriguingly, DTI abnormalities in the anterior superior longitudinal fasciculus have been associated with the severity of saccadic eye impairments [21], suggesting a role for this white matter tract and the associated cortical regions in this clinical sign, although further study will be needed to confirm this finding. The inferior fronto-occipital fasciculus can also be abnormal in PSPS, particularly in the patients with frontal cognitive symptoms [22].

In contrast to the relatively focal cortical patterns of atrophy, which are observed almost exclusively in the frontal lobe, DTI abnormalities have also been observed within the temporal lobes, involving the inferior longitudinal fasciculus. White matter tract abnormalities therefore appear to be more widespread than gray matter atrophy, perhaps suggesting that white matter tract degeneration may precede cortical atrophy in PSPS. Of note, the corticospinal tracts are typically spared in PSPS, which differentiates it from primary lateral sclerosis (PLS).

The diagnostic utility of these specific DTI tract measurements is currently unknown and will likely be limited by the fact that analysis requires sophisticated software that is not, at the moment, suitable for clinical use. However, manual measurements of midbrain and superior cerebellar peduncle diffusivity from diffusion-weighted imaging, which is routinely used clinically, show promise for helping to differentiate PSPS from PD and MSA, which do not show abnormalities in these regions.

Magnetic resonance spectroscopy

Magnetic resonance spectroscopy (MRS) findings in PSPS are heterogeneous. Levels of the neuronal marker NAA, when expressed as a ratio of Cr or Cho, have been observed to be reduced in the putamen and frontal cortex in patients with PSPS compared to controls. However, these findings are not consistent, with others failing to find any reductions. There is a suggestion that levels of NAA in PSPS differ from those observed in PD, which does not typically show any abnormal metabolites on MRS; although variability across patients and studies precludes any real utility of MRS in differential diagnosis [23].

Nuclear medicine

Patients with PSPS show well-characterized functional deficits on both FDG-PET and cerebral blood flow SPECT imaging, with hypometabolism and

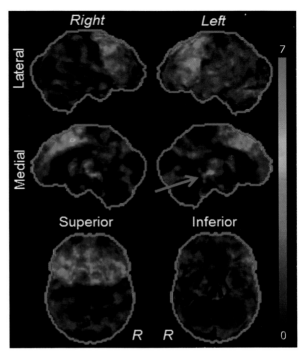

Figure 12.6 Statistical stereotactic surface projection maps showing patterns of FDG-PET hypometabolism in a patient with PSPS. Hypometabolism is observed in the posterior frontal lobe and midbrain (arrow). The z score values represent differences from a normal cohort and are color coded as indicated in the color scale (0 = normal; 7 = most abnormal).

hypoperfusion observed in the frontal lobes, striatum, thalamus, and midbrain; changes that can be observed early in the disease course. Frontal abnormalities are typically posterior, involving the premotor cortex, and do not tend to involve the prefrontal cortex heavily (Figure 12.6). Patterns of prefrontal hypometabolism or hypoperfusion would be more suggestive of FTD.

Striatal dopamine binding, measured using both dopamine transporter and D2 receptor ligands, has also been observed to be decreased in patients with PSPS. Decreased striatal dopamine binding is also observed in PD and MSA, although it is more severely affected in PSPS [24]. However, given the heterogeneity observed across patients, it is difficult to detect subtle differences across these diseases in individual patients. Dopamine imaging therefore appears to be very sensitive, but not specific, for PSPS.

The advantage of these nuclear medicine techniques, however, is that scans can be interpreted in individual patients, and therefore can be very useful in a clinical setting. It is much more difficult to get a clear picture of the regional distribution of atrophy on a single MRI scan.

Resting-state fMRI

Disruptions in functional connectivity within the brain have been observed in patients with PSPS [17]. Specifically, functional connectivity is reduced between the thalamus and a network of gray matter regions, including the lateral premotor cortex, supplementary motor area, prefrontal cortex, striatum, and cerebellum. These findings suggest that connectivity between regions along the dentatorubrothalamic tract is disrupted in these patients. Disrupted connectivity is likely due to degeneration of the white matter tracts which connect these structures. As discussed in the section on diffusion tensor imaging above, degeneration of the superior cerebellar peduncles is indeed observed in patients with PSPS. Degeneration of this tract may result in reduced connectivity within the thalamus.

Corticobasal syndrome
Structural MRI

Brain atrophy in patients with CBS typically targets the cortex and striatum, without any appreciable atrophy in the brainstem. Cortical atrophy is observed predominantly in posterior regions of the frontal lobe, including the medial and lateral premotor cortices, although additional atrophy is often noted in the superior parietal lobe (Figure 12.7). The temporal lobes may become involved in some patients. Cortical atrophy is also strikingly asymmetric in the majority of CBS patients (Figure 12.8), reflecting the asymmetric nature of the clinical symptoms. Greatest atrophy is observed in the hemisphere contralateral to the side of the more affected limb. The presence of cortical asymmetry and lack of midbrain atrophy differentiates CBS from PSPS [25].

Importantly, however, the pathology underlying the CBS is heterogeneous and the patterns of atrophy vary according to pathology (Figure 12.9) [26]. All patients, regardless of pathology, show atrophy in the premotor cortex, although greater additional involvement of the temporal and parietal lobes is predictive of underlying Alzheimer's disease (AD) pathology, and greater involvement of the prefrontal cortex is predictive of underlying frontotemporal lobar degeneration (FTLD) characterized by the protein TDP-43.

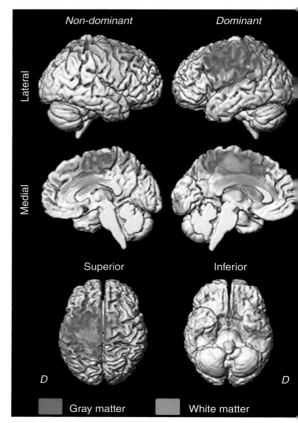

Figure 12.7 Three-dimensional renderings of the brain showing patterns of gray and white matter atrophy in a group of patients with CBS compared to a group of normal subjects. Gray and white matter atrophy is observed in posterior frontal and parietal lobes, with additional white matter atrophy in the body of the corpus callosum. Patterns of atrophy are asymmetric with more severe involvement of the dominant hemisphere. Analysis was performed using voxel-based morphometry and SPM5 software (http://www.fil ion.ucl.ac.uk/spm). All images were flipped so that the dominant hemisphere was on the same side of the image.

Generally, more widespread patterns of atrophy therefore point towards an underlying AD or FTLD, whereas more focal patterns predominantly involving the premotor cortex suggest an underlying tauopathy (CBD or PSP).

Diffusion tensor imaging

Patterns of white matter tract degeneration in CBS reflect the frontoparietal patterns of cortical atrophy, and predominantly involve frontoparietal association fibers, as well as intraparietal associative fibers and the body and splenium of the corpus callosum [27]. Degeneration of the frontoparietal association fibers, as well as parietal atrophy, may be involved in the

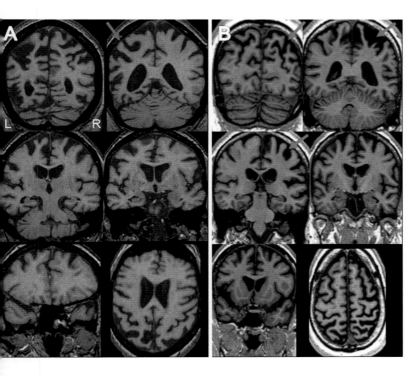

Figure 12.8 Volumetric MRI from two patients with CBS. Patient A is a 71-year-old female patient with pathological confirmation of CBD. Patient B is a 58-year-old male patient who was still alive. Both show asymmetric atrophy in the superior parietal and posterior frontal lobes, with a relative sparing of the temporal lobes and prefrontal cortex.

development of limb apraxia, a characteristic feature of CBS [27]. Degeneration of motor pathways, particularly the corticospinal tracts, has also been observed [28], which may reflect the fact that these patients do sometimes develop motor features such as the Babinski sign, hyperreflexia, and spasticity.

White matter tract degeneration is typically asymmetric, with greatest degeneration observed in the hemisphere that shows greatest atrophy. The presence of hemispheric asymmetry in measures of white matter diffusion allows excellent discrimination of CBS from PSPS and PD, neither of which typically displays asymmetry [29].

Magnetic resonance spectroscopy

Patients with CBS consistently show reductions in the ratio of NAA/Cr within a number of brain regions, including the putamen and frontal and parietal lobes, highlighting severe neuronal damage in these patients. Findings are often asymmetric, with hemispheric differences in the magnitude of 20% in the majority of patients. Asymmetry is typically observed in patients who are also asymmetric clinically. Reductions in NAA/Cr are typically worse than those

observed in MSA or PD [30], concordant with the fact that CBS also shows more widespread cortical atrophy compared to these other disorders.

Nuclear medicine

Patterns of hypometabolism on FDG-PET and hypoperfusion on cerebral blood flow SPECT imaging have been observed in patients with CBS, involving the lateral premotor cortex, supplementary motor area, prefrontal lobes, superior parietal lobes, striatum, and the thalamus (Figure 12.10). The temporal lobes are often normal, although not always. Patterns are more severe in the dominant hemisphere, with similar, albeit milder, patterns observed in the non-dominant hemisphere.

Findings on FDG-PET and SPECT are usually more severe and widespread than those observed in patients with PSPS, and tend to show particularly greater involvement of the parietal lobes, with less involvement of the midbrain. Patterns also have a greater tendency to be asymmetric in CBS. Visual assessment of these scans may be diagnostically helpful, although variability observed across patients can make it difficult. Some of the variability observed is

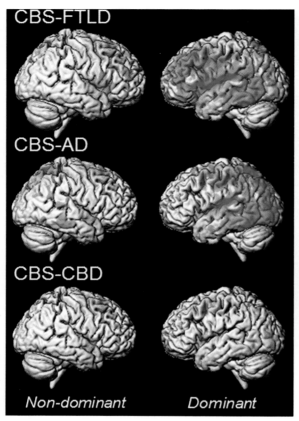

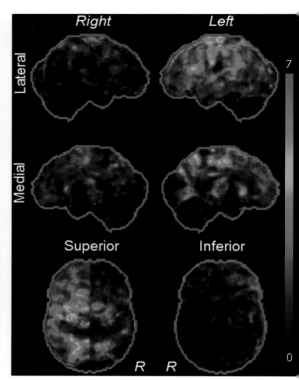

Figure 12.10 Statistical stereotactic surface projection maps showing patterns of FDG-PET hypometabolism in a patient with CBS. Hypometabolism is observed in the left posterior frontal lobes, parietal lobes and caudate nucleus. The z score values represent differences from a normal cohort and are color coded as indicated in the color scale (0 = normal; 7 = most abnormal).

Figure 12.9 Three-dimensional renderings of the brain demonstrating how patterns of gray matter atrophy differ in patients with CBS who have different underlying pathologies. Corticobasal syndrome patients with frontotemporal lobar degeneration (FTLD) pathology show widespread atrophy of the frontal and temporal lobes, whereas those with Alzheimer's disease (AD) show more temporoparietal patterns of atrophy. Less severe patterns of atrophy are observed in patients with CBD. However, all groups show atrophy in the premotor cortex.

likely explained by different underlying pathologies. For example, patterns of parietal hypoperfusion in CBS may be associated with AD, whereas more pronounced frontal patterns may be more associated with CBD [31].

Dopamine transporter imaging is typically abnormal in patients with CBS, with decreased uptake observed in the caudate and putamen and significant hemispheric asymmetry [32]. These abnormalities tend to be less pronounced than in PSPS. In contrast, patients with CBS rarely show reduced uptake with postsynaptic D2 receptors [33]. This contrasts with findings in patients with PSPS where postsynaptic D2 receptors are usually abnormal.

Progressive supranuclear palsy corticobasal syndrome hybrid

The differential diagnosis between PSPS and CBS is often difficult, and patients can present with clinical features of both syndromes, and hence meet clinical criteria for both syndromes. For example, falls and vertical supranuclear palsy can co-exist with asymmetric rigidity and ideomotor apraxia. In these cases, patients display the imaging features typical for both of these syndromes (Table 12.2 and Figure 12.11) [34]. Hence, atrophy is observed in the superior cerebellar peduncles and midbrain, similar to PSPS, with widespread cortical atrophy involving the frontal and parietal lobes which is typical of CBS. These hybrid patterns of atrophy explain the overlapping clinical features. Atrophy of the body of the corpus callosum and the caudate nuclei is also observed, similar to both PSPS and CBS.

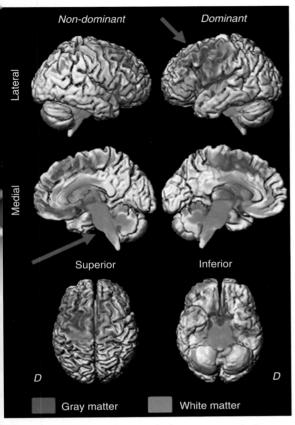

Figure 12.11 Patterns of gray and white matter atrophy in patients with the progressive supranuclear palsy corticobasal syndrome hybrid compared to controls. Patients show brainstem atrophy (longer arrow) typical for PSPS, and widespread cortical atrophy (shorter arrow) typical for CBS. Analysis was performed using voxel-based morphometry and SPM5 software (http://www.fil.ion.ucl.ac.uk/spm). All images were flipped so that the dominant hemisphere was on the same side of the image.

Primary progressive apraxia of speech

Patients with PPAOS show focal patterns of cortical abnormalities on MRI, with atrophy restricted to the supplementary motor area and lateral superior premotor cortex (Figure 12.12) [8]. White matter atrophy is observed in these same regions, although it also spreads into prefrontal and precentral regions. Patterns of atrophy are typically bilateral, although they can be asymmetric in some patients. When atrophy is asymmetric, patients are most likely to show greater involvement of the left hemisphere. Degeneration is observed in white matter tracts underlying these regions of atrophy, with abnormalities observed in premotor aspects of the superior longitudinal

fasciculus and body of the corpus callosum. Hypometabolism on FDG-PET is also typically observed in the lateral superior premotor cortex and supplementary motor area, although patterns are very mild and can be relatively normal in some patients.

Imaging in pathologically confirmed PSP and CBD

Predicting the presence of PSP or CBD pathology is difficult clinically, given that the clinical syndromes associated with these tauopathies overlap to a large degree. It is therefore important also to consider neuroimaging features that are associated with these pathological diagnoses, regardless of clinical syndrome [11].

Both PSP and CBD are associated with atrophy in the posterior superior frontal lobe, with involvement of the premotor cortex. However, the degree of cortical atrophy differs, with more widespread and severe atrophy observed in CBD [35]. Gray matter atrophy in CBD typically extends further forward into the prefrontal cortex, further backwards into the parietal lobe, and down into the inferior frontal gyri compared to PSP. Subcortical gray matter structures are also involved to a greater degree in CBD than PSP. Therefore, both CBD and PSP should be considered in the differential diagnosis if atrophy is focused on the posterior frontal lobes, although CBD pathology is more likely if severe patterns of gray matter atrophy are observed, particularly with involvement of the basal ganglia. Rates of whole brain atrophy observed over time are also significantly higher in patients with CBD (approximately 3% per year compared to 1% per year in PSP) [36], likely reflecting the more severe cortical atrophy.

While the posterior superior frontal lobe atrophy appears to be a consistent finding in both PSP and CBD, atrophy observed in other regions of the brain can vary across patients and give rise to differing clinical presentations. Patients with dementia typically show more severe involvement of the cortex than those with an extrapyramidal dominant syndrome for both PSP and CBD [35], reflecting a shifting of pathology to the cortex in those with dementia. For example, CBD patients with PCA show additional involvement of the parietal and occipital lobes and subjects with bvFTD show additional involvement of prefrontal cortices; patterns which are typically associated with these clinical syndromes.

157

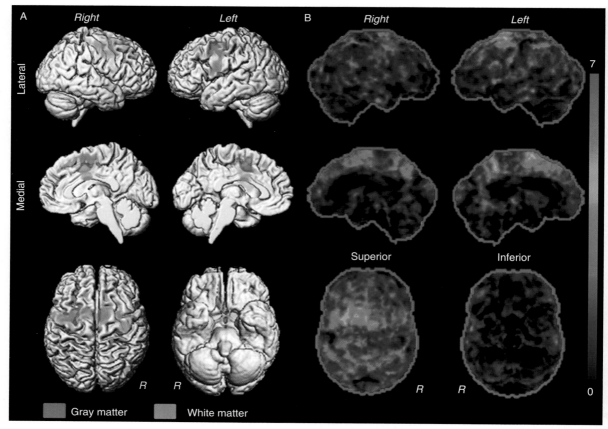

Figure 12.12 Imaging findings in PPAOS. (A) Three-dimensional renderings of the brain showing patterns of gray and white matter atrophy in a group of patients with PPAOS compared to a group of normal subjects. Analysis was performed using voxel-based morphometry and SPM5 software (http://www.fil.ion.ucl.ac.uk/spm). (B) Statistical stereotactic surface projection maps showing patterns of FDG-PET hypometabolism in a patient with PPAOS. Atrophy and hypometabolism particularly target the superior premotor cortex, with white matter atrophy also observed in the inferior premotor cortex and body of the corpus callosum.

Brainstem atrophy is typically involved to a greater degree in PSP than CBD, although it is unclear whether brainstem involvement is associated with PSP in general or with PSP presenting as PSPS. Brainstem atrophy is indeed worse in PSP patients that present with an extrapyramidal syndrome compared to a dementia syndrome, and one may suspect that a CBD patient with PSPS would show brainstem atrophy. Involvement of the brainstem may therefore be a better marker of PSPS, than PSP pathology.

Similarly, the presence of asymmetric patterns of atrophy appears to be a better marker of the presence of CBS, rather than CBD pathology, since CBD cases can be symmetric [37]. Symmetric CBD cases tend to present with more symmetric clinical syndromes, such as bvFTD or PSPS. The degree of asymmetry observed in groups of CBD cases will therefore

depend upon how cases are ascertained, and the proportion that show the typical asymmetric CBS.

Imaging in familial *MAPT* mutations
Structural MRI

Patterns of atrophy observed in patients with mutations in *MAPT* are strikingly different from those observed in PSP and CBD [11]. Atrophy most commonly affects the frontal and temporal lobes, although usually most severely targets the temporal lobes [38, 39] (Figure 12.13). Temporal lobe atrophy can be striking and is a consistent feature across different mutations, although the anteromedial temporal lobes are particularly targeted in some mutations, while others target the lateral temporal lobes

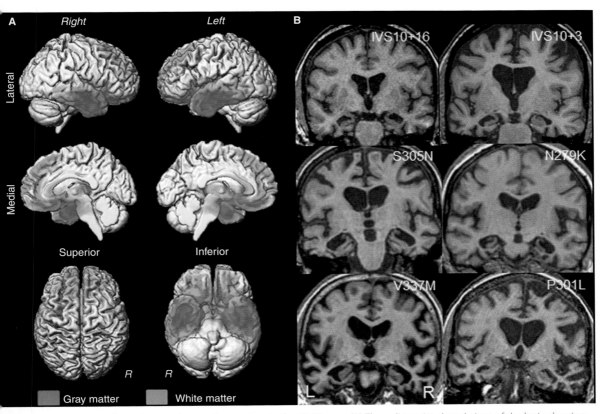

Figure 12.13 Patterns of atrophy in patients with mutations in the *MAPT* gene. (A) Three-dimensional renderings of the brain showing patterns of gray and white matter atrophy in a group of patients with *MAPT* mutations compared to a group of normal subjects. Gray and white matter atrophy is observed predominantly in the anterior temporal lobes, with some involvement of the frontal lobes. White matter atrophy is observed in the genu of the corpus callosum. Analysis was performed using voxel-based morphometry and SPM5 software (http://www.fil.ion.ucl.ac.uk/spm). (B) Coronal volumetric MRI from six patients with different *MAPT* mutations illustrating medial temporal or lateral temporal atrophy.

(Figure 12.13) [39]. Severe involvement of the temporal lobes explains why many patients show deficits in episodic and semantic memory, in addition to the typical behavioral and personality changes. Atrophy is also often observed in the orbitofrontal and insular cortices, with relative sparing of the parietal lobes. Although not necessarily a consistent finding, patients have also been reported with atrophy of the striatum and brainstem, likely reflecting the parkinsonian features that can be observed in *MAPT* patients.

Patterns of atrophy in *MAPT* patients are relatively symmetric (Figure 12.13), although asymmetry has been observed in individual patients, without any particular hemispheric preference. Regional patterns of atrophy can also be variable across patients with different mutations and even across patients within the same family. The basis for this neuroanatomical heterogeneity is not currently well understood.

Progressive brain atrophy is observed in patients with *MAPT* mutations, with rates of whole brain atrophy of between 1.5% and 2.5% per year and rates of hippocampal atrophy of approximately 8% per year [39–41]. These rates of hippocampal atrophy are even higher than those observed in DAT. Rates of whole brain atrophy are approximately linear over time in symptomatic patients [39, 41], meaning that the rates of atrophy will be approximately the same at any point in the disease and do not appear to accelerate or decelerate over the first few years after the patient has developed symptoms.

Importantly, many *MAPT* families are recruited and followed at institutions around the world, allowing for the assessment of family members that carry the mutation but have not yet developed any symptoms. This provides an invaluable opportunity to assess the earliest stages of the disease. Atrophy has

159

been observed during this presymptomatic phase of the disease, with rates of whole brain atrophy of 1.4% per year which accelerate as the patient becomes closer to symptom onset [38]. There is a suggestion that the medial temporal lobe, particularly the hippocampus, may be one of the earliest structures to become involved [42, 43]. It is, however, unclear how early atrophic changes can be detected. It is likely that the time that these changes are observed before symptom onset may vary across patients and mutations.

Diffusion tensor imaging

Little is currently known about the patterns of white matter tract degeneration associated with familial *MAPT* mutations. It is likely however, given the severe atrophy of the temporal lobes, that temporal lobe white matter tracts will also be affected, such as the inferior longitudinal fasciculus and the uncinate fasciculus. Degeneration of these tracts is indeed observed in patients with bvFTD, which is the most common clinical phenotype associated with *MAPT* mutations. Patients with bvFTD also show degeneration of the superior longitudinal fasciculus, anterior cingulate, and the genu of the corpus callosum, reflecting involvement of the frontal lobes.

Magnetic resonance spectroscopy

Only one study to date has assessed MRS in patients with *MAPT* mutations [44]. Symptomatic patients with *MAPT* mutations showed decreased NAA/Cr ratios and increased *myo*-Ins/Cr ratios in the medial parietal lobe compared to controls. As discussed previously, the NAA/Cr ratio provides a marker of neuronal integrity and likely reflects the presence of neuronal loss in these patients. The elevated *myo*-Ins/Cr ratio may suggest the additional presence of gliosis.

Interestingly, presymptomatic patients with *MAPT* mutations also showed elevated *myo*-Ins/Cr ratios, but did not show any abnormalities in the NAA/Cr ratio. These patients also did not show any hippocampal atrophy. These findings suggest that changes in *myo*-Ins/Cr may occur early in the disease process, and are followed later by changes in NAA/Cr and hippocampal atrophy. Microglial activation may therefore precede neuronal loss and atrophy in this tauopathy. Decreases in the NAA/Cr ratio and hippocampal volume also appear to be associated with

proximity to the age at symptom onset. These changes may therefore not be observed until shortly before symptom onset. It therefore seems as though it may be possible to detect biochemical abnormalities related to neurodegeneration years before symptom onset in patients with *MAPT* mutations. However, these observations all came from one study and will need to be replicated, with MRS findings assessed in other regions that are relevant to the disease process, such as the frontal and temporal lobes.

Resting-state fMRI

Disruptions in functional connectivity are associated with the clinical syndrome most commonly observed in patients with *MAPT* mutations, that is bvFTD. These patients commonly show reduced connectivity within the frontal lobe salience network [45, 46]; a network that plays a role in processing social-emotional and homeostatically relevant stimuli. These disruptions are observed in the frontoinsular cortex and anterior cingulate. However, regional disruptions are also observed within the default mode network, with reduced connectivity observed in the temporal lobes and medial prefrontal cortex [46], and increased connectivity observed in the medial parietal lobes [45, 46]. Patterns of reduced connectivity in both networks occur in regions that typically show atrophy and hypometabolic changes. The increases in connectivity in the medial parietal lobe reflect the fact that the salience network and default mode network are, in fact, anti-correlated to each other [45]. Therefore, impairment in the salience network is thought to alter the responses in the posterior default mode network, leading to enhanced parietal lobe connectivity. Interestingly, the reverse pattern is observed in DAT, whereby impairment in the posterior default mode network leads to enhanced connectivity in the salience network.

These changes in functional connectivity within the salience and default mode network have also been observed in symptomatic patients with mutations in the *MAPT* gene [46]. In addition, disrupted connectivity has been demonstrated in presymptomatic patients with *MAPT* mutations, with decreased connectivity observed in the temporal lobes and medial prefrontal cortex within the default mode network (Figure 12.14) [46]. These changes in connectivity occurred in the absence of any atrophy, showing, importantly, that changes in functional connectivity

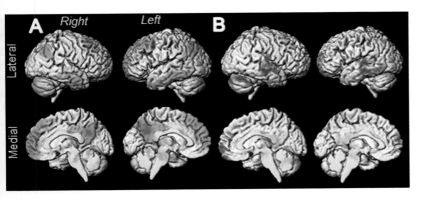

Figure 12.14 Resting-state fMRI findings in the default mode network in asymptomatic individuals with mutations in the *MAPT* gene. The default mode network is shown in A. Patterns of reduced (shown in purple) and increased (shown in orange) connectivity in the asymptomatic individuals are shown in B. Reduced connectivity is observed in the lateral temporal lobes, medial prefrontal cortex, and cerebellum. Increased connectivity is observed in the medial parietal lobes.

precede the occurrence of atrophy in these regions. These changes within the default mode network were more striking than changes in the salience network, likely reflecting the fact that *MAPT* mutations are associated with predominantly temporal lobe involvement, with less striking involvement of regions involved in the salience network. This explanation also fits with the fact that atrophic changes in presymptomatic individuals, if present, are usually observed within the temporal lobe. However, the presymptomatic individuals still showed enhanced connectivity in the posterior default mode network. The reason that this is observed, in the absence of decreased connectivity in the salience network, is not currently understood, although it may reflect measurement sensitivity or disrupted temporal sequencing of events in these patients.

Nuclear medicine

Hypometabolism on FDG-PET and hypoperfusion on cerebral blood flow SPECT imaging are predominantly observed in the temporal lobes, involving both lateral and medial regions, with additional involvement of the frontal lobes in patients with *MAPT* mutations (Figure 12.15) [43, 47]. Additional abnormalities in the parietal lobes and basal ganglia, and asymmetry, are also sometimes noted.

Dopamine transporter imaging shows strikingly reduced binding in both the caudate and putamen [48], with striatal uptake sometimes observed to be 37.5% of normal levels. In contrast, imaging of postsynaptic D2 receptors is typically normal, suggesting that dysfunction is likely occurring distal to the D2 receptors [48]. These findings have been

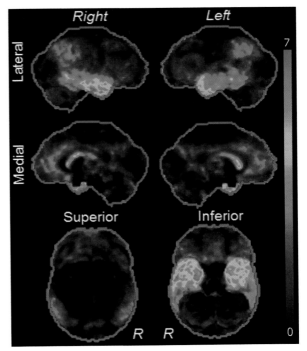

Figure 12.15 Statistical stereotactic surface projection maps showing patterns of FDG-PET hypometabolism in a patient with a *MAPT* mutation. The z score values represent differences from a normal cohort and are color coded as indicated in the color scale (0 = normal; 7 = most abnormal). Hypometabolism is symmetric and observed predominantly in the anterior temporal lobes and caudate nucleus, with milder involvement of the medial frontal and parietal lobes.

observed in the N279K and P301S mutations [48, 49]. These patterns contrast to those in PSPS where patients show reduced binding with both dopamine transporter and D2 receptors. The reduced dopamine transport binding in patients with *MAPT* mutations is also largely symmetric, which contrasts to the asymmetric findings observed in the CBS.

Abnormalities on FDG-PET, SPECT, and dopamine transporter imaging have been observed in presymptomatic patients with *MAPT* mutations, demonstrating that these imaging features predate the onset of clinical symptoms. Presymptomatic individuals show abnormalities particularly in the temporal lobes on FDG-PET, although abnormalities have also been observed in the frontal lobes [41]. Reduced dopamine transporter binding is observed predominantly in the putamen in presymptomatic individuals [42]. Interestingly, these abnormalities on dopamine transporter binding have even been observed up to 10 years before the onset of clinical symptoms [50], showing that these changes occur very early in the disease process. Additional abnormalities in microglial activation have also been observed on PET imaging in presymptomatic individuals with the N279K mutation [42], suggesting the presence of neuroinflammation.

Imaging in Pick's disease

PiD is a relatively rare tauopathy that can only be diagnosed pathologically, and hence imaging has only been reported in a handful of cases [11]. Atrophy on MRI is particularly striking in the prefrontal cortex, involving dorsolateral, medial, and orbital regions, as well as the anterior cingulate and insula (Figure 12.16) [51–53]. Frontal lobe atrophy can be asymmetric, often with greater involvement of the left hemisphere. Milder atrophy is also observed in the anteromedial temporal lobes, temporal pole, and striatum. Parietal atrophy is rarely observed and if present, is usually mild and observed later in the disease course. These patterns differ from those observed in the other tauopathies, with PiD showing greater prefrontal and anterior temporal atrophy than CBD patients that also present with bvFTD, and greater frontal atrophy than patients with mutations in *MAPT*.

Rare tauopathies

Argyrophilic grain disease

Argyrophilic grains (AGs) are characterized by the finding of 4R tau-positive spindle-shaped lesions in neuronal processes and coiled bodies in oligodendrocytes. They are often observed in patients that are otherwise pathologically normal, but can also occur in cases of PSP, CBD, and *MAPT* mutations. In

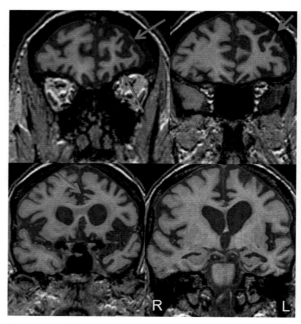

Figure 12.16 Coronal volumetric MRI showing patterns of striking left frontal atrophy in a 71-year-old male patient with PiD.

patients where AGs are the only pathological feature, dementia can be observed, although others are cognitively normal [54]. The dementia phenotype is often characterized by behavioral changes and memory loss, although apraxia and parkinsonism can be observed. The presence of AGs is not associated with atrophy, although hippocampal atrophy can be observed in those that are demented [54]. Whether the presence of AGs modifies the clinical and imaging features of PSP, CBD, and *MAPT* is currently unknown.

Globular glial tauopathy

There are a number of diseases where globular glial 4R tau has been reported, including PSP with corticospinal tract degeneration, sporadic multiple system tauopathy with dementia, and white matter tauopathy with globular glial inclusions. Cases of PSP with corticospinal tract degeneration commonly present with PSPS, CBS or PLS. Upper motor neuron signs, including spasticity, hyperreflexia, and the Babinski sign, are usually noted. Mild generalized cerebral atrophy is observed on MRI. Hypometabolism on FDG-PET and hypoperfusion on SPECT have been observed in the posterior frontal lobes, parietal lobes, and basal ganglia [55]. Upper motor neuron symptoms can also be present in white matter tauo-pathy with globular glial inclusions, although these patients, and patients with multiple system tauopathy, typically present with bvFTD. Generalized cerebral atrophy has been reported in multiple system tauopathy, with a particular focus in the temporal lobes [56].

Niemann–Pick disease type C

Niemann–Pick disease type C is a progressive disorder associated with dystonia, ataxia, and gaze palsy, and is characterized by the presence of tau-positive neuro-fibrillary tangles, distended neurons, and swollen neur-ites on pathology. It results from mutations in genes encoding the NPC1 and NPC2 proteins, and typically affects children and young adults. Atrophy is observed in adult patients on MRI. The only group study per-formed to date showed involvement of the medial temporal lobes, parietal operculum, thalamus, puta-men, cerebellum, and insula [57]. Except for some involvement of the parietal lobes, the cortex appears to be relatively spared. Cerebellar atrophy is not observed in all patients. Subtle atrophy of the midbrain has also been observed, with an 8% reduction in mid-brain area compared to controls, and some evidence that the ratio of midbrain to pons is related to duration of illness [58]. Widespread white matter tract degener-ation is observed on DTI [57], with involvement of the midbrain and superior cerebellar peduncles. Degener-ation of the corpus callosum is also observed. The midbrain changes observed on both MRI and DTI are similar to those observed in PSPS, although they appear to be less severe. MRS metabolite ratios can also be abnormal, with reduced NAA/Cr and increased Cho/Cr in the frontal lobes and centrum semiovale.

Hypometabolism on FDG-PET is consistently observed in the frontal cortex and thalamus. Abnor-malities have also been observed in the parieto-occipital cortex and cerebellum, although the nature of these findings is inconsistent, with hypometabo-lism observed in some patients and hypermetabolism observed in others. There is also some evidence for decreased binding of D2 dopamine receptors in pos-terior regions of the striatum.

Postencephalitic parkinsonism

PEP (also known as von Economo disease), a chronic complication of encephalitis lethargica, is a tauopathy characterized by multisystem neuronal loss and gliosis with widespread neurofibrillary lesions. Patients develop parkinsonism, including rigidity, which can occur up to 20–40 years after encephalitis. Imaging features that have been reported in cases of PEP include striatal hyperintensities, and atrophy of the caudate and putamen on MRI [59]. Abnormalities are also observed on FDG-PET and dopamine trans-port imaging, whereby decreased binding can be observed in the putamen.

Subacute sclerosing panencephalitis

SSPE is a rare progressive, inflammatory neurodegen-erative disease caused by defective measles virus in children. Patients typically present with myoclonus, extrapyramidal dysfunction, altered behavior, cogni-tive impairment, seizures, and abnormal vision. Abnormalities on MRI are usually first identified in the white matter, with hyperintensities observed in the parietal, occipital, and frontal lobes on T_2-weighted images [58]. Early changes are usually periventricular or involve subcortical white matter. Cortical involvement and atrophy, often observed in the frontal lobes, are not typically observed until later in the disease course. Involvement of the thalamus, pons, brainstem, cerebellar peduncles, basal ganglia, and corpus callosum can be observed, but rarely. However, MRI can still be normal even in advanced stages of the disease, and, conversely, severe atrophy has been observed in early-stage cases.

However, abnormalities in other modalities have been observed in patients with normal-appearing white matter on T_2-weighted MRI. White matter changes have been observed on DTI, with symmetric abnormalities observed in the corpus callosum, corticospinal tracts, superior longitudinal fasciculus, inferior longitudinal fasciculus, and thalamic radiation in patients both with normal and abnormal T_2-weighted MRI [60]. Abnormal MRS metabolites have also been observed in the normal-appearing white matter, with increased Cho/Cr and *myo*-Ins/Cr, yet normal NAA/Cr ratios. Hypometabolism on FDG-PET and hypoperfusion on SPECT in the thalamus, cerebellum, and occipital lobe can also be observed.

Tangle-dominant dementia

Tangle-dominant dementia is a sporadic form of late-onset dementia in which neuropathology shows dif-fuse cerebral atrophy with neurofibrillary tangles, often ghost tangles, and neuropil threads, almost limited to limbic areas with only rare and mild involvement of the neocortex, basal ganglia, and brainstem [61]. Amyloid deposits are absent. These cases are extremely rare and tend to be associated with predominant medial temporal atrophy.

Summary

Tauopathies are associated with widely ranging patterns of structural and functional imaging abnormalities, demonstrating that the deposition of abnormal tau is not associated with one specific neuroimaging signature. Each specific tauopathy is, however, associated with characteristic imaging abnormalities that have the potential to be diagnostically useful during life. Heterogeneity across other regions of the brain explains the clinical heterogeneity that can be associated with these tauopathies. Future work will need to focus on assessing the more recent techniques of DTI and resting-state fMRI in pathologically confirmed cohorts in order to determine whether these modalities could provide sensitive and specific biomarkers of these tauopathies.

References

1. Dickson DW, Kouri N, Murray ME, Josephs KA. Neuropathology of frontotemporal lobar degeneration-tau (FTLD-tau). J Mol Neurosci. 2011;45(3):384–9.

2. Josephs KA, Hodges JR, Snowden JS, et al. Neuropathological background of phenotypical variability in frontotemporal dementia. Acta Neuropathol. 2011;122(2):137–53.

3. Josephs KA. Frontotemporal dementia and related disorders: deciphering the enigma. Ann Neurol. 2008;64(1):4–14.

4. Forman MS, Farmer J, Johnson JK, et al. Frontotemporal dementia: clinicopathological correlations. Ann Neurol. 2006;59(6):952–62.

5. Hodges JR, Davies RR, Xuereb JH, et al. Clinicopathological correlates in frontotemporal dementia. Ann Neurol. 2004;56(3):399–406.

6. Josephs KA, Petersen RC, Knopman DS, et al. Clinicopathologic analysis of frontotemporal and corticobasal degenerations and PSP. Neurology. 2006;66(1):41–8.

7. Kertesz A, McMonagle P, Blair M, Davidson W, Munoz DG. The evolution and pathology of frontotemporal dementia. Brain. 2005;128(Pt 9):1996–2005.

8. Josephs KA, Duffy JR, Strand EA, et al. Characterizing a neurodegenerative syndrome: primary progressive apraxia of speech. Brain 2012;135(Pt 5):1522–36.

9. van Swieten J, Spillantini MG. Hereditary frontotemporal dementia caused by Tau gene mutations. Brain Pathol. 2007;17(1):63–73.

10. Wszolek ZK, Pfeiffer RF, Bhatt MH, et al. Rapidly progressive autosomal dominant parkinsonism and dementia with pallido-ponto-nigral degeneration. Ann Neurol. 1992;32(3):312–20.

11. Whitwell JL, Josephs KA. Neuroimaging in frontotemporal lobar degeneration – predicting molecular pathology. Nat Rev. 2012;8(3):131–42.

12. Longoni G, Agosta F, Kostic VS, et al. MRI measurements of brainstem structures in patients with Richardson's syndrome, progressive supranuclear palsy-parkinsonism, and Parkinson's disease. Mov Disord. 2011;26(2):247–55.

13. Cosottini M, Ceravolo R, Faggioni L, et al. Assessment of midbrain atrophy in patients with progressive supranuclear palsy with routine magnetic resonance imaging. Acta Neurol Scand. 2007;116(1):37–42.

14. Whitwell JL, Xu J, Mandrekar J, et al. Imaging measures predict progression in progressive supranuclear palsy. Mov Disord. 2012;27(14):1801–4.

15. Paviour DC, Price SL, Stevens JM, Lees AJ, Fox NC. Quantitative MRI measurement of superior cerebellar peduncle in progressive supranuclear palsy. Neurology 2005;64(4):675–9.

16. Quattrone A, Nicoletti G, Messina D, et al. MR imaging index for differentiation of progressive supranuclear palsy from Parkinson disease and the Parkinson variant of multiple system atrophy. Radiology 2008;246(1):214–21.

17. Whitwell JL, Avula R, Master A, et al. Disrupted thalamocortical connectivity in PSP: a resting state fMRI, DTI, and VBM study. Parkinsonism Relat Disord. 2011;17(8):599–605.

18. Josephs KA, Whitwell JL, Eggers SD, Senjem ML, Jack CR, Jr. Gray matter correlates of behavioral severity in progressive supranuclear palsy. Mov Disord. 2011;26(3):493–8.

19. Looi JC, Macfarlane MD, Walterfang M, et al. Morphometric analysis of subcortical structures in progressive supranuclear palsy: In vivo evidence of neostriatal and mesencephalic atrophy. Psychiatry Res. 2011;194(2):163–75.

20. Padovani A, Borroni B, Brambati SM, et al. Diffusion tensor imaging and voxel based morphometry study in early progressive supranuclear palsy. J Neurol Neurosurg Psychiatry 2006;77(4):457–63.

21. Whitwell JL, Master AV, Avula R, et al. Clinical correlates of white matter tract degeneration in PSP. Arch Neurol 2011;68(6):753–60.

22. Kvickstrom P, Eriksson B, van Westen D, et al. Selective frontal neurodegeneration of the inferior fronto-occipital fasciculus in progressive supranuclear palsy (PSP) demonstrated by diffusion tensor tractography. BMC Neurol. 2011;11:13.

23. Clarke CE, Lowry M. Systematic review of proton magnetic resonance spectroscopy of the striatum in parkinsonian syndromes. Eur J Neurol. 2001;8(6):573–7.

24. Brooks DJ, Ibanez V, Sawle GV, et al. Differing patterns of striatal 18F-dopa uptake in Parkinson's disease, multiple system atrophy, and progressive supranuclear palsy. Ann Neurol. 1990;28(4):547–55.

25. Soliveri P, Monza D, Paridi D, et al. Cognitive and magnetic resonance imaging aspects of corticobasal degeneration and progressive supranuclear palsy. Neurology. 1999;53(3):502–7.

26. Whitwell JL, Jack CR, Jr., Boeve BF, et al. Imaging correlates of pathology in corticobasal syndrome. Neurology. 2010;75(21):1879–87.

27. Borroni B, Garibotto V, Agosti C, et al. White matter changes in corticobasal degeneration syndrome and correlation with limb apraxia. Arch Neurol. 2008 65(6):796–801.

28. Boelmans K, Kaufmann J, Bodammer N, et al. Involvement of motor pathways in corticobasal syndrome detected by diffusion tensor tractography. Mov Disord. 2009;24(2):168–75.

29. Rizzo G, Martinelli P, Manners D, et al. Diffusion-weighted brain imaging study of patients with clinical diagnosis of corticobasal degeneration, progressive supranuclear palsy and Parkinson's disease. Brain. 2008;131(Pt 10):2690–700.

30. Abe K, Terakawa H, Takanashi M, et al. Proton magnetic resonance spectroscopy of patients with parkinsonism. Brain Res Bull 2000;52(6):589–95.

31. Hu WT, Rippon GW, Boeve BF, et al. Alzheimer's disease and corticobasal degeneration presenting as corticobasal syndrome. Mov Disord. 2009;24(9):1375–9.

32. Cilia R, Rossi C, Frosini D, et al. Dopamine transporter SPECT imaging in corticobasal syndrome. PloS One 2011;6(5):e18301.

33. Klaffke S, Kuhn AA, Plotkin M, et al. Dopamine transporters, D2 receptors, and glucose metabolism in corticobasal degeneration. Mov Disord. 2006;21(10):1724–7.

34. Josephs KA, Eggers SD, Jack CR, Jr., Whitwell JL. Neuroanatomical correlates of the progressive supranuclear palsy corticobasal syndrome hybrid. Eur J Neurol. 2012;19(11):1440–6. doi:10.1111/j.1468-1331.2012.03726.

35. Josephs KA, Whitwell JL, Dickson DW, et al. Voxel-based morphometry in autopsy proven PSP and CBD. Neurobiol Aging 2008;29(2):280–9.

36. Whitwell JL, Jack CR, Jr., Parisi JE, et al. Rates of cerebral atrophy differ in different degenerative pathologies. Brain. 2007;130(Pt 4):1148–58.

37. Hassan A, Whitwell JL, Boeve BF, et al. Symmetric corticobasal degeneration (S-CBD). Parkinsonism Relat Disord. 2010;16(3):208–14.

38. Whitwell JL, Jack CR, Jr., Boeve BF, et al. Atrophy patterns in IVS10+16, IVS10+3, N279K, S305N, P301L, and V337M MAPT mutations. Neurology. 2009;73(13):1058–65.

39. Whitwell JL, Weigand SD, Gunter JL, et al. Trajectories of brain and hippocampal atrophy in FTD with mutations in MAPT or GRN. Neurology. 2011;77(4):393–8.

40. Rohrer JD, Ridgway GR, Modat M, et al. Distinct profiles of brain atrophy in frontotemporal lobar degeneration caused by progranulin and tau mutations. Neuroimage. 2010;53(3):1070–6.

41. Spina S, Farlow MR, Unverzagt FW, et al. The tauopathy associated with mutation +3 in intron 10 of Tau: characterization of the MSTD family. Brain. 2008;131(Pt 1):72–89.

42. Miyoshi M, Shinotoh H, Wszolek ZK, et al. In vivo detection of neuropathologic changes in presymptomatic MAPT mutation carriers: a PET and MRI study. Parkinsonism Relat Disord. 2010;16(6):404–8.

43. Arvanitakis Z, Witte RJ, Dickson DW, et al. Clinical-pathologic study of biomarkers in FTDP-17 (PPND family with N279K tau mutation). Parkinsonism Relat Disord. 2007;13(4):230–9.

44. Kantarci K, Boeve BF, Wszolek ZK, et al. MRS in presymptomatic MAPT mutation carriers: a potential biomarker for tau-mediated pathology. Neurology. 2010;75(9):771–8.

45. Zhou J, Greicius MD, Gennatas ED, et al. Divergent network connectivity changes in behavioural variant frontotemporal dementia and Alzheimer's disease. Brain. 2010;133(Pt 5):1352–67.

46. Whitwell JL, Josephs KA, Avula R, et al. Altered functional connectivity in asymptomatic MAPT subjects: a comparison to bvFTD. Neurology. 2011;77(9):866–74.

47. Seelaar H, Papma JM, Garraux G, et al. Brain perfusion patterns in familial frontotemporal lobar degeneration. Neurology. 2011;77(4):384–92.

165

48. Pal PK, Wszolek ZK, Kishore A, *et al.* Positron emission tomography in pallido-ponto-nigral degeneration (PPND) family (frontotemporal dementia with parkinsonism linked to chromosome 17 and point mutation in tau gene). *Parkinsonism Relat Disord.* 2001;7(2):81–8.

49. Sperfeld AD, Collatz MB, Baier H, *et al.* FTDP-17: an early-onset phenotype with parkinsonism and epileptic seizures caused by a novel mutation. *Ann Neurol.* 1999;46(5):708–15.

50. Kishore A, Wszolek ZK, Snow BJ, *et al.* Presynaptic nigrostriatal function in genetically tested asymptomatic relatives from the pallido-ponto-nigral degeneration family. *Neurology.* 1996;47(6):1588–90.

51. Rankin KP, Mayo MC, Seeley WW, *et al.* Behavioral variant frontotemporal dementia with corticobasal degeneration pathology: phenotypic comparison to bvFTD with Pick's disease. *J Mol Neurosci.* 2011;45(3):594–608.

52. Whitwell JL, Jack CR, Jr., Parisi JE, *et al.* Imaging signatures of molecular pathology in behavioral variant frontotemporal dementia. *J Mol Neurosci.* 2011;45(3):372–8.

53. Rohrer JD, Lashley T, Schott JM, *et al.* Clinical and neuroanatomical signatures of tissue pathology in frontotemporal lobar degeneration. *Brain.* 2011;134(Pt 9):2565–81.

54. Mukherjee O, Wang J, Gitcho M, *et al.* Molecular characterization of novel progranulin (GRN) mutations in frontotemporal dementia. *Hum Mutat.* 2008;29(4):512–21.

55. Josephs KA, Katsuse O, Beccano-Kelly DA, *et al.* Atypical progressive supranuclear palsy with corticospinal tract degeneration. *J Neuropathol Exp Neurol.* 2006;65(4): 396–405.

56. Bigio EH, Lipton AM, Yen SH, *et al.* Frontal lobe dementia with novel tauopathy: sporadic multiple system tauopathy with dementia. *J Neuropathol Exp Neurol.* 2001;60(4):328–41.

57. Walterfang M, Fahey M, Desmond P, *et al.* White and gray matter alterations in adults with Niemann-Pick disease type C: a cross-sectional study. *Neurology.* 2010;75(1):49–56.

58. Walterfang M, Macfarlane MD, Looi JC, *et al.* Pontine-to-midbrain ratio indexes ocular-motor function and illness stage in adult Niemann-Pick disease type C. *Eur J Neurol.* 2012;19(3):462–7.

59. Espay AJ, Henderson KK. Postencephalitic parkinsonism and basal ganglia necrosis due to Epstein-Barr virus infection. *Neurology.* 2011;76(17):1529–30.

60. Rutherford NJ, Zhang YJ, Baker M, *et al.* Novel mutations in TARDBP (TDP-43) in patients with familial amyotrophic lateral sclerosis. *PLoS Genet.* 2008;4(9): e1000193.

61. Jellinger KA, Bancher C. Senile dementia with tangles (tangle predominant form of senile dementia). *Brain Pathol.* 1998;8(2):367–76.

Chapter 13

Magnetic resonance imaging of multiple system atrophy

Klaus Seppi, Christoph Mueller, Gregor K. Wenning, and Michael Schocke

Introduction

Multiple system atrophy (MSA) is an adult-onset, sporadic, progressive neurodegenerative disorder, which involves both the central and autonomic nervous systems, presenting a much faster disease progression and worse prognosis than Parkinson's disease (PD). Diagnosis during life can be challenging, especially in early stages of the disease, and distinction between MSA and other neurodegenerative parkinsonian disorders – especially PD – can be difficult on clinical grounds alone. Nevertheless, an early diagnosis and differentiation between PD and atypical parkinsonian disorders (APDs) are crucial, because of prognostic and therapeutic implications. Despite the increasing clinical recognition of MSA, only a few epidemiological studies exist, which report a prevalence rate below 5 and an incidence rate of about 1 in 100 000 [1, 2]. Onset is usually in the sixth decade followed by progression, with death occurring after an average of 9 years of disease.

Two major motor presentations can be distinguished clinically: patients presenting with predominant parkinsonism (MSA-P, Parkinson variant); and patients presenting with predominant cerebellar signs (MSA-C, cerebellar variant). MSA-P reflects the neuropathological features of striatonigral degeneration (SND), and MSA-C those of olivopontocerebellar atrophy (OPCA) [3]. Two large MSA series showed different distribution rates of the clinical subtypes, with a predominance of MSA-P in Europe and of MSA-C in Japan [4, 5].

From a clinical standpoint MSA is currently defined by parkinsonian features, cerebellar ataxia, autonomic failure, urogenital dysfunction, and pyramidal signs. Progressive autonomic failure is the cardinal feature in almost all patients with MSA, and is clinically dominated by urogenital and neurogenic orthostatic hypotension. Rarely, cognitive dysfunction and even dementia may occur [6].

To date, three levels of certainty for the diagnosis of MSA are established according to the Gilman criteria: possible, probable, and definite MSA [7]. Definite MSA requires neuropathological findings and autopsy demonstration of typical histological features; probable MSA requires clinical signs of autonomic failure, parkinsonism, and ataxia (see Table 13.1);

Table 13.1. Criteria for the diagnosis of probable MSA

A sporadic, progressive, adult-onset disease characterized by
Autonomic failure involving urinary incontinence or an orthostatic decrease of blood pressure within 3 minutes of standing by at least 30 mm Hg systolic or 15 mm Hg diastolic
AND
Poorly levodopa-responsive parkinsonism (bradykinesia with rigidity, tremor, or postural instability)
OR
A cerebellar syndrome (gait ataxia with cerebellar dysarthria, limb ataxia, or cerebellar oculomotor dysfunction)
MSA, multiple system atrophy. Gilman *et al.* [7].

Magnetic Resonance Imaging in Movement Disorders, ed. Paul Tuite and Alain Dagher. Published by Cambridge University Press. © Cambridge University Press 2013.

Table 13.2. Criteria for the diagnosis of possible MSA

A sporadic, progressive, adult-onset disease characterized by
Parkinsonism (bradykinesia with rigidity, tremor, or postural instability)
OR
A cerebellar syndrome (gait ataxia with cerebellar dysarthria, limb ataxia, or cerebellar oculomotor dysfunction)
AND
At least one feature suggesting autonomic dysfunction (urinary urgency, frequency or incomplete bladder emptying, erectile dysfunction in males, or significant orthostatic blood pressure decline that does not meet the level required in probable MSA)
AND
At least one of the additional features shown in Table 13.3

MSA, multiple system atrophy.
Gilman et al. [7].

Table 13.3. Additional features of possible MSA

Possible MSA-P	Possible MSA-C
Additional clinical features	
<ul><li>Babinski sign with hyperreflexia</li><li>Stridor</li><li>Rapidly progressive parkinsonism</li><li>Poor response to levodopa</li><li>Postural instability within 3 years of motor onset</li><li>Gait ataxia, cerebellar dysarthria, limb ataxia, or cerebellar oculomotor dysfunction</li><li>Dysphagia within 5 years of motor onset</li></ul>	<ul><li>Babinski sign with hyperreflexia</li><li>Stridor</li><li>Parkinsonism (bradykinesia and rigidity)</li></ul>
Additional imaging features	
<ul><li>Atrophy on MRI of putamen, middle cerebellar peduncle, pons, or cerebellum</li><li>Hypometabolism on FDG-PET in putamen, brainstem, or cerebellum</li></ul>	<ul><li>Atrophy on MRI of putamen, middle cerebellar peduncle, or pons</li><li>Hypometabolism on FDG-PET in putamen</li><li>Presynaptic nigrostriatal dopaminergic denervation on SPECT or PET</li></ul>

MSA, multiple system atrophy; MSA-P, Parkinson variant of MSA; MSA-C, cerebellar variant of MSA; MRI, magnetic resonance imaging; FDG, ^{18}F-fluorodeoxyglucose; PET, positron emission tomography; SPECT, single-photon emission computed tomography.
Gilman et al. [7].

and possible MSA defines patients with suspected disease defined by a spectrum of features as listed in Tables 13.2 and 13.3.

Neuropathologically, MSA is defined by glial cytoplasmic inclusions (GCIs) formed by fibrillar α-synuclein in oligodendroglial cells and selective neuronal loss with varying degrees of demyelination and atrophy in multiple areas of the central nervous system (CNS). Therefore, MSA is classified as a synucleinopathy, which also includes conditions such as PD and dementia with Lewy bodies (DLB). Major sites of pathology include the nigrostriatal system, cerebellum, pons, medulla, and olivopontocerebellar pathways as well as the intermediolateral cell columns of the spinal cord and other parts of the central autonomic nervous system [5]. To date it is widely accepted that MSA is a distinct sporadic disease that is characterized by well-defined clinical features reflecting underlying SND, OPCA, and central autonomic degeneration. Neurodegeneration in MSA is driven by GCIs that can be observed throughout the white matter and that are also detectable in the basal ganglia, cerebellum, and brainstem [8].

The neurodegenerative processes mentioned above may lead to signal changes on MRI in affected brain areas. Using conventional magnetic resonance imaging (cMRI), regional cell loss may illustrate atrophy of specific brain structures. Reactive gliosis may lead to signal changes in T_2 sequences, fluid-attenuated inversion recovery (FLAIR) sequences, and the apparent diffusion coefficients (ADC), and increased iron deposition results in signal abnormalities in iron-sensitive MR sequences, including T_2-, T_2^*-, gradient echo (GRE)-, and susceptibility-weighted imaging (SWI) sequences. Therefore, brain MRI changes may help confirm a clinical diagnosis of MSA and are able to provide additional information on regional changes in tissue volume and signal abnormalities. Indeed, the revised Gilman diagnostic criteria for MSA have incorporated imaging criteria (see Table 13.3) [7, 9]. Although MRI might show specific structural and signal changes in patients with MSA, its main role remains in the differential diagnosis of neurodegenerative parkinsonism. Moreover, the longitudinal assessment of serial MRI-derived parameters offers the opportunity for robust inferences regarding the progression of MSA. MR scanners with 1.5 tesla (T) field strengths are the most commonly used technique applied in clinical routine and for which most data in MSA are obtainable. Therefore, in this chapter, the reader should assume the study referenced utilized a 1.5T magnet, unless otherwise stated.

This chapter focuses on structural MR techniques such as cMRI including standard T_1- and T_2-weighted as well as FLAIR sequences, and different advanced MR techniques including methods to assess regional cerebral atrophy quantitatively, such as magnetic resonance volumetry (MRV), diffusion-weighted imaging and diffusion tensor imaging (DWI/DTI), as well as magnetization transfer imaging (MTI). Except for MR spectroscopy (MRS), functional MR techniques including perfusion MRI, blood oxygen level-dependent fMRI, and arterial spin labeling will not be covered here, as there are no data available in patients with MSA.

Structural MRI in MSA

Since 1986, with the publication of two MRI studies on neurodegenerative "Parkinson plus syndromes" [10, 11], structural MRI has shown great potential for the differential diagnosis of neurodegenerative parkinsonism over the past 25 years. cMRI has the ability to show changes in the basal ganglia, cortical, or infratentorial structures for the discrimination of APDs and PD. Due to its high spatial and contrast resolution, cMRI at 1.5T with T_1-, T_2-, and proton density-weighted sequences offers in vivo visualization of changes in the striatum, brainstem, and cerebellum that have been described as diagnostic pointers for MSA and are summarized in Table 13.4. The most striking imaging features are putaminal atrophy, hypointensity of the putamen, and "slit-like" marginal hyperintensity (hyperintense putaminal rim) in T_2-weighted sequences (Figure 13.1). This hypointensity reflects high iron content, whereas the hyperintense foci are caused by gliosis; resulting in inhomogeneous visualization of the putamen, especially in the dorsolateral portion. Although putaminal atrophy seems to be quite specific and appears to distinguish between MSA and PD, T_2 putaminal hypointensity and the hyperintense putaminal rim may also occur in PD [12–14].

Infratentorial abnormalities in MSA include atrophy of the lower brainstem, pons, medulla oblongata, inferior olives, middle cerebellar peduncle (MCP), and cerebellum as well as hyperintensities in the pons, MCP, and cerebellum (Figure 13.2). T_2 signal hyperintensities within the pons and both MCPs reflect degeneration of pontocerebellar fibers; whereas the median raphe, transverse pontocerebellar fibers ventral to the tegmentum, and anterior and anterolateral contours of the pons show no signal changes. Taken together these changes may resemble a pattern designated the "hot cross bun" sign (see Figure 13.1A). This sign is highly suggestive of MSA but is also found in non-degenerative parkinsonism and in spinocerebellar ataxia (SCA) [15, 16]. When comparing MSA-P with MSA-C, the supratentorial structural and signal changes at 1.5T mentioned above appear more often and earlier in MSA-P than in MSA-C; on the other hand infratentorial abnormalities appear more often and earlier in MSA-C than in MSA-P[17].

Overall, putaminal and infratentorial findings detected by MRI at 1.5T demonstrate high specificity for distinguishing MSA from PD and healthy

Table 13.4. MRI findings in MSA at 1.5T

Conventional MRI at 1.5T	
Supratentorial	Putaminal atrophy and T_2 hypointensity, "slit-like" marginal hyperintensity (hyperintense putaminal rim)
Infratentorial	Atrophy and/or hyperintensities of lower brainstem, MCP, cerebellum, and the pons (possible "hot cross bun sign"); dilation of the fourth ventricle
MRI-based quantitative assessment	
Planimetry	Decreased MCP width, smaller pontine area; increased m/p-ratio and decreased MRPI distinguish PSP from MSA
Volumetry	Volume loss of supratentorial and infratentorial brain structures, including striatum, brainstem, and cerebellum
Diffusion-weighted imaging	Increased diffusivity values in the putamen (posterior > anterior) and MCP in patients with MSA-P Increased diffusivity values in the putamen, MCP, pons, and cerebellar white matter in patients with MSA-C

MRI, magnetic resonance imaging; MSA, multiple system atrophy; T, Tesla; MCP, middle cerebellar peduncle; m/p-ratio, midbrain-to-pontine ratio; MRPI, magnetic resonance parkinsonism index; PSP, progressive supranuclear palsy; MSA-P, Parkinson variant of MSA; MSA-C, cerebellar variant of MSA.

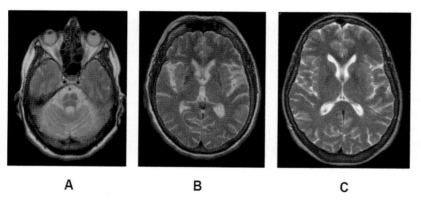

A   B   C

Figure 13.1 (A) Hot cross bun sign in a patient with MSA-C (female 62 years; disease duration 3 years; Hoehn and Yahr stage 3) on T_2-weighted (T_2w) images (1.5T). (B) Putaminal changes (hyperintense rim, putaminal hypointensity in comparison with the globus pallidus, and putaminal atrophy) at both sides in a patient with MSA-P (female; age 66 years; disease duration 4 years; Hoehn and Yahr stage 3) on T_2w images (1.5T). (C) No relevant abnormalities in the basal ganglia in a patient with Parkinson's disease (female; age 61 years; disease duration 6 years; Hoehn and Yahr stage 2) on T_2w images (1.5T).

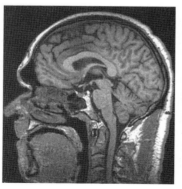 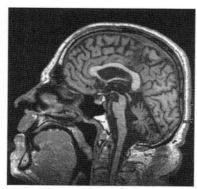

A   B

Figure 13.2 (A) No relevant brainstem atrophy in a patient with Parkinson's disease (male; age 60 years; disease duration 5 years; Hoehn and Yahr stage 2) on sagittal T_1-weighted (T_1w) images (1.5T). (B) Infratentorial atrophy (pons and cerebellum) in a patient with MSA-P (male; age 63 years; disease duration 4 years; Hoehn and Yahr stage 3) on sagittal T_1w images (1.5T).

controls, while specificity of the putaminal changes is inadequate to differentiate MSA from other forms of APDs. The diagnostic values of reported abnormalities in cMRI are summarized in Table 13.5. Especially in the early course of the disease, sensitivity of the characteristic findings is suboptimal and inconsistent in the literature. Indeed, about 60% of patients with MSA-P had neither putaminal nor infratentorial changes within 2 years from disease onset as reported by a previous paper, in which MRI findings at the first hospital visit were analyzed for 139 patients with MSA, including 54 patients with MSA-P [4]. Generally, sensitivity of signal alterations can be improved by modifying technical aspects such as spatial resolution by using thinner slices or modifying relaxation contrast by using $T_2{}^*$-weighted GRE sequences (see the section on iron-sensitive MRI) [18–20]. By applying a 3-mm-thin section conventional spin echo protocol, Righini and coworkers found a substantial increase in MR sensitivity for the differential diagnosis between MSA-P and PD [18].

A new MRI rating scale which has been used in a multicenter study includes the evaluation of 32 different basal ganglia and infratentorial abnormalities using a MRI protocol consisting of two-dimensional sagittal and axial T_1-, axial proton density-, and axial and coronal T_2-weighted acquisitions [21]. The scale has been validated in 297 patients with progressive supranuclear palsy (PSP) and 330 patients with MSA, showing it can reliably and consistently measure MRI abnormalities in patients with established PSP and MSA. Diagnostic accuracy of the scale and the items has not been provided. Moreover, the scale has not been validated for PD, the most common condition that is confused with MSA-P [22].

Signal abnormalities seem to be influenced by the applied magnetic field strength, as shown in a study using brain MRI at 0.35T, 1.5T, and 3T in patients with MSA and PD [23]. With increasing field strength putaminal hyperintensity became less frequent, whereas the occurrence of hypointensity at the dorsolateral putaminal margin increased in patients with MSA. The frequency of the hot cross bun sign and hyperintensity in the MCP was no different between magnetic field strengths. Overall, the role of signal changes for the differential diagnosis of MSA on T_2-weighted sequences at 3T is unclear. Interestingly, one study suggested that a T_2 hyperintense putaminal rim might be a non-specific, normal finding at 3T [24]. Therefore, studies evaluating the diagnostic accuracy using structural MRI at 3T in patients with MSA are lacking.

Evidence supporting a role for cMRI in the differential diagnosis of MSA from other cerebellar disorders is scarce. Bürk and coworkers [25] investigated the discriminative validity of cMRI at 1.5T in patients with sporadic cerebellar ataxia including patients with MSA-C and patients with idiopathic cerebellar ataxia and parkinsonism (IDCA-P). Patients with MSA-C were characterized by a higher frequency and severity of MRI abnormalities (atrophic changes and additional hyperintense signal changes) of the MCP and pons. The presence of these MRI features thus points to the diagnosis of MSA-C and helps differentiate MSA-C from other types of sporadic cerebellar ataxia with extracerebellar features.

Methods to assess regional cerebral atrophy quantitatively

As an indirect method of measuring regional brain atrophy, groups have applied simple quantitative measures of diameters, areas, and volumes including region of interest (ROI)-based assessment of various structures on MRI for differential diagnostic purposes. A summary of these methods and their diagnostic accuracy for MSA is listed in Table 13.6 and includes the following techniques: MR-planimetry, -volumetry, and voxel-based morphometry (VBM).

Planimetry

In terms of infratentorial atrophy, several studies have demonstrated that MSA is associated with a relatively greater pontine and MCP atrophy compared to PSP and PD, whereas patients with PSP have a relatively greater midbrain and superior cerebellar peduncle (SCP) atrophy compared to MSA and PD [26–31]. Consistent with the atrophy of the MCP in MSA, the average MCP width was shown to be significantly smaller in patients with MSA than in those with PD or control subjects. The average MCP width was 6.1 mm in MSA compared to 9.3 mm and 9.8 mm in PD and controls, respectively, without any overlap between MSA patients and PD patients or healthy subjects using a cutoff value of 8 mm [30]. The separation of MSA from PSP patients, however, was incomplete [30, 31]. Additionally, MSA patients with the hot cross bun sign showed a significantly smaller

Table 13.5. Diagnostic accuracy of conventional MRI for the diagnosis of MSA

Reference	Cohort size	Main results	Discriminator	Sensitivity,%	Specificity,%
Konagaya et al., 1994 [110]	MSA 28 PD 25	Slit-hyperintensity in the outer margin of the putamen on T_2w images in MSA	Putaminal rim	61 (MSA)	100 (vs. PD)
Kraft et al., 1999 [111]	MSA-P 15 PSP 10 PD 65	Hyperintense lateral rim and a dorsolateral hypointense signal attenuation on T_2w images within the putamen in MSA-P	Putaminal rim and hypointense putamen	60 (MSA-P)	100 (vs. PD and PSP)
			Hypointense putamen	33 (MSA-P)	91 (vs. PD) 60 (vs. PSP)
Bhattacharya et al., 2002 [13]	MSA-P 14 MSA-C 4 PD 21	Brainstem atrophy in MSA-P and MSA-C Putaminal atrophy in MSA-P Putaminal hypointensity and lateral slit-like hyperintensity in PD, MSA-P, and mild in PD Cerebellar abnormalities in MSA-C/ MSA-P and in some PD patients	Putaminal atrophy	43 (MSA-P)	100 (vs. PD and MSA-C)
		Significant differences in MSA-P and PD, including putaminal atrophy, putaminal hypointensity, atrophy of midbrain, pons, and medulla as well as hot cross bun sign	Putaminal hypointensity (moderate/severe)	43 (MSA-P)	100 (vs. PD and MSA-C)
		No significant differences between MSA-P and MSA-C	Putaminal rim (moderate/severe)	36 (MSA-P)	96 (vs. PD and MSA-C)
			Midbrain atrophy	36 (MSA-P)	100 (vs. PD)
			Pontine atrophy	43 (MSA-P)	100 (vs. PD)
			Atrophy medulla oblongata	43 (MSA-P)	100 (vs. PD)
			Signal increase MCP	21 (MSA-P)	100 (vs. PD)
			Hot cross bun sign	7 (MSA-P)	100 (vs. PD)
Righini et al., 2002 [18]	MSA-P 24 PD 27	Significant abnormal putaminal T_2 hypointensity and proton density hyperintensity in MSA compared to PD	T_2 putaminal hypo- or hyperintensity (FSE 5 mm)	45 (MSA)	100 (vs. PD)
			Proton density putaminal hyperintensity (CSE 3 mm)	88 (MSA)	88 (vs. PD)
			T_2 putaminal hypointensity (CSE 3 mm)	83 (MSA)	100 (vs. PD)
Schocke et al., 2002 [14]	MSA-P 10 PD 11 HC 7	Putaminal atrophy and T_2 hyperintense putaminal rim in MSA-P	Putaminal atrophy	60 (MSA-P)	100 (vs. PD and HC)
			Putaminal rim	80 (MSA-P)	91 (vs. PD) 100 (vs. HC)

Table 13.5. *(cont.)*

Reference	Cohort size	Main results	Discriminator	Sensitivity,%	Specificity,%
Lee *et al.*, 2004 [112]	MSA-P 36 MSA-C 27 PD 30	Hyperintense rim and putaminal atrophy, signal increase in MCP and cerebellum as well as atrophy of MCP and cerebellum	Putaminal hypointensity	90 (MSA-P) 82 (MSA-C)	70 (vs. PD)
			Putaminal atrophy	83 (MSA-P)	87 (vs. PD)
			Putaminal rim	72 (MSA-P)	90 (vs. PD)
			Dilation of fourth ventricle	78 (MSA-P) 93 (MSA-C)	87 (vs. PD)
			MCP atrophy	75 (MSA-P) 100 (MSA-C)	87 (vs. PD)
			Pontine atrophy	100 (MSA-C)	87 (vs. PD)
			Cerebellar atrophy	96 (MSA-C)	90 (vs. PD)
			Signal increase cerebellum	82 (MSA-C)	97 (vs. PD)
			Signal increase MCP	85 (MSA-C)	100 (vs. PD)
Bürk *et al.*, 2005 [25]	MSA-C 30 IDCA-P 11	Significant more frequent atrophy of brainstem and MCP in MSA-C compared to IDCA-P	MCP atrophy	93 (MSA-C)	82 (vs. IDCA-P)
		Significant more hyperintensities of infratentorial structures (MCP, pons) in MSA-C compared to IDCA-P	Brainstem atrophy	100 (MSA-C)	82 (vs. IDCA-P)
		No significant differences in hypointensities or hyperintensities of basal ganglia structures between groups	Hypointensity dentate nuclei	57 (MSA-C)	100 (vs. IDCA-P)
			Hot cross bun sign	97 (MSA-C)	100 (vs. IDCA-P)
			Hyperintensity MCP	87 (MSA-C)	100 (vs. IDCA-P)
Nicoletti *et al.*, 2006 [30]	MSA 16 (MSA-P 13, MSA-C 3) PD 26 HC 14	All MSA patients showed at least one MR feature (putaminal hypointensity, putaminal rim, hot cross bun sign), whereas all HC and all but one PD patient showed normal MRI	Putaminal hypointensity	38 (MSA)	100 (vs. PD and HC)
			Putaminal rim	56 (MSA)	96 (vs. PD) 90 (vs. HC)
			Hot cross bun sign	50 (MSA)	100 (vs. PD and HC)
			Presence of at least one of the abnormal features mentioned above	100 (MSA)	96 (vs. PD) 100 (vs. HC)

Table 13.5. (*cont.*)

Reference	Cohort size	Main results	Discriminator	Sensitivity,%	Specificity,%
Seppi et al., 2006 [44]	MSA-P 15 PD 20 HC 11	Significant higher rate of putaminal slit-like hyperintensity, putaminal signal hypointensity relative to the globus pallidum, and putaminal atrophy in MSA-P compared to PD and HC	Putaminal rim (moderate/severe)	47 (MSA-P)	100 (vs. PD and HC)
			Putaminal hypointensity (moderate/severe)	47 (MSA-P)	100 (vs. PD and HC)
			Putaminal atrophy	67 (MSA-P)	100 (vs. PD and HC)
Ito et al., 2007 [113]	MSA-P 9 MSA-C 24 PD 38 HC 27	Significant higher occurrence of putaminal linearization in MSA-P compared to MSA-C, PD, and HC Significantly smaller adjusted putaminal area in MSA-P compared to MSA-C, PD, and HC	Putaminal linearization	89 (MSA-P)	91 (vs. MSA-C, PD, and HC)
von Lewinski et al., 2007 [20]	MSA 52 PD 88 HC 29	Hyperintense lateral putaminal rim on FLAIR sequences at 1T in MSA	Hyperintense putaminal rim	48 (MSA)	93 (vs. PD and HC)
Paviour et al., 2007 [50]	MSA-P 11 PD 12 PSP 20 HC 7	Significant increased signal intensity in the pons and MCP in MSA-P compared to PSP, PD, and HC using T_2w FSE sequences	Putaminal hypointensity	27 (MSA-P)	100 (vs. PD) 80 (vs. PSP)
		Differences in putaminal hypointensity and hyperintense putaminal rim among groups	Putaminal rim	55 (MSA-P)	83 (vs. PD) 90 (vs. PSP)
			Signal increase pons	45 (MSA-P)	100 (vs. all groups)
			Signal increase MCP	36 (MSA-P)	100 (vs. all groups)
Kwon et al., 2008 [114]	MSA-P 24 PD 8	Putaminal atrophy and hyperintense rim in posterolateral portion of the putamen, hot cross bun sign, pontine atrophy, fourth ventricle dilation, hyperintense MCP, and cerebellar atrophy	Putaminal findings	58 (MSA-P)	100 (vs. PD)
			Putaminal and infratentorial findings	79 (MSA-P)	100 (vs. PD)
Ito et al., 2009 [115]	MSA-P 17 PSP 11 PD 37 HC 16	Significant greater mean putaminal atrophy in MSA-P compared to PSP, PD, and HC	Putaminal atrophy	88 (MSA-P)	93 (vs. HC and PSP) 95 (vs. PD)
		Significant greater mean putaminal high-intensity T_2 signal in MSA-P compared to PSP, PD, and HC	Putaminal high-intensity T_2 signal	81 (MSA-P)	93 (vs. all groups)

Table 13.5. (cont.)

Reference	Cohort size	Main results	Discriminator	Sensitivity,%	Specificity,%
		Significant greater mean putaminal low-intensity T_2 signal in MSA-P compared to PD and HC	Putaminal low-intensity T_2 signal	61 (MSA-P)	98 (vs. HC and PSP) 96 (vs. PD)
		Significant greater mean putaminal high-intensity T_1 signal in MSA-P compared to PSP, PD, and HC	Putaminal high-intensity T_1 signal	93 (MSA-P)	99 (vs. PSP) 98 (vs. PD) 94 (vs. HC)
Lim et al., 2009 [116]	MSA 63 (MSA-P 18, MSA-C 45) HC 63	Significant higher median grading score of white matter hyperintensity in MSA compared to HC *Diagnostic accuracy values not given*			
Sakurai et al. 2011 [117]	MSA-P 19 PD 15 HC 15	More conspicuous detection of hyperintense putaminal rim in MSA-P using FLAIR imaging compared to T_2w imaging	Putaminal rim (FLAIR)	89	87
			Putaminal rim (T_2w)	58	93
Kasahara et al., 2012 [118]	MSA-C 16	Significant higher grade of hot cross bun sign observed using PDw imaging than T_2w imaging in MSA-C *Diagnostic accuracy values not given*			
Massey et al., 2012 [75]	MSA 13 PSP 22 PD 7 CBD 6 HC 9	Sensitivity, specificity, and accuracy of radiological diagnosis of PSP were 72.7%, 94.3%, and 86.0%, respectively Sensitivity, specificity, and accuracy of radiological diagnosis of MSA were 76.9%, 100%, and 94.7%, respectively	Putaminal atrophy	50 (MSA)	89 (vs. HC) 80 (vs. PD and CBD) 44 (vs. PSP) 65 (vs. all groups)
			Midbrain atrophy	86 (PSP) 33 (MSA)	67 (vs. MSA and HC) 14 (vs. PSP)
			Absence of midbrain atrophy	67 (MSA)	87 (vs. PSP)
			Hummingbird sign	68 (PSP)	100 (vs. MSA, CBD and HC)
			Absence of hummingbird sign	100 (MSA)	68 (vs. PSP)
			MCP atrophy	33 (MSA)	100 (vs. HC)
			MCP hyperintensity	50 (MSA)	100 (vs. PSP and HC)
			Hot cross bun sign	58 (MSA)	100 (vs. CBD and HC)

MSA, multiple system atrophy; MSA-P, Parkinson variant of MSA; MSA-C, cerebellar variant of MSA; PD, Parkinson's disease; PSP, progressive supranuclear palsy; HC, healthy controls; IDCA-P, idiopathic cerebellar ataxia with extracerebellar presentation not corresponding to MSA-C; CBD, corticobasal degeneration; MRI, magnetic resonance imaging; MCP, middle cerebellar peduncle; CSE, conventional spin echo; FSE, fast spin echo; FLAIR, fluid attenuated inversion recovery; PDw, proton density-weighted; T_2w, T_2-weighted.

Table 13.6. Diagnostic accuracy of the quantitative assessment of regional cerebral atrophy including MR-planimetry, -volumetry, and VBM for the diagnosis of MSA.

Reference	Cohort size	Main results	Discriminator	Sensitivity,%	Specificity,%
Schulz et al., 1999 [35]	MSA-P 12 MSA-C 17 PD 11 PSP 6 HC 16	Significant reductions in mean striatal and brainstem volumes in patients with MSA-P, MSA-C, and PSP, whereas patients with MSA-C and MSA-P also showed a reduction in cerebellar volume Patients with PD could not be separated from HC and patients with MSA-P could not be separated from patients with PSP	Volumes of brainstem, caudate nucleus, putamen, and cerebellum using MRV (stepwise linear discrimination)*	67 (MSA-P)	100 (vs. PD 100 (vs. HC) 67 (vs. PSP)
				76 (MSA-C)	100 (vs. PD) 82 (vs. HC) 100 (vs. PSP)
Brenneis et al., 2003 [58]	MSA-P 14 PD 14	Significant progression of brain atrophy in subcortical (striatum, mesencephalon, thalamus, and cerebellum) and cortical areas (supplementary motor area, medial frontal gyrus, middle frontal gyrus, orbitofrontal cortex, insula, and hippocampus) of both hemispheres as well as left primary sensorimotor cortex, left lateral premotor cortex, and the left posterior parietal cortex in MSA-P within 1 year No significant progression of brain atrophy in PD within 1.4 years *Diagnostic accuracy values not given*			
Bürk et al., 2004 [39]	MSA-C 33 IDCA-P 13 HC 16	Significant reduction of standardized cerebellar and brainstem volumes in all cerebellar groups compared to HC Brainstem atrophy was most prominent in MSA-C, while cerebellar atrophy did not differ between MSA-C and IDCA-P Mean volumes of caudate and putamen were not significantly different in HC and cerebellar patients	Volumes of cerebellum, brainstem, caudate nucleus, and putamen using MRV (stepwise linear discrimination)**	82	100
Hauser et al., 2006 [119]	MSA-C 14 HC 16	Significant loss of gray matter volume in the cerebellar hemispheres, vermis, dorsal parts of the mesencephalon, putamen, and the caudate nucleus Significant reduction of white matter in the cerebellum, cerebellar peduncles, pons, and internal capsule *Diagnostic accuracy values not given*			
Nicoletti et al., 2006 [30]	MSA 16 (MSA-P 13, MSA-C 3) PD 26 HC 14	Significant smaller average MCP width in MSA compared to PD/HC using T_1w sequences	MCP width	100 (MSA)	100 (vs. PD and HC)

Table 13.6. (*cont.*)

Reference	Cohort size	Main results	Discriminator	Sensitivity,%	Specificity,%
Paviour *et al.*, 2006 [36]	MSA-P 9 PSP 18 PD 9 HC 9	Significant lower midbrain and SCP volumes in PSP compared to MSA-P, PD, and HC Significant lower frontal volume in PSP compared to PD and HC, but not to MSA-P Significant greater third ventricle in PSP compared to HC, but not to MSA-P and PD Significant lower cerebellar, pontine, and posterior inferior volumes in MSA-P compared to PD and HC Significant lower midbrain volume in MSA-P compared to HC No significant differences between PD and HC	Midbrain, SCP, frontal, third ventricle, and whole brain volumes	89 (PSP)***	97 (vs. MSA-P, PD, and HC)
			SCP, midbrain, pons, and cerebellar volumes	94 (PSP)***	89 (vs. MSA-P)
Minnerop *et al.*, 2007 [59]	MSA 48 (MSA-P 16, MSA-C 32) HC 46	Significant gray matter reduction in the basal parts of the cerebellum in MSA-C compared to MSA-P Significant white matter reduction in the brainstem in MSA-C compared to MSA-P Significant R_2 decrease in the cerebellum, brainstem, and several small cortical regions in MSA-C compared to MSA-P Gray matter loss in the cerebellum, right thalamus, both putamina, and several cortical regions including insular cortex in MSA-C compared to HC Decreased relaxation rate R_2 in the cerebellum, pontine brainstem, and cortical regions including insular cortex in MSA-C compared to HC Gray matter reduction in the cerebellum, dorsal midbrain, both putamina, and several cortical regions including the insular cortex in MSA-P compared to HC *Diagnostic accuracy values not given*			
Quattrone *et al.*, 2008 [31]	MSA-P 19 PD 108 PSP 33 HC 50	Significant smaller midbrain area and SCP width in PSP compared to PD, MSA-P, and HC with some overlap of values between groups Significant larger P/M and MCP/SCP ratios in PSP compared to PD, MSA-P, and HC with some overlap of values between groups Significant larger MR parkinsonism index in PSP compared to PD, MSA-P, and HC without any overlap of values among groups	P/M ratio	95 (PSP)***	97 (vs. PD, MSA-P, and HC)
			MCP/SCP ratio	90 (PSP)***	94 (vs. PD, MSA-P, and HC)

Table 13.6. (cont.)

Reference	Cohort size	Main results	Discriminator	Sensitivity,%	Specificity,%
			MRPI = (P/M) × (MCP/SCP)	100 (PSP)***	100 (vs. PD, MSA-P, and HC)
Hussl et al., 2010 [32]	MSA-P 26 PSP 22 PD 75	Significant smaller m/p-ratios and higher MRPI values in PSP compared to MSA-P, PD, and HC	m/p-ratio	64 (PSP)***	92 (vs. non-PSP) 95 (vs. PD) 85 (vs. MSA-P)
			MRPI	82 (PSP)***	80 (vs. non-PSP) 76 (vs. PD) 92 (vs. MSA-P)
Minnerop et al., 2010 [102]	MSA 14 (MSA-P 4, MSA-C 10) HC 14	Significant less gray matter in the cerebellum and cerebral cortex in MSA compared to HC at baseline Significant less white matter in the cerebellar peduncles and brainstem in MSA compared to HC at baseline Significant thinner callosal regions in MSA compared to HC at baseline Significant decreased thickness of the corpora callosa in MSA compared to HC at follow-up *Diagnostic accuracy values not given*			
Tzarouchi et al., 2010 [57]	MSA-P 11 HC 11	Significant decreased gray matter in the putamen, caudate nuclei, thalami, anterior cerebellar lobes, and cerebral cortex in MSA-P compared to HC Significant decreased white matter atrophy in the pons, midbrain, and peduncles in MSA-P compared to HC *Diagnostic accuracy values not given*			
Kashihara et al., 2011 [120]	MSA 28 PSP 11 CBD 10 PD 80 SCA 9 Controls 54	Significant lower neuromelanin-positive SNc volumes in MSA, PSP, CBD, and PD compared to controls No significant decrease of neuromelanin-positive SNc volumes in SCA compared to controls *Diagnostic accuracy values not given*			
Messina et al., 2011 [38]	MSA-P 15 PSP 32 PD 72 HC 46	No significant differences in brain volumes between PD and HC Significant reduced volumes of the cerebellum, thalamus, putamen, pallidum, hippocampus, and brainstem in MSA-P and PSP compared to PD and HC Significant larger ventricular system in MSA-P and PSP compared to PD and HC Significant smaller thalamus volume in PSP compared to MSA-P *Diagnostic accuracy values not given*			

* No PD patient was classified as having MSA-P or vice versa; however, three of the PD patients were classified as having MSA-C or PSP; discrimination of patients with MSA from PSP was poor.
** There was substantial cerebellar atrophy in both cerebellar groups while additional brainstem atrophy was significantly more pronounced in MSA-C patients. Absolute caudate and putamen atrophy was found to be restricted to single MSA-C individuals while group comparisons of mean volumes did not yield significant differences from controls. One control subject (6%) and six MSA-C patients (18%) were classified as IDCA-P.
*** Diagnostic accuracy values for planimetric measurements of regional brain structures are highest in PSP; therefore, sensitivity values were primarily given for PSP.
MSA, multiple system atrophy; MSA-P, Parkinson variant of MSA; MSA-C, cerebellar variant of MSA; PD, Parkinson's disease; PSP, progressive supranuclear palsy; HC, healthy controls; SCA, spinocerebellar ataxia; CBD, corticobasal degeneration; VBM, voxel-based morphometry; MRV, magnetic resonance volumetry; IDCA-P, idiopathic cerebellar ataxia with extracerebellar presentation not corresponding to MSA-C; P/M, pons/midbrain; MCP, middle cerebellar peduncle; SCP, superior cerebellar peduncle; MRPI, magnetic resonance parkinsonism index; SNc, substantia nigra pars compacta; T_1w, T_1-weighted.

MCP width than MSA patients without this MR feature [30]. On the other hand, the area of the pons measured on midsagittal T_1-weighted MR images has been shown to be smaller in MSA-P patients compared to patients with PD and PSP as well as healthy controls; however, there was some overlap at the individual level [26, 31]. As single measurements of these infratentorial structures have been shown not to distinguish adequately between neurodegenerative parkinsonian disorders, especially MSA and PSP, the ratio between midbrain area and pontine area (m/p-ratio) was found to be significantly smaller in patients with PSP compared to other groups [26]. Furthermore, the so-called MR parkinsonism index (MRPI), calculated as the product of the ratio of pons area to midbrain area in midsagittal expanse multiplied by the ratio of the width of MCPs and SCPs ([area pons/area midbrain] × [width MCP/width SCP]), has been shown to discriminate patients with PSP from those with PD, those with MSA, and control subjects, on an individual basis [31–33]. In comparing the MRPI and the m/p-ratio, the MRPI seems to better differentiate PSP from MSA-P, while the m/p-ratio is a better discriminator between PSP and PD [32]. Both a decreased m/p-ratio as well as a decreased MRPI seem to distinguish PSP from MSA, PD, and healthy controls; however, there are some overlapping individual values [26, 31–34].

Volumetry

Manual or semi-automated ROI techniques have been performed to characterize regional brain volume differences in parkinsonian patients. Indeed, volume loss of different supratentorial and infratentorial brain structures, measured by MR volumetry (MRV) with semi-automatic segmentation techniques on an ROI approach, has been reported in patients with APDs. Significant volume loss has been described in the striatum, brainstem, and cerebellum in patients with MSA [35–37]. On the basis of individual structure volumetry, differentiation of MSA from other parkinsonian disorders is difficult. Application of a stepwise discriminant analysis in patients with MSA, PSP, PD, and healthy controls separated all 12 patients with MSA-P and 15 of 17 patients with MSA-C from the PD patients and healthy controls, whereas differentiation of patients with MSA from PSP was poor [35]. More recently, measurements of midbrain, SCP, frontal, third ventricle, and whole brain volumes

adequately discriminate PSP from MSA-P, PD, and healthy controls (sensitivity 89%, specificity 97%) [36]. Furthermore, the best separation between PSP and MSA-P was achieved by using midbrain, SCP, pons, and cerebellar volumes, resulting in a sensitivity of 94% and specificity of 89%. A recent study evaluated 72 patients with PD, 15 with MSA-P, 32 with PSP, and 46 control subjects, assessing the volume of several brain regions, including the cerebellar cortex, thalamus, putamen, pallidum, hippocampus, lateral ventricles, third and fourth ventricles, and brainstem with MRI-based fully automated segmentation software (FreeSurfer) [38]. For this purpose, images have to be subdivided directly into a series of neuroanatomically defined structures with a-priori knowledge of their individual intensity properties, atlas location, and location relative to each other. No volumetric differences were found between PD and controls, while volumes of the cerebellum, putamen, pallidum, hippocampus, and brainstem were significantly reduced in MSA-P and PSP compared to patients with PD and control subjects. PSP and MSA-P patients only differed in thalamic volumes, which were significantly smaller in the PSP group compared to the other groups. On the other hand, ventricular volumes were significantly larger in PSP and MSA-P compared to PD and controls. In this study, no diagnostic accuracy values were given. Bürk and colleagues [39] used MRV on an ROI approach to study the atrophy of the cerebellum, brainstem, caudate nucleus, and putamen in patients with sporadic cerebellar ataxia (including patients with MSA-C and IDCA-P) compared with control subjects. Cerebellar and brainstem volumes were significantly reduced in all cerebellar groups compared to healthy controls, depicting brainstem atrophy as the most prominent in MSA-C, while cerebellar atrophy did not differ between MSA-C and IDCA-P. By application of stepwise discriminant analysis, diagnosis could be correctly predicted in 94% of the controls, 82% of the MSA-C patients, and 100% of the IDCA-P patients.

Quantitative structural MR-based techniques

DWI is sensitive to the random Brownian motion of water molecules, quantified by the calculation of the apparent diffusion coefficient (ADC). Although diffusion is generally restricted alongside fiber tracts, microstructural damage might widen the space between intact fibers, increasing the mobility of water molecules and resulting in higher ADC values. DWI measured in only one direction can lead to an underestimation of diffusion-related pathological changes because the fiber tracts are not orientated in the same direction. The trace of diffusion tensor Trace(D) is given by the average of ADCs (averaged ADC) measured in three orthogonal directions and is by definition independent of anisotropy [40]. The term diffusivity used in this chapter includes Trace(D), averaged ADCs, and mean diffusivity (MD). MTI is based on energy transfer between mobile protons in free water and highly bound protons within structures. The extent of magnetization transfer – correlating with the degree of myelination and axonal density – can be quantified by the calculation of the magnetization transfer ratio (MTR). Paramagnetic ions such as iron accumulate in the brain with increasing age, decreasing the MR signal intensity by creating local magnetic field inhomogeneities. Iron-sensitive MR sequences include T_2-weighted sequences, T_2^*-weighted GRE sequences, SWI, and quantitative measures, such as R_2 and R_2^* maps (relaxation time) as well as phase values on SWI [41].

Although neuronal loss and gliosis may explain alterations obtained by studies using DWI/DTI and MTI, changes are notoriously difficult to interpret due to an insufficient understanding of the structural underpinnings of these changes.

Diffusion-weighted and diffusion tensor imaging

Over the past decade, there has been growing interest in the use of DWI/DTI for the differential diagnosis of APDs from PD. The most relevant studies are summarized in Table 13.7. Several studies performed on an ROI basis found that DWI discriminates MSA-P in early disease stages from PD as well as healthy subjects on the basis of putaminal diffusivity measures values [14, 40, 42–48]. Two studies compared the diagnostic value of striatal ADCs or putaminal diffusivity to either dopamine D2 receptor binding IBZM-SPECT ([^{123}I]-iodobenzamide – single-photon emission computed tomography) [43], or cardiac MIBG ([^{123}I]-meta-iodobenzylguanidine uptake) [48]. Putaminal diffusivity measures were more accurate compared with IBZM-SPECT and cardiac MIBG. In line with the known underlying neuropathology in MSA-P, a more severe involvement of posterior

compared with anterior putaminal diffusivity was found in patients with MSA-P (Figure 13.3) [44, 47].

Importantly, PD subjects with a longer disease duration and concomitant white matter changes might also have increased putaminal diffusivity [49]. Although most reports have found increased putaminal diffusivity in MSA-P at 1.5T [14, 40, 44–47], one study did not confirm this finding [50]. Methodological reasons (putaminal ROI contains parts of the globus pallidus as demonstrated by a published figure in the article) and a longer disease duration in the PD group might explain this discrepancy [42, 45, 46, 51]. The same study also failed to demonstrate diffusivity changes in the SCP of PSP patients – again in contrast with previous reports showing significantly increased diffusivity measures in the SCP in PSP patients at 1.5T [45, 51, 52]. Abnormal diffusivity measures in the MCP have been reported for MSA [45, 47, 50, 51, 53], and abnormal diffusivity measures in the SCP for PSP [51, 52, 54]. The majority of these studies reported a good differentiation between PSP and MSA [50, 54], as well as from controls and PD [47, 52, 54]. However, while diffusivity in the MCP has been reported to have a high diagnostic accuracy for MSA-P in some publications [45, 50], this could not be confirmed by others [47, 51].

Kanazawa and colleagues showed significant increased ADC values in the pons, MCP, cerebellar white matter, and putamen of patients with MSA-C compared to healthy controls [53].

A recent study determined the diagnostic value of fractional anisotropy (FA) for the early diagnosis of MSA [55]; for this reason, 21 patients with MSA-C as well as 14 healthy controls underwent MRI scans. The results revealed reduced FA and white matter atrophy in the MCP, the inferior cerebellar peduncle, and the ventral pons in patients with MSA-C, showing an FA decrease during the first few years after onset as well. Although an overlap of FA values between some MSA-C patients and controls was evident, sensitivity and specificity were 98% and 93%, respectively, for discriminating early MSA-C from normal controls. Therefore, the authors suggested FA measurements may help make an early diagnosis and monitor progression in MSA-C patients. A more recent study evaluated the use of DTI in 19 patients with MSA-C, 12 with MSA-P, 20 with PD as well as 20 healthy controls [56]. Results showed a significant increase in diffusivity values in the MCP and cerebellum, and a decrease in FA in the pyramidal tract, MCP, and

Table 13.7. Diagnostic accuracy of quantitative structural MR-based techniques including DWI, MTI, and iron-sensitive sequences for the diagnosis of MSA

Reference	Cohort size	Main results	Discriminator	Sensitivity,%	Specificity,%
DWI/DTI*					
Schocke et al., 2002 [14]	MSA-P 10 PD 11 HC 7	Significant increased putaminal diffusivity values in MSA-P compared to PD and HC No significant group differences of diffusivity values in the other ROIs Significant correlation between UPDRS III and putaminal diffusivity values	Putaminal diffusivity	100 (MSA-P)	100 (vs. PD and HC)
Seppi et al., 2003 [42]	MSA-P 12 PD 13 PSP 10	Significant increased diffusivity values in putamen, globus pallidus, and caudate nucleus in PSP compared to PD No differences of diffusivity values of the different ROIs between PSP and MSA-P	Putaminal diffusivity	100 (MSA-P)	100 (vs. PD)
Kanazawa et al., 2004 [53]	MSA-C 12 HC 11	Significant increased diffusivity values in the MCP, pons, putamen, and cerebellar white matter in patients with MSA-C compared to HC Significant correlation of disease duration with diffusivity values in the MCP, pons, and cerebellar white matter *Diagnostic accuracy values not given*			
Schocke et al., 2004 [40]	MSA-P 11 PD 17 HC 10	Significant higher putaminal and pallidal diffusivity values in MSA-P compared to both PD patients and healthy volunteers Complete discrimination between MSA-P vs. PD and HC with putaminal diffusivity values in y- and (z-) direction Significant correlation between UPDRS III and putaminal diffusivity values	Putaminal diffusivity	100 (MSA-P)	100 (vs. PD and HC)
Seppi et al., 2004 [43]	MSA-P 15 PD 17 HC 10	Significant lower S/FC ratios and higher striatal diffusivity values in MSA-P compared to both PD and HC No significant differences in S/FC ratios and striatal diffusivity values between PD and HC Higher overall predictive accuracy of striatal diffusivity values (97%) compared to IBZM S/FC ratio (75%)	Striatal diffusivity	93 (MSA-P)	100 (vs. PD and HC)
			IBZM S/FC ratio	80 (MSA-P)	71 (vs. PD and HC)

181

Table 13.7. (cont.)

Reference	Cohort size	Main results	Discriminator	Sensitivity,%	Specificity,%
Shiga et al., 2005 [121]	MSA 11 (8 MSA-C, 3 MSA-C) HC 10	Significant decreased FA values in MCP, basis pontis, and internal capsule Significant negative correlation of MCP FA values with ataxia scores	FA in MCP	100 (MSA-P and MSA-C)	100 (vs. HC)
Blain et al., 2006 [51]	MSA-P 10 MSA-C 7 PD 12 PSP 17 HC 12	Significant increased diffusivity values and decreased FA values in MCP in MSA compared to PSP, PD, and HC Significant increased pontine diffusivity values in MSA compared to PSP, PD, and HC Significant increased SCP diffusivity values in PSP compared to MSA, PD, and HC, and significant decreased SCP FA values in PSP compared to PD Significant correlation between ataxia and diffusivity values in MCP and pons in MSA	MCP diffusivity	100 (only MSA-C)	100 (vs. all groups)
Nicoletti et al., 2006 [45]	MSA-P 16 PD 16 PSP 16 HC 15	Significant increased putaminal diffusivity values in MSA-P compared to PD and HC Significant increased MCP diffusivity values in MSA-P not only compared to PD and HC but also compared to PSP	MCP diffusivity	100 (MSA-P)	100 (vs. all groups)
			Putaminal diffusivity	100 (MSA-P)	100 (vs. PD and HC) 81 (vs. PSP)
Seppi et al., 2006 [44]	MSA-P 15 PD 20 HC 11	Significant increased diffusivity values in the entire, anterior, and posterior putamen in MSA-P compared to PD and HC Significant higher diffusivity values in the posterior compared to the anterior putamen in MSA-P No significant differences between posterior and anterior putamen in PD and HC	Putaminal diffusivity	93 (MSA-P)	100 (vs. PD and HC)
			Posterior putaminal diffusivity	100 (MSA-P)	100 (vs. PD and HC)
Ito et al., 2007 [46]	MSA 20 (MSA-P 10, MSA-C 10) PD 21 HC 20	Significant higher diffusivity values and significant lower FA values in the pons, cerebellum, and putamen in MSA compared to PD and HC	Diffusivity pons	70 (MSA-P)	70 (vs. PD)

Table 13.7. (*cont.*)

Reference	Cohort size	Main results	Discriminator	Sensitivity,%	Specificity,%
		No difference in the diffusivity and FA values of the different regions between MSA-P and MSA-C	Diffusivity cerebellum	60 (MSA-P)	88 (vs. PD)
		All patients that had both significant low FA and high diffusivity values in each of the three regions were MSA-P cases, and those that had both normal FA and diffusivity values in the pons were all PD cases	Diffusivity putamen	70 (MSA-P)	64 (vs. PD)
			FA pons	70 (MSA-P)	100 (vs. PD)
			FA cerebellum	70 (MSA-P)	64 (vs. PD)
			FA putamen	70 (MSA-P)	88 (vs. PD)
			Both low FA and high diffusivity values in any of the three areas	90 (MSA-P)	100 (vs. PD)
Köllensperger et al., 2007 [48]	MSA-P 9 PD 9 HC 16	Significant increased putaminal diffusivity values in MSA-P compared to PD and HC No significant differences of blood pressure response to passive tilt between PD and MSA-P DWI was superior to both tilt table testing and MIBG scintigraphy in the differential diagnosis of MSA-P versus the other groups	Putaminal diffusivity	100 (MSA-P)	100 (vs. all groups)
		Significant lower H/M ratios in PD compared to HC with considerable overlap between MSA-P and PD	MIBG H/M ratio	56 (MSA-P)	89 (vs. all groups)
Nilsson et al., 2007 [122]	MSA-P 4 PD 2 PSP 3 HC 2	Degeneration of the MCP and pontine crossing tracts, with decreased FA and increased diffusivity values in advanced MSA Selective degeneration of the SCP in PSP, such as reduction of cortical projection fibers *Diagnostic accuracy values not given*			
Paviour et al., 2007 [50]	MSA-P 11 PD 12 PSP 20 HC 7	Significant higher diffusivity values in the MCP and rostral pons in MSA-P compared to PSP and PD Significant correlation between diffusivity values in rostral pons and H & Y in MSA-P	MCP diffusivity	91 (MSA-P)	82 (vs. all groups) 84 (vs. PSP)

Table 13.7. (cont.)

Reference	Cohort size	Main results	Discriminator	Sensitivity,%	Specificity,%
		Significant correlation between globus pallidum diffusivity values and H & Y and UPDRS II and III			
Nicoletti et al., 2008 [54]	MSA-P 15 PD 16 PSP 28 HC 15	Significant higher SCP diffusivity values in PSP compared to MSA-P, PD, and HC Assessment of diffusivity values in the SCP was not possible in 2 patients due to methodological reasons	SCP diffusivity	100 (PSP)	93 (vs. PD and HC)
			SCP diffusivity	97 (PSP)	93 (vs. MSA-P)
Oishi et al., 2009 [55]	MSA-C 21 HC 14	Significant FA reduction and white matter atrophy in ventral pons, MCP, and ICP in MSA-C patients compared to HC	FA MCP	98 (MSA-C)	93 (vs. HC)
					AUC = 0.9769
Pellecchia et al., 2009 [47]	MSA-P 9 MSA-C 12 HC 11	Significant increased diffusivity values in entire and anterior putamen in MSA-P compared to MSA-C and HC Significant increased diffusivity values in posterior putamen in MSA-P compared to HC Significant increased diffusivity values in MCP and cerebellar white matter in MSA-C compared to MSA-P and HC Significant increased pontine diffusivity values in MSA-C compared to HC Significant higher diffusivity values in the posterior compared to the anterior putamen in MSA-P and MSA-C, but not in PD and HC Significant correlation of disease duration with cerebellar diffusivity values in MSA-C and pontine diffusivity values in MSA-P Significant correlation of UMSARS and UPDRS with diffusivity values in posterior and entire putamen Diagnostic accuracy values not given			
Tir et al., 2009 [82]	MSA-P 14 PD 19 HC 14	VBM: significant lower density of GM in MSA-P in a motor-related circuit: especially in the left primary motor cortex, relative to PD, and in the left supplementary motor area, relative to HC Voxel-wise FA analysis: significant reduced FA in the left primary motor cortex and the right cerebellum No clinicoradiological correlation with FA values Diagnostic accuracy values not given			
Tha et al., 2010 [77]	MSA-C 16 HC 16	Significant reduction of FA values and elevation of diffusivity values in supra- and infratentorial white matter structures in MSA compared to HC No significant abnormalities in supratentorial white matter using T_2w and proton density images Diagnostic accuracy values not given			
Pellecchia et al., 2011 [103]	MSA 11 (MSA-P 7, MSA-C 4)	Significant increase of diffusivity values in the putamen, pons, cerebellar white matter, thalamus, and frontal white matter between baseline and 1-year follow-up Diagnostic accuracy values not given			

Table 13.7. (cont.)

Reference	Cohort size	Main results	Discriminator	Sensitivity,%	Specificity,%
Wang et al., 2011 [56]	MSA 31 (MSA-P 12, MSA-C 19) PD 20 HC 20	Significant increased diffusivity values in the MCP and cerebellum in MSA-P and MSA-C compared to HC Significant decreased FA values in the pyramidal tract, MCP, and white matter of the cerebellum in MSA-C and MSA-P compared to HC No significant diffusivity changes in PD compared to HC	Diffusivity cerebellum	95 (MSA-C) 75 (MSA-P)	85 (vs. PD and HC)
			FA cerebellum	95 (MSA-C) 83 (MSA-P)	80 (vs. PD and HC)
			Diffusivity cerebellum	58 (MSA-C)	100 (vs. PD and HC)
			Diffusivity basal ganglia	52 (MSA)	90 (vs. HC)
Tsukamoto et al., 2012 [61]	MSA 25 (MSA-P 5, MSA-C 20) PSP 20 PD 17 HC 18	Significant higher regional diffusivity values in the pons, MCP, cerebellar white matter, and dentate nucleus in MSA compared to PSP, PD, and HC Significant higher regional diffusivity values in the posterior putamen in MSA compared to PSP and HC Significant higher regional diffusivity values in the globus pallidus and midbrain in PSP compared to MSA, PD, and HC Significant higher regional diffusivity values in the caudate nucleus and SCP in PSP compared to MSA and HC Significant higher regional diffusivity values in the entire putamen, posterior part of putamen, entire globus pallidus, lateral part of globus pallidus, and head of caudate nucleus in MSA-P compared to MSA-C Significant higher regional diffusivity values in the pons, MCP, and cerebellar white matter in MSA-C compared to MSA-P No significant differences in regional diffusivity values in PD compared to MSA, PSP, and HC in all regions *Diagnostic accuracy values not given*			
MTI					
Naka et al., 2002 [63]	MSA 12 HC 11	Significant lower MTRs in the pontine base, MCP, putamen, and white matter of the precentral gyrus in MSA compared to HC *Diagnostic accuracy values not given*			
Eckert et al., 2004 [62]	MSA 12 PD 15 PSP 10 HC 20	Change of MTR in the globus pallidus, putamen, caudate nucleus, SN, and white matter**			
		Model including MTRs of globus pallidus, putamen, and caudate nucleus (using stepwise linear discrimination model)		58 (MSA)	100 (vs. PD and HC) 90 (vs. PSP)

Table 13.7. *(cont.)*

Reference	Cohort size	Main results	Discriminator	Sensitivity,%	Specificity,%
Da Rocha *et al.*, 2007 [64]	MSA 10 HC 25	Complete differentiation of MSA patients and HC by detecting corticospinal tract degeneration using T_1 SE/MTC FLAIR sequences are useless in distinguishing patients from HC		100 (MSA)	100 (vs. HC)
Iron					
Kraft *et al.*, 2002 [19]	MSA 15 PD 40 HC 17	Significant differences for relative putaminal hypointensities in T_2*w GRE sequences in MSA compared to PD No significant differences for relative putaminal hypointensities in T_2w FSE in MSA compared to PD *Diagnostic accuracy values not given*			
von Lewinski *et al.*, 2007 [20]	MSA 52 PD 88 HC 29	Signal loss of the dorsolateral putamen on T_2* GRE sequences at 1.0T in MSA	Signal loss dorsolateral putamen	69 (MSA)	91 (vs. PD and HC)
		Hyperintense lateral putaminal rim on FLAIR sequences at 1T in MSA	Hyperintense putaminal rim	48 (MSA)	93 (vs. PD and HC)
			Signal loss dorsolateral putamen and hyperintense putaminal rim	42 (MSA)	97 (vs. PD and HC)
			SI PUT/CAUD	65 (MSA)	95 (vs. PD)
				Diagnostic accuracy 82%	
Arabia *et al.*, 2010 [123]	MSA 20 PSP 41 PD 189 HC 150	Significant higher frequencies of putaminal hypointensities in MSA-P and PSP compared to PD and HC using T_2* GRE sequences with 15 ms echo time	Putaminal hypointensities	55 (MSA) 25 (PD) 44 (PSP)	93 (vs. HC)
Gupta *et al.*, 2010 [66]	MSA-P 12 PSP 12 PD 11	Significant higher red nucleus hypointensity in PSP compared to MSA-P and PD using SWI Significant higher putaminal hypointensity in PSP compared to PD using SWI No significant differences in putaminal hypointensity between PSP and MSA-P or MSA-P and PD using SWI	SWI hypointensity score >2 (red nucleus)	67 (PSP)	82 (vs. PD) 83 (vs. MSA-P)
			SWI hypointensity score >2 (putamen)	50 (PSP)	91 (vs. PD)

Table 13.7. (cont.)

Reference	Cohort size	Main results	Discriminator	Sensitivity,%	Specificity,%
Sakurai et al., 2010 [67]	MSA-P 10 PD 14 HC 10	Significant higher grade of putaminal hypointensity in MSA-P compared to PD and HC on all 3D-PRESTO, T_2*w, and T_2w sequences	Putaminal hypointensity (3D PRESTO)	90 (MSA-P)	79 (vs. PD) 70 (vs. HC)
		Significant differences in the mean grade of putaminal hypointensity in MSA-P among 3D-PRESTO, T_2*w, and T_2w sequences	Putaminal atrophy (3D PRESTO)	70 (MSA-P)	100 (vs. PD and HC)
Wang et al., 2012 [68]	MSA-P 10 PD 21 HC 54	Significant higher iron deposition in the putamen and pulvinar thalamus in MSA-P compared to PD using SWI More sensitivity in differentiating MSA-P from PD by means of the high-iron-deposition-percentage area than the average phase shift *Diagnostic accuracy values not given*	Putamen	AUC = 0.88 (high-iron-deposition-percentage area) AUC = 0.78 (average phase shift)	
			Pulvinar thalamus	AUC = 0.79 (high-iron-deposition-percentage area) AUC = 0.62 (average phase shift)	
			Lower inner region of the putamen	AUC = 0.92 (high-iron-deposition-percentage area) AUC = 0.91 (average phase shift)	

* In the studies by Schocke et al. [14] Seppi et al. [42, 43] and Kanazawa et al. [53] ADC was measured in z-slice direction only, in the other studies ADCs were averaged (ADCave) over three orthogonal measurements, thus representing the Trace(D) or MD.
** The main finding in this study was a change in the MTR in the globus pallidus, putamen, caudate nucleus, substantia nigra, and white matter in PD, MSA, and PSP patients, matching the pathological features of the underlying disorder. MTRs were significantly reduced in the putamen in MSA patients compared to PD patients and healthy controls as well as in the substantia nigra in patients with PSP, MSA, and PD. MSA, multiple system atrophy; MSA-P, Parkinson variant of MSA; MSA-C, cerebellar variant of MSA; PD, Parkinson's disease; PSP, progressive supranuclear palsy; HC, healthy controls; S/FC, striatal to frontal cortex uptake; H/M, heart/mediastinum; MRI, magnetic resonance imaging; T, Tesla; GM, gray matter; ICP, inferior cerebellar peduncle; MCP, middle cerebellar peduncle; SCP, superior cerebellar peduncle; SN, substantia nigra; GRE, gradient echo; FLAIR, fluid-attenuated inversion recovery; AUC, area under the curve; ROI, region of interest; FA, fractional anisotropy; H & Y, Hoehn and Yahr Scale; DWI, diffusion-weighted imaging; DTI, diffusion tensor imaging; SWI, susceptibility weighted imaging; FSE, fast spin echo; MTI, magnetization transfer imaging; MD, mean diffusivity; Trace(D), trace of diffusion tensor; MTR, magnetization transfer ratio; SI $_{PUT/CAUD}$, signal intensity dorsolateral putamen/signal intensity head of caudate nucleus; T_1 SE/MTC, T_1 spin-echo with an additional magnetization transfer contrast pulse; PRESTO, principles of echo shifting with a train of observations; T_2w, T_2-weighted; T2*w, T_2*-weighted; VBM, voxel-based morphometry; IBZM, [123I]-iodobenzamide; MIBG, [123I]-meta-iodobenzylguanidine; UMSARS, Unified Multiple System Atrophy Rating Scale; UPDRS, Unified Parkinson's Disease Rating Scale.

white matter of the cerebellum in patients with MSA-P and MSA-C compared to controls. Furthermore, significant reduction of gray matter was only found in the cerebellar hemispheres in patients with MSA-C, whereas no significant atrophy of either gray or white matter was found in patients with MSA-P or PD compared to healthy controls, which is discordant to other MR studies [57–59].

There are few 3T DWI studies and the results are inconsistent; possibly due to increased signal-to-noise

187

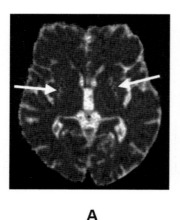
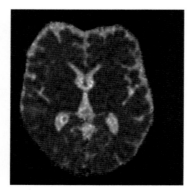

A   **B**

Figure 13.3 Axial mean diffusivity maps at the level of mid-striatum in a patient with MSA-P (A; female; age 68 years; disease duration 2 years; Hoehn and Yahr stage 2) and a patient with Parkinson's disease (B; male; age 69 years; disease duration 4 years; Hoehn and Yahr stage 2). Note the diffuse hyperintensity – corresponding to increased mean diffusivity values – in the putamen (arrows) in the patient with MSA-P.

ratios, increased magnetic susceptibility effects, and increased echo-planar image distortion at 3T that may affect DWI/DTI findings compared to 1.5T. Diffusivity values in the pons, cerebellum, and putamen at 3T were found to be significantly higher and FA values lower in MSA than in PD or controls. In differentiating MSA-P from PD using FA and diffusivity values, there was similar sensitivity (70%) and higher specificity (100%) in the pons than in the putamen and cerebellum. In addition, all patients that had both significantly low FA and high diffusivity values in each of these three areas were MSA-P cases, and those that had both normal FA and diffusivity values in the pons were all PD cases [46]. Focke and colleagues [60] found a significant increase of diffusivity values in the globus pallidus and substantia nigra (SN) bilaterally in PSP patients versus PD patients and controls. Furthermore, diffusivity values in the SN were higher in the PSP group compared to patients with MSA-P, and DTI showed no significant predictive power in patients with MSA-P. However, by contrast to all other reports, the authors of this study used a stimulated echo acquisition mode (STEAM)-based DTI compared to the conventional echo-planar imaging (EPI)-based DTI, used in other publications [40, 42]. A more recent study evaluated the utility of regional diffusivity values at 3T in patients with neurodegenerative parkinsonism [61]. In the MSA group, diffusivity was significantly higher in the posterior putamen, midbrain, pons, MCP, and cerebellar white matter, which is in line with the characteristic lesions in MSA. For the differentiation of MSA from PSP, diffusivity in the posterior putamen achieved levels of significance.

Magnetization transfer imaging

Using MTI, basal ganglia abnormalities have been reported in patients with MSA. One study revealed significantly decreased MTRs in the putamen, globus pallidus, and SN in MSA patients [62]. With stepwise discriminant analysis there was a good discrimination of PD patients and controls from the MSA and PSP patients, as only one out of 12 MSA patients was wrongly classified into the control group. On the other hand, separation between PD patients and controls as well as between MSA and PSP patients was insufficient. Naka and coworkers revealed significant MTR reductions in the putamen and the white matter of precentral gyrus compared to controls [63]. Another study evaluated pyramidal involvement in ten patients with probable MSA [64]. They detected the presence of spasticity, hyperreflexia, and a Babinski sign, as well as abnormal MTR values of the pyramidal tract and primary motor cortex in all of the patients, showing a correlation between MTR abnormalities and clinical features of pyramidal tract dysfunction. A recent multimodal MRI study showed reduced MTR values in the putamen of patients with MSA-P; however, this finding did not allow for a differentiation between parkinsonian conditions [60]. Due to the limited evidence of MTI in neurodegenerative parkinsonism, its use remains experimental. Diagnostic accuracy values of the studies mentioned above are listed in detail in Table 13.7.

Iron-sensitive MRI

Well-known histopathological findings indicate increased iron deposition in the putamen of patients with MSA, and several MRI techniques are able to demonstrate changes that are reflective of this increased iron accumulation [65]. While an earlier paper focused on the visual assessment or semi-quantitative grading of signal changes on iron-sensitive MRI sequences [19, 20, 66], more recently published work assessed quantitative changes on iron-sensitive MR sequences. Quantitative parameters on iron-sensitive MR sequences used in MSA include T_2^*, SWI, SWI phase images, R_2 and R_2^*, whereas R_2^* offers a higher sensitivity compared to R_2. Diagnostic accuracy values of iron-sensitive MR series are summarized in Table 13.7.

Using T_2^*-weighted GRE sequences instead of T_2-weighted fast spin echo (FSE) images, hypointense putaminal signal changes were reported to be more frequent in MSA than in PD patients [19]. However, this finding is not seen in all cases of clinically diagnosed MSA patients. Sensitivity in this study was 73%: 4 of 15 MSA patients did not have a hypointense signal of the putamen on T_2^*-weighted GRE sequences. On the other hand, putaminal hypointensity on T_2^*-weighted GRE sequences was seen in 13 of 40 PD patients, indicating that this finding is of limited utility in differentiating MSA from PD patients [19]. A study evaluating putaminal paramagnetic susceptibility changes on T_2^*-weighted GRE sequences at 1T in patients with MSA and PD as well as controls reported a high specificity of 91% with a sensitivity of 69% for signal loss of the dorsolateral putamen on T_2^*-weighted GRE sequences in detecting MSA. The combination of hypointensity with a hyperintense lateral rim in FLAIR sequences increased the specificity to 97% by reducing sensitivity to 42%. Quantitative assessment of signal intensities on an ROI basis in the T_2^*-weighted GRE sequences revealed that the quotient of mean signal intensities in the dorsolateral putamen and the head of the caudate nucleus could discriminate MSA from PD with an accuracy of 82%, which was higher than using the putaminal ROI alone [20]. Principles of echo shifting with a train of observations (PRESTO) sequences provide high sensitivity to susceptibility changes from iron accumulation and have been evaluated for detecting putaminal hypointensity in patients with MSA-P and differentiating MSA-P from PD [67]. Putaminal hypointensity was seen more often in MSA-P than PD and controls in all three, 3D-PRESTO, T_2^*-weighted, and T_2-weighted sequences. The 3D-PRESTO sequence was more sensitive for detecting the putaminal hypointensity in MSA-P than

the T_2^*-weighted sequence, reflecting the susceptibility changes caused by iron depositions in the putamen. For putaminal hypointensity, sensitivity was 90% and specificity was 79% (versus PD) and 70% (versus controls); whereas for putaminal atrophy sensitivity was 70% and specificity was 100% (versus PD and controls). Because of physiological age-related iron accumulation a similar hypointensity can be seen in healthy subjects [65].

A recent study applied SWI phase images for the determination of different iron-deposition patterns in several gray nuclei in 16 patients with idiopathic PD, 8 patients with MSA-P, and 44 age-matched healthy controls [68]. For this reason, different phase shifts as well as the high iron percentage of the area were evaluated in the entire putamen, four subregions of the putamen (upper inner region, upper outer region, lower inner region, lower outer), the pulvinar thalamus, the SN, the red nucleus, the caudate nucleus, the thalamus, and the globus pallidus. The MSA-P cohort had significantly higher iron deposition in the putamen and the pulvinar of the thalamus compared with the PD and control group, while iron deposition in the SN was similar between the MSA-P and PD groups, which was significantly higher compared to controls. Area under the curve (AUC) of receiver operating characteristic (ROC) curve analysis showed higher sensitivity in differentiating MSA-P from PD, by means of the high-iron-deposition-percentage area than the average phase shift. Moreover, the lower inner region of the putamen was the most valuable subregion in differentiating MSA-P from PD among the four putaminal subregions [68]. A recent study could show higher values in R_2 and R_2^* maps within the basal ganglia in patients with MSA-P compared to patients with PD [60]. The most marked findings, however, resulted from R_2^* measurements, where the best separation could be achieved in the putamen, showing bilaterally significant R_2^* increases; whereas R_2 mapping of the MSA-P group compared to PD showed a trend but was not statistically significant (Figure 13.4).

Multimodal imaging

Multimodal imaging is an approach to measure MR parameters sensitive to complementary tissue characteristics. Several multimodal imaging studies in PD, using combinations of volumetry, R_2^*, MD, or FA [69–71], showed that a combination of different methods sensitive to complementary tissue characteristics may provide better discrimination compared to single techniques. In MSA, Focke and colleagues performed a multimodal MRI study using a comprehensive quantitative MRI protocol, including R_2^*-, R_2-, and R_1-mapping, magnetization transfer, and DTI measures at 3T in 12 patients with PD, 10 with MSA-P, 9 with PSP, and 13 healthy controls [60]. The best separation of MSA from PD could be achieved by using R_2^* sequences in the putamen, resulting in a sensitivity of 77.8% and specificity of 100%, presenting the best predictive power (AUC ≤ 0.96). DTI showed no differences in patients with MSA-P compared to PD, PSP, and healthy controls; most likely because this study used STEAM-based DTI, which is known to have lower signal intensity-to-noise ratio compared to EPI-based DTI. MTR values were reduced in the putamen in patients with MSA-P, resulting in statistically significant predictive power for distinguishing MSA-P from PD. In summary, although there were some differences between MSA-P and PSP, the findings did not achieve significance.

Radiological correlations with pathological and clinical data using cMRI and DWI/DTI

Watanabe and colleagues investigated disease progression and survival along with MRI assessments of 85 patients with MSA-C and 54 with MSA-P [4]. According to the clinical phenotype, putaminal abnormalities were more frequent in MSA-P, whereas pontine abnormalities were more common in MSA-C. Furthermore, this cross-sectional study reported an increase in MRI findings in advancing disease, showing a frequency of a T_2 hyperintense putaminal rim of 38% within 2 years, 65% within 4 years, and 77% more than 4 years after disease onset. Paviour and coworkers studied clinical–radiological correlations in patients with PSP (n = 18), MSA-P (n = 9), and PD (n = 9), as well as healthy controls (n = 18), using volumetric measurements of whole brain and regional volumes, including cerebellum, pons, midbrain, SCP, and ventricular volumes as well as frontal and posterior-inferior cerebral regions [36]. They revealed that motor disability in MSA-P is associated with a smaller pontine volume, whereas midbrain volume was not associated with motor deficits. While in this

study more severe midbrain atrophy was associated with postural instability in patients with PSP, there was not an association between falls or postural stability and the regional atrophy in MSA-P.

Over 15 years ago, Kraft and colleagues first correlated hypointense and hyperintense signal changes on T_2-weighted MRI with neuronal loss, reactive microgliosis and astrogliosis, as well as iron content in the putamen of two postmortem confirmed patients with MSA [72]. They suggested that putaminal hypointensity might reflect increased iron deposition as well as the presence of reactive microglial and astroglial cells. More recently, Matsusue and colleagues compared postmortem T_2-weighted images at 1.5T with histological findings in seven autopsy-proved cases with MSA. They concluded that putaminal atrophy histologically reflects neuronal loss and gliosis, and diffuse ferritin and iron deposition are correlates for putaminal T_2 hypointensity. Furthermore, the hyperintense putaminal rim seems to reflect degeneration of the lateral margin of the putamen or degeneration of the external capsule, whereas tissue rarefaction was associated with neuronal loss and gliosis [73]. Cerebellar atrophy and degeneration was found more severely in the cerebellar white matter than in the cerebellar cortices. Cerebellar hyperintensity was associated with loss of myelinated fibers and gliosis, whereas dentate nucleus hypointensity depicted diffusive ferritin deposition in dentate nuclei and white matter both within and surrounding the nuclei [74]. A recent study assessed cMRI abnormalities – blinded to clinical details – in 48 neuropathologically confirmed cases, consisting of 22 patients with PSP, 13 with MSA, 7 with PD, 6 with corticobasal degeneration (CBD), and 9 healthy controls [75]. Additionally, diagnostic values of clinical and radiological diagnosis were explored. Sensitivity and specificity of the clinical diagnosis of PSP in this study were 91% and 83%, respectively, whereas values for MSA were found to be 62% and 98%, respectively. In contrast, sensitivity and specificity of radiological diagnosis were 73% and 94% for PSP, and 77% and 100% for MSA, respectively. Specificity of reported MRI findings, including the "hummingbird" and "morning glory" sign as well as atrophy and hyperintensity of MCP and the "hot cross bun" sign for PSP and MSA, respectively, was quite high but sensitivity was suboptimal.

Using DWI/DTI, several studies have found a correlation of diffusivity measures of the entire and

Patient 1

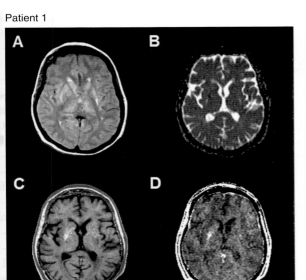

Patient 2

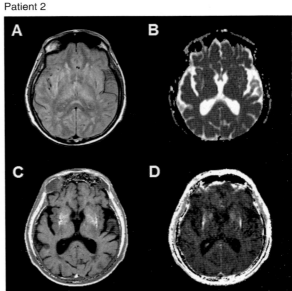

Figure 13.4 Axial MRI scans at 1.5T in two MSA-P patients (**patient 1**: female, disease duration 1 year; **patient 2**: male, disease duration 2 years). (A) Proton density weighted image. (B) Mean diffusivity. (C) R_2 map. (D) R_2^* map. **Patient 1 shows** high diffusivity in the putamen bilaterally (B) and low iron levels (D) **and patient 2 shows** high iron levels (D) with increased putaminal diffusivity (B).

posterior putamen with disease severity as assessed with the UPDRS (Unified Parkinson's Disease Rating Scale) and UMSARS (Unified Multiple System Atrophy Rating Scale) [12, 14, 40, 47]. Significant correlations between disease duration with cerebellar ADC values in MSA-C and pontine ADC values in MSA-P were reported by Pellecchia and coworkers [47].

Prakash and colleagues [76] suggested that DTI reductions of white matter integrity in the cerebellar peduncles correlate better to clinical features of patients with sporadic and hereditary ataxias than cMRI measures of pontocerebellar atrophy, although diagnostic accuracy values were not given. In all subjects, mainly patients with MSA-C and SCA-1, average FA values were significantly decreased in the MCP, SCP, and inferior cerebellar peduncle (ICP), showing correlation with disease severity as well. Furthermore, patients with MSA-C showed significantly reduced FA values in left cerebellar white matter, right pyramidal tract, left internal capsule, the midline transverse pontine fibers, and the right MCP, compared to controls.

Another study [77] revealed widespread FA reductions and MD elevations in several infra- and supratentorial white matter structures, such as

MCP, pontine base, periaqueductal area, lateral midbrain as well as portions of the internal and external capsule, in patients with MSA-C. In addition, several significant correlations between areas with FA and/or MD alterations and clinical data were observed, including Barthel index score, SARA score (Scale for the Assessment and Rating of Ataxia), severity of orthostatic hypotension, and disease duration.

Voxel-based analysis

Voxel-based analyses of quantitative data such as volumetric T_1 maps, R_2 maps, or DWI/DTI maps permit an unbiased, operator-independent, and semi-automated detection of significant differences in different tissue types of the whole brain, avoiding a-priori ROI selection [78]. Advantages of voxel-based analysis include independence from operators due to automated detection; since it involves group-wise comparisons it is not appropriate for evaluation of individual patients. Furthermore, in performing a voxel-based study many methodological options are available and there are known pitfalls, which are summarized in a very recent review [79].

191

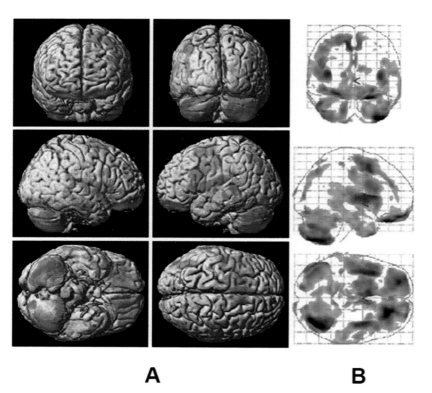

A　　　　　　　　**B**

Figure 13.5 Progression of brain atrophy in MSA-P in comparison with PD – highlighted in red (A) and gray (B) – involving several cortical areas: motor cortex, posterior parietal cortex, middle frontal, medial frontal, and orbitofrontal cortex, insula as well as the cerebellum. (A) overlay onto a rendered brain surface; (B) glass brain view.

In patients with MSA-P and MSA-C, VBM [54] confirmed ROI-based volumetric findings that demonstrated basal ganglia and infratentorial volume losses and additionally revealed volume reduction in several cortical regions. VBM has also been used to investigate the progression of cortical and subcortical atrophy patterns in MSA-P compared to PD and revealed early degeneration of the basal ganglia followed by later-onset cortical atrophy (see Figure 13.5) [80]. Voxel-based relaxometry (VBR) has recently been used to study brain morphology in MSA-C versus MSA-P and healthy volunteers as well [59, 81]. In accordance with the VBM analysis in MSA-C, which showed reductions of gray and white matter in the cerebellum and brainstem, VBR analysis of the same patients revealed reduction of the relaxation rate R_2 in the same regions due to an increased content of cerebrospinal fluid in the respective voxels, reflecting infratentorial brain atrophy [81]. In addition, R_2 was increased in the putamen, a region in which VBM did not show abnormalities, thus suggesting that the combination of VBR and VBM may provide convergent and complementary information

about the brain morphology of MSA-C [81]. Using VBM and VBR, direct comparison of MSA-C and MSA-P showed differences only in infratentorial brain regions, where structural abnormalities were more pronounced in MSA-C than in MSA-P. In MSA-C, there was greater volume loss of gray matter in the basal parts of the cerebellum and of white matter in the brainstem as well as a stronger reduction of the relaxation rate R_2 in the cerebellum and brainstem [59]. In several studies, VBM analysis revealed decreased gray matter in the basal ganglia and the cerebral cortex in MSA-P patients compared to healthy controls [57–59]. In a recent study, VBR analysis showed prolonged T_2 in various cortical regions and a negative correlation between T_2 and cerebral volume could be demonstrated [57].

Oishi and coworkers performed a voxel-based FA analysis and VBM in patients with early MSA-C [55]. In this study, white matter atrophy without gray matter atrophy was revealed as a characteristic finding related to FA reduction. This contrasts to previous reports demonstrating volume loss in both the gray and white matter, and may be due to the fact that the patients included were in early stages of disease and did not fulfill diagnostic criteria. Using a combination of VBM and whole brain voxel-based DTI, patients with MSA-P, PD, and healthy controls were evaluated regarding motor-related circuit dysfunction [82]. In VBM analysis, MSA-P patients showed reduced gray matter density in motor-related circuits, including the left primary motor cortex (PMC) and the left supplementary area, compared to PD patients and control subjects, respectively. Using the volumetric diffusion technique, MSA-P patients had lower FA values in the left PMC and the right posterior cerebellum compared to controls. There was no difference between MSA-P patients, PD patients, and controls in terms of ADC values. The authors suggested that MSA-P is characterized by both macro- and microstructural changes in the sensorimotor circuit.

Magnetic resonance spectroscopy

In proton magnetic resonance spectroscopy (^{1}H MRS), protons chemically bound to different molecules can be differentiated by characteristic imprints of spectral resonances, the so-called chemical shifts [83]. The main resonances in brain ^{1}H MRS relate to N-acetylaspartate (NAA) as an indirect expression of the integrity and function of neurons, choline (Cho)-containing compounds as a marker for cell membrane turnover indicating glial activity, creatine (Cr), including phosphocreatine, as a marker for energy metabolism, as well as lactate as an indicator for anaerobic glycolysis detected under pathological conditions [84, 85]. The N-acetylaspartate to creatine ratio (NAA/Cr) is considered a metabolic marker reflecting the integrity and function of neurons and axons in the brain, with a decrease indicating neuronal or axonal dysfunction. Studies using ^{1}H MRS revealed reduced NAA/Cr and NAA/Cho ratios in the lentiform nucleus or striatum not only in APD [86–89], but also in PD [84, 90, 91], as opposed to previously published results that suggested reduced NAA/Cr ratios in striatal structures in MSA but not PD [86–89]. Mostly technical factors including the application of different echo- and relaxation times, voxel sizes, and pulse sequences may account for some of the contradictory results [84, 90]. By increasing sensitivity and dispersion of the chemical shift, use of higher magnetic field strengths in ^{1}H MRS may render this technique more important in the differential diagnosis of parkinsonian disorders, even though

greater magnetic susceptibility may diminish this benefit. A recent study applied multiple regional single-voxel ^{1}H MRS of the putamen, pontine basis, and cerebral white matter at 3T in 24 patients with MSA compared to 11 PD patients and 18 healthy controls [92]. In both MSA-C and MSA-P significant NAA/Cr reductions were observed in the pontine basis, while reduced putaminal NAA/Cr was found in the patients with MSA-P. There was a significant NAA/Cr reduction in the pontine basis as well as in the putamen in patients with MSA-P compared with both controls and PD, which suggests that the combined assessment of NAA/Cr in the pontine basis and putamen may help distinguish MSA-P from PD [92]; however, diagnostic accuracy values were not given. Magnetic resonance spectroscopic imaging (MRSI) is an advanced ^{1}H MRS technique, which acquires spectra simultaneously over a large brain region from multiple voxels during the same sequence, allowing not only the spatial location of the voxels to be changed (without loss of quality) by sub-voxel shifts during post-processing, but allowing also individual voxels to be aligned with anatomical features and allowing an absolute quantification of metabolites such as NAA to be performed [93]. Quantitative analysis techniques have advantages over the alternative ratio-based methods, as the most commonly used standards, Cr and Cho, have been found to vary in concentration in some circumstances, making interpretation of ratios difficult in studies using ^{1}H MRS and being one of the reasons for the conflicting results of ^{1}H MRS studies in neurodegenerative parkinsonism in the past [90]. A recent study using MRSI at 1.5T in 11 patients with PD, 11 with MSA-P, 6 with MSA-C, 13 with PSP, and 18 controls revealed lower NAA concentrations in the pallidum, putamen, and lentiform nucleus in patients with PSP and MSA-P compared to healthy controls and patients with PD [93]. Mainly due to the conflicting results, the limited specificity, and technical challenges of ^{1}H MRS, its use in the field of neurodegenerative parkinsonism is mainly experimental [94].

Progression studies with MRI

Compared with patients with PD, there is faster disease progression in MSA, with death occurring on average 8–10 years after disease onset [95]. Past neuropathological studies of MSA brains have reported structural changes that are reflective of advanced stages of disease [96]. Imaging allows for prospective monitoring of these changes even in early stages of disease and how they evolve over time. Unfortunately longitudinal studies have been rarely performed in MSA [17, 97]. Evolution of MSA pathology has been shown in a study using cMRI at 0.2T [17]. Only 50% of MSA-P patients were reported to have putaminal slit changes on T_2 within 3 years after symptom onset, and 86% within 6 years after symptom onset. In contrast, 71% of patients with MSA-C showed complete "hot cross bun" sign within 5 years, and even 100% of patients within 7 years after symptom onset [17].

Automated methods for the longitudinal assessment of volumetric MR studies are based on an automated definition of tissue type in each voxel, thus being operator independent. VBM is applied to groups of scans, highlighting atrophy patterns in groups of patients over time. By contrast, methods using registration of serial imaging are applied to individual scan pairs with accurate registration of follow-up and baseline scan, thus determining rates of atrophy rather than atrophy patterns [98]. Several imaging studies revealed progression in MSA using volumetric measurements [80, 99, 100]. Fluid registration of serial MRI scans was used to demonstrate regional atrophy in one MSA patient with subsequent pathological confirmation (Figure 13.6) [101]. The two scans revealed several differences between regions of increasing atrophy: the most prominent atrophy was found to be in the pons and MCP, as well as in the midbrain, medulla, vermis, cerebellar white matter, superior and inferior cerebellar peduncles, tegmentum, and olives. Annual whole and regional brain atrophy rates were assessed in 9 patients with PD, 17 with PSP, 9 with MSA-P, and 18 healthy controls [99]. Annual regional atrophy rates in MSA-P were greatest in the pons and cerebellum, depicting values of up to 3.2% and 1.9% atrophy per year, which was reported significantly different to those in PD and controls. Moreover, pontine and cerebellar atrophy rates were significantly higher than whole brain atrophy rates in MSA-P. Annual whole brain atrophy rates are 0.6% in PD, 0.4% in healthy controls, 1.0% in MSA-P, and 1.2% in PSP, and although higher in MSA-P and PSP compared to PD and controls in this study, the difference of the annual atrophy rates was significant only for the comparison of PSP versus healthy controls.

VBM was applied to two consecutive MR images of 14 patients with probable MSA-P in comparison to

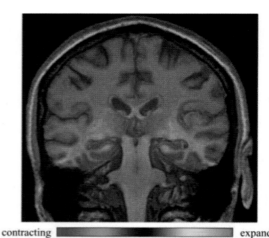

contracting ▬▬▬▬▬ expanding

Figure 13.6 Coronal MRI scan with voxel-compression-mapping overlay to demonstrate areas undergoing atrophy in an MSA patient. Greatest rates of atrophy are found to be in the pons, MCP, midbrain and medulla. Increased atrophy, but at a slower rate, is seen in the upper midbrain and lower medulla. Even slower, but definitely pathological, atrophy rates are seen in both temporal lobes. Ventricular enlargement is also shown.

14 patients with PD to determine the evolution of the regional brain atrophy. For this reason, the follow-up images were compared with the baseline investigation by paired t-tests including the scan interval as a covariate (MSA: 1.4 years; PD: 1.0 year). Subsequently, statistical parametric mapping (SPM) of MSA progression was compared with that of PD patients to exclude age and PD-related atrophy and to determine an MSA-specific progression pattern. This study revealed no progression of brain atrophy in the PD cohort and marked progression of brain atrophy in the MSA-P cohort in regions including the striatum, mesencephalon, thalamus, and cerebellum, as well as cortical regions such as the primary sensorimotor cortex, supplementary motor area, lateral premotor cortex, medial frontal gyrus, middle frontal gyrus, orbitofrontal cortex, insula, posterior parietal cortex, and hippocampus. A short disease duration was correlated with greater progression of atrophy in the striatum, whereas a longer disease duration was correlated with increasing atrophy in the cortical areas and cerebellar hemispheres, thus suggesting that early degeneration of the basal ganglia drives subsequent cortical atrophy [80]. A more recent study used VBM applying six-parameter (rigid body) transformations to the corpus callosum to measure progression of callosal tissue loss in MSA [102]. In patients with

194

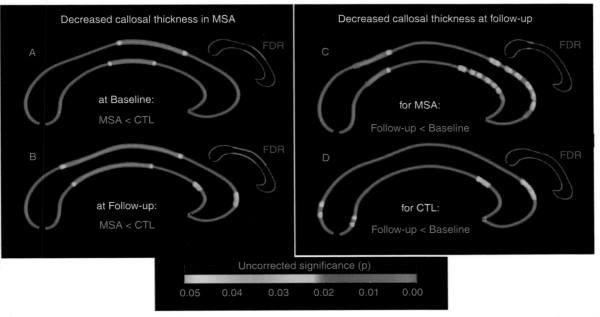

Figure 13.7 Differences in callosal thickness. The left part illustrates the decreased callosal thickness in MSA patients compared with controls at baseline (A) and at follow-up (B). The right part illustrates the decreased callosal thickness at follow-up compared with baseline in MSA patients (C) and in controls (D). Spectral colors indicate uncorrected significance (large callosal maps); red indicates false discovery rate (FDR)-corrected significance (small callosal maps).

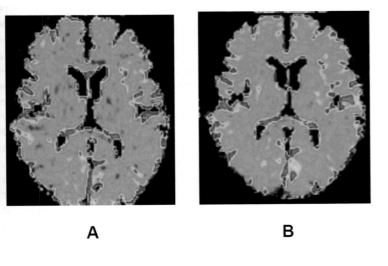

A   **B**

Figure 13.8 Axial mean diffusivity images spatially normalized into the Montreal Neurological Institute (MNI) space obtained at the level of the putamen in a patient at baseline (A) and at follow-up (B). Compared with baseline, the mean diffusivity is increased at the follow-up study, mostly in the putamen.

MSA, there was decreased callosal thickness compared to controls at baseline and follow-up; mainly involving the anterior and posterior body at baseline and additionally the isthmus at follow-up (Figure 13.7). Moreover, callosal thickness declined over time in MSA, mainly in the isthmus, which did not occur in the controls, suggesting that this pattern of callosal tissue loss may reflect a disease-specific pattern of neurodegeneration and cortical atrophy, fitting well with the predominant impairment of motor functions in MSA.

Using DWI, a significant increase of putaminal diffusivity over time has been demonstrated in two longitudinal DWI studies (Figures 13.8 and 13.9) [12, 103]. Seppi and coworkers [12] showed a marked increase of the diffusivity in the putamen of ten

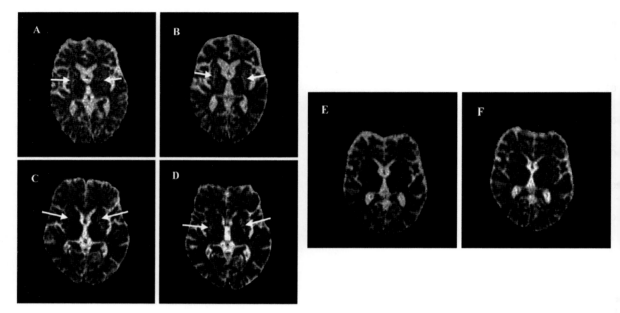

Figure 13.9 Mean diffusivity maps at the level of mid-striatum in individual patients with MSA-P (n = 2; A, baseline; B, follow-up in one patient; C, baseline; D, follow-up in another patient) and PD (E, baseline; F, follow-up). Note the diffuse hyperintensity – corresponding to increased mean diffusivity values – in the putamina of the patients with MSA-P (arrows in A, B, C, and D) which is increased at follow-up (B, D) compared to baseline examination (A, C). The PD patient shows no increased mean diffusivity values in the putamen, neither at baseline (E) nor at follow-up (F).

MSA-P patients, whereas none of the diffusivity values in the basal ganglia regions in ten PD patients changed significantly at follow-up compared to baseline. Over 15 months, there was a rapid increase in putaminal diffusivity in MSA-P, including a correlation with motor progression as assessed by the UPDRS. On the other hand, no progression of any putaminal abnormalities was shown using semi-quantitative ratings of abnormalities on structural MRI. The second serial DWI study tried to assess the evolution of diffusion properties not only in striatal, but also extrastriatal brain regions in seven patients with MSA-P and four patients with MSA-C [103]. After 1 year, the most prominent increase in diffusivity values was observed in the putamen. Further increases of diffusivity were found in the pons, cerebellar white matter, thalamus, and frontal white matter.

Imaging applications to clinical trials

In recent years, brain MRI has increasingly become part of clinical trials for assessing treatment outcome in neurological disorders such as Alzheimer's disease, stroke, and multiple sclerosis. The demonstration of MRI-derived parameters that show its relevance to the pathogenesis and progression of disease may help in monitoring outcomes in clinical trials.

It is hoped that MRI may help determine outcomes in such studies by reducing the sample size or shortening the duration of the trial. Rates of progression derived from longitudinal studies with serial neuroimaging are available for volumetric MRI using registration of serial imaging and DWI. Paviour and coworkers [100] reported that sample size calculations based on brainstem atrophy rates reduced the required cohorts by three to five times compared to those based on whole brain atrophy rates. The smallest sample sizes in MSA-P were achieved using cerebellar and pontine atrophy rates. Pellecchia and colleagues [103] calculated sample size estimates based on Trace(D) value changes over 1 year and suggested that the number of MSA patients might be diminished when using regions showing the most significant DWI changes, such as the putamen and pons rather than others.

Figure 13.10 demonstrates sample size estimates based on established progression rates of clinical and neuroimaging markers with identical requirements for the power calculation of the different markers [100, 103–106].

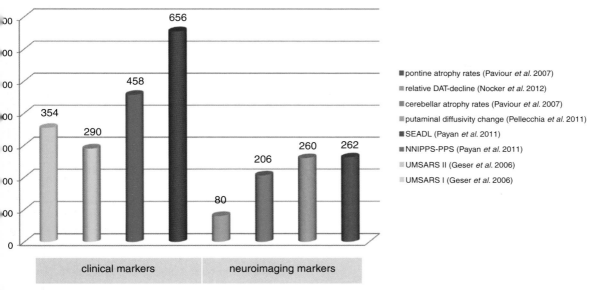

Figure 13.10 Sample size estimates based on established progression rates of clinical and neuroimaging markers. The bar graphs illustrate the number of patients needed in a trial, to detect the effect of a drug with an anticipated ability to reduce the rate of progression of the clinical or neuroimaging marker by 30% over 1 year with a power of 90%. Paviour et al. 2007 refers to [100]; Pellecchia et al. 2011 refers to [103]; Nocker et al. 2012 refers to [104]; Geser et al. 2006 refers to [105]; Payan et al. 2011 refers to [106]. SEADL: Schwab and England Activities of Daily Living; NNIPPS-PPS: Natural History and Neuroprotection in Parkinson Plus Syndromes – Parkinson Plus Scale (NNIPPS = phase III randomized placebo-controlled trial of riluzole in PSP and MSA); UMSARS I+II: part one (functional evaluation) and part two (motor examination) of the Unified Multiple System Atrophy Rating Scale.

To date, three MSA clinical trials used MRI as a secondary outcome measure. An efficacy and safety study on lithium in MSA (NCT00997672) compared micro- and macrostructural MR parameters before and after the treatment, including VBM, resting-state fMRI, DTI, and MRS, but was terminated due to 80% adverse events. The MSA-RAS-202 study (EudraCT 2009–014644–11), testing the clinical effect of rasagiline on subjects with MSA-P, tried to determine and compare rates of progression of putaminal abnormalities and abnormalities of other brain regions as assessed by DWI in an imaging substudy in MSA-P patients treated with rasagiline versus those with placebo. The imaging results are in accordance with previous studies, showing increased putaminal ADC values over time, while there were no differences between the active and control groups [107]. A recent study (NCT00911365) on mesenchymal stem cells (MSC) in patients with MSA tried to estimate change in cerebral glucose metabolism and gray matter density as determined using FDG-PET and MRI-based morphometry as secondary outcome measures. The results revealed greater reductions in cerebral glucose metabolism and gray matter density at 360 days relative to baseline in the cerebellum and

the cerebral cortical areas in the placebo group compared with the MSC group [108].

In summary, brain MRI might be a sensitive, reliable, and reproducible companion to clinical measures for assessing the progression of neurological diseases [109]. Future research will reveal the best neuroimaging method or methods for application in MSA clinical trials.

Limitations

Presently the diagnostic accuracy as well as sensitivity and specificity of imaging methods for MSA are based on neuroimaging study participants classified by using clinical diagnostic criteria as the golden standard without pathological confirmation. As clinical diagnostic certainty increases with disease progression, most of the studies have included patients in advanced disease stages, thus making the clinical diagnosis of the patients more reliable. Nevertheless, since diagnosis is based on clinical and not pathological criteria it cannot be certain that all enrolled subjects have definite MSA [7]. Moreover, most of the studies have enrolled 10 to 30 subjects per disease entity, therefore limiting the validity of the findings.

197

Ultimately it would be more helpful to have larger studies of early parkinsonian subjects and follow their imaging and clinical features to determine correlations over time between measures and the evolving diagnosis. Indeed, evidence of early MR-based signal changes and structural abnormalities for the differential diagnosis of neurodegenerative parkinsonism is scarce and would be of important research interest. Further major limitations of MR-based neuroimaging studies in MSA include heterogeneous MRI protocols, and different segmentations of brain areas using ROIs or whole ROIs, thus limiting comparability between studies. Therefore, standardization of protocols and algorithms of various MR techniques should be an important research focus for MSA studies.

Summary

Neuroimaging has become more important for MSA clinically as well as in research studies. Indeed, the revised MSA consensus criteria include several imaging features for the diagnostic category of possible MSA [7]. Atrophy on cMRI of the putamen, MCP, pons, or cerebellum or hypometabolism on FDG-PET in putamen, brainstem, or cerebellum were included as additional features for possible MSA-P; and atrophy on cMRI of putamen, MCP, or pons or hypometabolism on FDG-PET in putamen or presynaptic nigrostriatal dopaminergic denervation on SPECT or PET were included as additional features for possible MSA-C [9]. Thus, the diagnosis of MSA is made on clinical features with supportive MRI findings. However, the MR features, while supportive, are not present in all individuals with MSA and may not necessarily be specific and thus do not allow for a separation of various APDs. Specifically the findings include supratentorial and infratentorial signal changes for MSA at 1.5T, such as the hyperintense putaminal rim, the pontine hot cross bun sign, and hyperintensity in the MCP. The presence of these findings at 3 or 7T remains uncertain. MRI-based quantitative assessment of atrophy of different brain structures including planimetry and volumetry may depict decreased MCP width and smaller pontine area as well as volume loss of supratentorial and infratentorial brain structures in MSA. DWI and DTI at 1.5T seem promising candidates since they may detect diffusion abnormalities, especially in the putamen but also in infratentorial structures such as the pons and MCP in patients with MSA even at early disease stages and are widely available on clinical MR scanners. Moreover, studies using iron-sensitive MR approaches have shown changes in the putamen in patients with MSA-P compared to PD patients and controls. There is however a lack of evidence for most of these MRI techniques, including structural MRI, imaging of brain iron, DTI, arterial spin labeling, perfusion imaging, rotating frame imaging, and MRS at higher magnetic fields of 3T or higher, to demonstrate specific brain alterations in MSA as opposed to other parkinsonian conditions. However, further large-scale prospective studies are warranted to identify which one of these MRI modalities or combinations provides the most robust diagnostic marker in patients with neurodegenerative parkinsonism.

Beside diagnostic aspects, serial neuroimaging studies with volumetric approaches and DTI have the potential to study progression in MSA in vivo.

As different MR sequences provide unique insights into tissue changes, multimodal imaging may discriminate MSA from other parkinsonian conditions, allow for studies of progression of disease topography as well as provide insights into pathogenic and pathophysiological aspects of MSA.

Acknowledgements

Portions of the text and tables are similar to other reviews authors have written (Mahlknecht et al. Neurodegener Dis. 2010;7(5):300–18; Seppi et al. Neuroimaging Clin N Am. 2010;20(1):29–55; Seppi et al J Neural Transm. 2005;112(12):1625–34; Seppi et al Curr Opin Neurol. 2005;18(4):370–5; Brooks et al Mov Disord. 2009;24(7):949–64) and are modified and updated as appropriate.

References

1. Vanacore N, Bonifati V, Fabbrini G, et al. Epidemiology of multiple system atrophy. ESGAP Consortium. European Study Group on Atypical Parkinsonisms. Neurol Sci. 2001;22(1):97–9.

2. Schrag A, Ben-Shlomo Y, Quinn NP. Prevalence of progressive supranuclear palsy and multiple system atrophy: a cross-sectional study. Lancet. 1999;354 (9192):1771–5.

3. Wenning GK, Litvan I, Tolosa E Milestones in atypical and secondary Parkinsonisms. Mov Disord. 2011;26(6):1083–95.

4. Watanabe H, Saito Y, Terao S, *et al.* Progression and prognosis in multiple system atrophy: an analysis of 230 Japanese patients. *Brain.* 2002;**125**(Pt 5):1070–83.

5. Wenning GK, Tison F, Ben Shlomo Y, Daniel SE, Quinn NP. Multiple system atrophy: a review of 203 pathologically proven cases. *Mov Disord.* 1997;**12**(2):133–47.

6. Kawai Y, Suenaga M, Takeda A, *et al.* Cognitive impairments in multiple system atrophy: MSA-C vs MSA-P. *Neurology.* 2008;**70**(16 Pt 2):1390–6.

7. Gilman S, Wenning GK, Low PA, *et al.* Second consensus statement on the diagnosis of multiple system atrophy. *Neurology.* 2008;**71**(9):670–6.

8. Trojanowski JQ, Revesz T; Neuropathology Working Group on MSA. Proposed neuropathological criteria for the post mortem diagnosis of multiple system atrophy. *Neuropathol Appl Neurobiol.* 2007;**33**(6):615–20.

9. Brooks DJ, Seppi K; Neuroimaging Working Group on MSA. Proposed neuroimaging criteria for the diagnosis of multiple system atrophy. *Mov Disord.* 2009;**24**(7):949–64.

10. Drayer BP, Olanow W, Burger P, *et al.* Parkinson plus syndrome: diagnosis using high field MR imaging of brain iron. *Radiology.* 1986;**159**(2):493–8.

11. Pastakia B, Polinsky R, Di Chiro G, *et al.* Multiple system atrophy (Shy-Drager syndrome): MR imaging. *Radiology.* 1986; **159**(2):499–502.

12. Seppi K, Schocke MF, Mair KJ, *et al.* Progression of putaminal degeneration in multiple system atrophy: a serial diffusion MR study. *Neuroimage.* 2006;**31**(1):240–5.

13. Bhattacharya K, Saadia D, Eisenkraft B, *et al.* Brain magnetic resonance imaging in multiple-system atrophy and Parkinson disease: a diagnostic algorithm. *Arch Neurol.* 2002;**59**(5):835–42.

14. Schocke MF, Seppi K, Esterhammer R, *et al.* Diffusion-weighted MRI differentiates the Parkinson variant of multiple system atrophy from PD. *Neurology.* 2002;**58**(4):575–80.

15. Muqit MM, Mort D, Miskiel KA, Shakir RA. "Hot cross bun" sign in a patient with parkinsonism secondary to presumed vasculitis. *J Neurol Neurosurg Psychiatry.* 2001;**71**(4):565–6.

16. Lee YC, Liu CS, Wu HM, *et al.* The 'hot cross bun' sign in the patients with spinocerebellar ataxia. *Eur J Neurol.* 2009;**16**(4):513–16.

17. Horimoto Y, Aiba I, Yasuda T, *et al.* Longitudinal MRI study of multiple system atrophy – when do the findings appear, and what is the course? *J Neurol.* 2002;**249**(7):847–54.

18. Righini A, Antonini A, Ferrarini M, *et al.* Thin section MR study of the basal ganglia in the differential diagnosis between striatonigral degeneration and Parkinson disease. *J Comput Assist Tomogr.* 2002;**26**(2):266–71.

19. Kraft E, Trenkwalder C, Auer DP. T2*-weighted MRI differentiates multiple system atrophy from Parkinson's disease. *Neurology.* 2002;**59**(8):1265–7.

20. von Lewinski F, Werner C, Jörn T, *et al.* T2*-weighted MRI in diagnosis of multiple system atrophy. A practical approach for clinicians. *J Neurol.* 2007; **254**(9):1184–8.

21. Rolland Y, Vérin M, Payan CA, *et al.* A new MRI rating scale for progressive supranuclear palsy and multiple system atrophy: validity and reliability. *J Neurol Neurosurg Psychiatry.* 2011;**82**(9):1025–32.

22. Osaki Y, Wenning GK, Daniel SE, *et al.* Do published criteria improve clinical diagnostic accuracy in multiple system atrophy? *Neurology.* 2002;**59**(10):1486–91.

23. Watanabe H, Ito M, Fukatsu H, *et al.* Putaminal magnetic resonance imaging features at various magnetic field strengths in multiple system atrophy. *Mov Disord.* 2010;**25**(12):1916–23.

24. Lee WH, Lee CC, Shyu WC, Chong PN, Lin SZ. Hyperintense putaminal rim sign is not a hallmark of multiple system atrophy at 3T. *AJNR Am J Neuroradiol.* 2005;**26**(9): 2238–2242.

25. Bürk K, Bühring U, Schulz JB, *et al.* Clinical and magnetic resonance imaging characteristics of sporadic cerebellar ataxia. *Arch Neurol.* 2005;**62**(6):981–5.

26. Oba H, Yagishita A, Terada H, *et al.* New and reliable MRI diagnosis for progressive supranuclear palsy. *Neurology.* 2005;**64**(12):2050–5.

27. Righini A, Antonini A, DeNotaris R, *et al.* MR imaging of the superior profile of the midbrain: differential diagnosis between progressive supranuclear palsy and Parkinson disease. *AJNR Am J Neuroradiol.* 2004; **25**(6):927–32.

28. Warmuth-Metz M, Naumann M, Csoti I, Solymosi L. Measurement of the midbrain diameter on routine magnetic resonance imaging: a simple and accurate method of differentiating between Parkinson disease and progressive supranuclear palsy. *Arch Neurol.* 2001;**58**(7):1076–9.

29. Paviour DC, Price SL, Stevens JM, Lees AJ, Fox NC. Quantitative MRI measurement of superior cerebellar peduncle in progressive supranuclear palsy. *Neurology.* 2005;**64**(4):675–9.

30. Nicoletti G, Fera F, Condino F, *et al.* MR imaging of middle cerebellar peduncle width: differentiation of multiple system atrophy from Parkinson disease. *Radiology.* 2006;**239**(3):825–30.

31. Quattrone A, Nicoletti G, Messina D, *et al.* MR imaging index for

199

differentiation of progressive supranuclear palsy from Parkinson disease and the Parkinson variant of multiple system atrophy. *Radiology*. 2008;**246**(1):214–21.

32. Hussl A, Mahlknecht P, Scherfler C, *et al*. Diagnostic accuracy of the magnetic resonance Parkinsonism index and the midbrain-to-pontine area ratio to differentiate progressive supranuclear palsy from Parkinson's disease and the Parkinson variant of multiple system atrophy. *Mov Disord*. 2010;**25**(14):2444–9.

33. Morelli M, Arabia G, Salsone M, *et al*. Accuracy of magnetic resonance parkinsonism index for differentiation of progressive supranuclear palsy from probable or possible Parkinson disease. *Mov Disord*. 2011;**26**(3):527–33.

34. Longoni G, Agosta F, Kostić VS, *et al*. MRI measurements of brainstem structures in patients with Richardson's syndrome, progressive supranuclear palsy-parkinsonism, and Parkinson's disease. *Mov Disord*. 2011;**26**(2):247–55.

35. Schulz JB, Skalej M, Wedekind D, *et al*. Magnetic resonance imaging-based volumetry differentiates idiopathic Parkinson's syndrome from multiple system atrophy and progressive supranuclear palsy. *Ann Neurol*. 1999;**45**(1):65–74.

36. Paviour DC, Price SL, Jahanshahi M, Lees AJ, Fox NC. Regional brain volumes distinguish PSP, MSA-P, and PD: MRI-based clinico-radiological correlations. *Mov Disord*. 2006;**21**(7):989–96.

37. Seppi K, Poewe W. Brain magnetic resonance imaging techniques in the diagnosis of parkinsonian syndromes. *Neuroimaging Clin N Am*. 2010;**20**(1):29–55.

38. Messina D, Cerasa A, Condino F, *et al*. Patterns of brain atrophy in

Parkinson's disease, progressive supranuclear palsy and multiple system atrophy. *Parkinsonism Relat Disord*. 2011;**17**(3):172–6.

39. Bürk K, Globas C, Wahl T, *et al*. MRI-based volumetric differentiation of sporadic cerebellar ataxia. *Brain*. 2004;**127**(Pt 1):175–81.

40. Schocke MF, Seppi K, Esterhammer R, *et al*. Trace of diffusion tensor differentiates the Parkinson variant of multiple system atrophy and Parkinson's disease. *Neuroimage*. 2004;**21**(4):1443–51.

41. Haacke EM, Xu Y, Cheng YC, Reichenbach JR. Susceptibility weighted imaging (SWI). *Magn Reson Med*. 2004;**52**(3):612–18.

42. Seppi K, Schocke MF, Esterhammer R, *et al*. Diffusion-weighted imaging discriminates progressive supranuclear palsy from PD, but not from the parkinson variant of multiple system atrophy. *Neurology*. 2003;**60**(6):922–7.

43. Seppi K, Schocke MF, Donnemiller E, *et al*. Comparison of diffusion-weighted imaging and [123I]IBZM-SPECT for the differentiation of patients with the Parkinson variant of multiple system atrophy from those with Parkinson's disease. *Mov Disord*. 2004;**19**(12):1438–45.

44. Seppi K, Schocke MF, Prennschuetz-Schuetzenau K, *et al*. Topography of putaminal degeneration in multiple system atrophy: a diffusion magnetic resonance study. *Mov Disord*. 2006;**21**(6):847–52.

45. Nicoletti G, Lodi R, Condino F, *et al*. Apparent diffusion coefficient measurements of the middle cerebellar peduncle differentiate the Parkinson variant of MSA from Parkinson's disease and progressive supranuclear palsy. *Brain*. 2006;**129** (Pt 10):2679–87.

46. Ito M, Watanabe H, Kawai Y, *et al*. Usefulness of combined

fractional anisotropy and apparent diffusion coefficient values for detection of involvement in multiple system atrophy. *J Neurol Neurosurg Psychiatry*. 2007;**78**(7):722–8.

47. Pellecchia MT, Barone P, Mollica C, *et al*. Diffusion-weighted imaging in multiple system atrophy: a comparison between clinical subtypes. *Mov Disord*. 2009;**24**(5):689–96.

48. Köllensperger M, Seppi K, Liener C, *et al*. Diffusion weighted imaging best discriminates PD from MSA-P: a comparison with tilt table testing and heart MIBG scintigraphy. *Mov Disord*. 2007;**22**(12):1771–6.

49. Hussl A, Esterhammer R, Schocke M, *et al*. Putaminal diffusivity in 1.5T MR imaging for the differential diagnosis of neurodegenerative parkinsonism. *Mov Disord*. 2011;**26** Suppl 2:S244

50. Paviour DC, Thornton JS, Lees AJ, Jäger HR. Diffusion-weighted magnetic resonance imaging differentiates Parkinsonian variant of multiple-system atrophy from progressive supranuclear palsy. *Mov Disord*. 2007;**22**(1):68–74.

51. Blain CR, Barker GJ, Jarosz JM, *et al*. Measuring brain stem and cerebellar damage in parkinsonian syndromes using diffusion tensor MRI. *Neurology*. 2006;**67** (12):2199–205.

52. Rizzo G, Martinelli P, Manners D, *et al*. Diffusion-weighted brain imaging study of patients with clinical diagnosis of corticobasal degeneration, progressive supranuclear palsy and Parkinson's disease. *Brain*. 2008;**131**(Pt 10):2690–700.

53. Kanazawa M, Shimohata T, Terajima K, *et al*. Quantitative evaluation of brainstem involvement in multiple system atrophy by diffusion-weighted MR imaging. *J Neurol*. 2004;**251**(9):1121–4.

54. Nicoletti G, Tonon C, Lodi R, *et al.* Apparent diffusion coefficient of the superior cerebellar peduncle differentiates progressive supranuclear palsy from Parkinson's disease. *Mov Disord.* 2008;**23**(16):2370–6.

55. Oishi K, Konishi J, Mori S, *et al.* Reduced fractional anisotropy in early-stage cerebellar variant of multiple system atrophy. *J Neuroimaging.* 2009;**19**(2):127–31.

56. Wang PS, Wu HM, Lin CP, Soong BW. Use of diffusion tensor imaging to identify similarities and differences between cerebellar and Parkinsonism forms of multiple system atrophy. *Neuroradiology.* 2011;**53**(7):471–81.

57. Tzarouchi LC, Astrakas LG, Konitsiotis S, *et al.* Voxel-based morphometry and voxel-based relaxometry in parkinsonian variant of multiple system atrophy. *J Neuroimaging.* 2010;**20**(3):260–6.

58. Brenneis C, Seppi K, Schocke MF, *et al.* Voxel-based morphometry detects cortical atrophy in the Parkinson variant of multiple system atrophy. *Mov Disord.* 2003;**18**(10):1132–8.

59. Minnerop M, Specht K, Ruhlmann J, *et al.* Voxel-based morphometry and voxel-based relaxometry in multiple system atrophy – a comparison between clinical subtypes and correlations with clinical parameters. *Neuroimage.* 2007;**36**(4):1086–95.

60. Focke NK, Helms G, Pantel PM, *et al.* Differentiation of typical and atypical Parkinson syndromes by quantitative MR imaging. *AJNR Am J Neuroradiol.* 2011;**32** (11):2087–92.

61. Tsukamoto K, Matsusue E, Kanasaki Y, *et al.* Significance of apparent diffusion coefficient measurement for the differential diagnosis of multiple system atrophy, progressive supranuclear palsy, and Parkinson's disease: evaluation by 3.0-T MR imaging. *Neuroradiology.* 2012;**54**(9):947–55.

62. Eckert T, Sailer M, Kaufmann J, *et al.* Differentiation of idiopathic Parkinson's disease, multiple system atrophy, progressive supranuclear palsy, and healthy controls using magnetization transfer imaging. *Neuroimage.* 2004;**21**(1):229–35.

63. Naka H, Imon Y, Ohshita T, *et al.* Magnetization transfer measurements of brain structures in patients with multiple system atrophy. *Neuroimage.* 2002;**17**(3):1572–8.

64. da Rocha AJ, Maia AC, da Silva CJ, *et al.* Pyramidal tract degeneration in multiple system atrophy: the relevance of magnetization transfer imaging. *Mov Disord.* 2007;**22**(2):238–44.

65. Stoessl AJ, Martin WW, McKeown MJ, Sossi V. Advances in imaging in Parkinson's disease. *Lancet Neurol.* 2011;**10**(11): 987–1001.

66. Gupta D, Saini J, Kesavadas C, Sarma PS, Kishore A. Utility of susceptibility-weighted MRI in differentiating Parkinson's disease and atypical parkinsonism. *Neuroradiology.* 2010; **52**(12):1087–94.

67. Sakurai K, Kawaguchi T, Kawai T, *et al.* Usefulness of 3D-PRESTO imaging in evaluating putaminal abnormality in parkinsonian variant of multiple system atrophy. *Neuroradiology.* 2010;**52**(9):809–14.

68. Wang Y, Butros SR, Shuai X, *et al.* Different iron-deposition patterns of multiple system atrophy with predominant parkinsonism and idiopathic Parkinson diseases demonstrated by phase-corrected susceptibility-weighted imaging. *AJNR Am J Neuroradiol.* 2012;**33**(2):266–73.

69. Menke RA, Scholz J, Miller KL, *et al.* MRI characteristics of the substantia nigra in Parkinson's disease: a combined quantitative T1 and DTI study. *Neuroimage.* 2009;**47**(2):435–41.

70. Péran P, Cherubini A, Assogna F, *et al.* Magnetic resonance imaging markers of Parkinson's disease nigrostriatal signature. *Brain.* 2010;**133**(11):3423–33.

71. Du G, Lewis MM, Styner M, *et al.* Combined R2* and diffusion tensor imaging changes in the substantia nigra in Parkinson's disease. *Mov Disord.* 2011;**26**(9):1627–32.

72. Schwarz J, Weis S, Kraft E, *et al.* Signal changes on MRI and increases in reactive microgliosis, astrogliosis, and iron in the putamen of two patients with multiple system atrophy. *J Neurol Neurosurg Psychiatry.* 1996;**60**(1):98–101.

73. Matsusue E, Fujii S, Kanasaki Y, *et al.* Putaminal lesion in multiple system atrophy: postmortem MR-pathological correlations. *Neuroradiology.* 2008;**50**(7):559–67.

74. Matsusue E, Fujii S, Kanasaki Y, *et al.* Cerebellar lesions in multiple system atrophy: postmortem MR imaging-pathologic correlations. *AJNR Am J Neuroradiol.* 2009;**30**(9):1725–30.

75. Massey LA, Micallef C, Paviour DC, *et al.* Conventional magnetic resonance imaging in confirmed progressive supranuclear palsy and multiple system atrophy. *Mov Disord.* 2012;**27**(14):1754–62.

76. Prakash N, Hageman N, Hua X, *et al.* Patterns of fractional anisotropy changes in white matter of cerebellar peduncles distinguish spinocerebellar ataxia-1 from multiple system atrophy and other ataxia syndromes. *Neuroimage.* 2009;**47** Suppl 2: T72–81.

77. Tha KK, Terae S, Yabe I, *et al.* Microstructural white matter abnormalities of multiple system atrophy: in vivo topographic

illustration by using diffusion-tensor MR imaging. *Radiology.* 2010;**255**(2):563–9.

78. Seppi K, Schocke MF. An update on conventional and advanced magnetic resonance imaging techniques in the differential diagnosis of neurodegenerative parkinsonism. *Curr Opin Neurol.* 2005;**18**(4):370–5.

79. Ridgway GR, Henley SM, Rohrer JD, *et al.* Ten simple rules for reporting voxel-based morphometry studies. *Neuroimage.* 2008;**40**(4):1429–35.

80. Brenneis C, Egger K, Scherfler C, *et al.* Progression of brain atrophy in multiple system atrophy. A longitudinal VBM study. *J Neurol.* 2007;**254**(2):191–6.

81. Specht K, Minnerop M, Müller-Hübenthal J, Klockgether T. Voxel-based analysis of multiple-system atrophy of cerebellar type: complementary results by combining voxel-based morphometry and voxel-based relaxometry. *Neuroimage.* 2005;**25**(1):287–93.

82. Tir M, Delmaire C, le Thuc V, *et al.* Motor-related circuit dysfunction in MSA-P: usefulness of combined whole-brain imaging analysis. *Mov Disord.* 2009;**24**(6):863–70.

83. Trabesinger AH, Meier D, Boesiger P. In vivo 1H NMR spectroscopy of individual human brain metabolites at moderate field strengths. *Magn Reson Imaging.* 2003;**21**(10):1295–302.

84. Firbank MJ, Harrison RM, O'Brien JT. A comprehensive review of proton magnetic resonance spectroscopy studies in dementia and Parkinson's disease. *Dement Geriatr Cogn Disord.* 2002;**14**(2):64–76.

85. Schocke MF, Berger T, Felber SR, *et al.* Serial contrast-enhanced magnetic resonance imaging and spectroscopic imaging of acute multiple sclerosis lesions under high-dose methylprednisolone therapy. *Neuroimage.* 2003;**20**(2):1253–63.

86. Federico F, Simone IL, Lucivero V, *et al.* Proton magnetic resonance spectroscopy in Parkinson's disease and atypical parkinsonian disorders. *Mov Disord.* 1997; **12**(6):903–9.

87. Federico F, Simone IL, Lucivero V, *et al.* Proton magnetic resonance spectroscopy in Parkinson's disease and progressive supranuclear palsy. *J Neurol Neurosurg Psychiatry.* 1997; **62**(3):239–42.

88. Federico F, Simone IL, Lucivero V, *et al.* Usefulness of proton magnetic resonance spectroscopy in differentiating parkinsonian syndromes. *Ital J Neurol Sci.* 1999;**20**(4):223–9.

89. Davie CA, Wenning GK, Barker GJ, *et al.* Differentiation of multiple system atrophy from idiopathic Parkinson's disease using proton magnetic resonance spectroscopy. *Ann Neurol.* 1995;**37**(2):204–10.

90. Clarke CE, Lowry M. Systematic review of proton magnetic resonance spectroscopy of the striatum in parkinsonian syndromes. *Eur J Neurol.* 2001;**8**(6):573–7.

91. Chaudhuri KR, Lemmens GM, Williams SC, *et al.* Proton magnetic resonance spectroscopy of the striatum in Parkinson's disease patients with motor response fluctuations. *Parkinsonism Relat Disord.* 1996;**2**(2):63–7.

92. Watanabe H, Fukatsu H, Katsuno M, *et al.* Multiple regional 1H-MR spectroscopy in multiple system atrophy: NAA/Cr reduction in pontine base as a valuable diagnostic marker. *J Neurol Neurosurg Psychiatry.* 2004;**75**(1):103–9.

93. Guevara CA, Blain CR, Stahl D, *et al.* Quantitative magnetic resonance spectroscopic imaging in Parkinson's disease, progressive supranuclear palsy and multiple system atrophy. *Eur J Neurol.* 2010;**17**(9):1193–202.

94. Mahlknecht P, Hotter A, Hussl A, *et al.* Significance of MRI in diagnosis and differential diagnosis of Parkinson's disease. *Neurodegener Dis.* 2010;**7**(5):300–18.

95. Wenning GK, Colosimo C, Geser F, Poewe W. Multiple system atrophy. *Lancet Neurol.* 2004;**3**(2):93–103.

96. Wenning GK, Seppi K, Tison F, Jellinger K. A novel grading scale for striatonigral degeneration (multiple system atrophy). *J Neural Transm.* 2002;**109**(3):307–20.

97. Klockgether T, Faiss J, Poremba M, Dichgans J. The development of infratentorial atrophy in patients with idiopathic cerebellar ataxia of late onset: a CT study. *J Neurol.* 1990;**237**(7):420–3.

98. Wild EJ, Fox NC. Serial volumetric MRI in Parkinsonian disorders. *Mov Disord.* 2009;**24** Suppl 2:S691–8.

99. Paviour DC, Price SL, Jahanshahi M, Lees AJ, Fox NC. Longitudinal MRI in progressive supranuclear palsy and multiple system atrophy: rates and regions of atrophy. *Brain.* 2006;**129**(Pt 4):1040–9.

100. Paviour DC, Price SL, Lees AJ, Fox NC. MRI derived brain atrophy in PSP and MSA-P. Determining sample size to detect treatment effects. *J Neurol.* 2007;**254**(4):478–81.

101. Schott JM, Simon JE, Fox NC, *et al.* Delineating the sites and progression of in vivo atrophy in multiple system atrophy using fluid-registered MRI. *Mov Disord.* 2003;**18**(8):955–8.

102. Minnerop M, Lüders E, Specht K, *et al.* Callosal tissue loss in multiple system atrophy – a one-year follow-up study. *Mov Disord.* 2010;**25**(15):2613–20.

103. Pellecchia MT, Barone P, Vicidomini C, et al. Progression of striatal and extrastriatal degeneration in multiple system atrophy: a longitudinal diffusion-weighted MR study. Mov Disord. 2011;26(7):1303–9.

104. Nocker M, Seppi K, Donnemiller E, et al. Progression of dopamine transporter decline in patients with the Parkinson variant of multiple system atrophy: a voxel-based analysis of [123I]β-CIT SPECT. Eur J Nucl Med Mol Imaging. 2012;39(6):1012–20.

105. Geser F, Wenning GK, Seppi K, et al. Progression of multiple system atrophy (MSA): a prospective natural history study by the European MSA Study Group (EMSA SG). Mov Disord. 2006;21(2):179–86.

106. Payan CA, Viallet F, Landwehrmeyer BG, et al. Disease severity and progression in progressive supranuclear palsy and multiple system atrophy: validation of the NNIPPS–Parkinson Plus Scale. PLoS One 2011;6(8):e22293.

107. Poewe W, Barone P, Giladi N, et al. A randomized, placebo-controlled clinical trial to assess the effects of rasagiline in patients with multiple system atrophy of the parkinsonian subtype. Mov Disord. 2012;27 Suppl. 1:S390.

108. Lee PH, Lee JE, Kim HS, et al. A randomized trial of mesenchymal stem cells in multiple system atrophy. Ann Neurol. 2012;72(1):32–40.

109. Ciumas C, Montavont A, Ryvlin P. Magnetic resonance imaging in clinical trials. Curr Opin Neurol. 2008;21(4):431–6.

110. Konagaya M, Konagaya Y, Iida M. Clinical and magnetic resonance imaging study of extrapyramidal symptoms in multiple system atrophy. J Neurol Neurosurg Psychiatry. 1994;57(12):1528–31.

111. Kraft E, Schwarz J, Trenkwalder C, et al. The combination of hypointense and hyperintense signal changes on T2-weighted magnetic resonance imaging sequences: a specific marker of multiple system atrophy? Arch Neurol. 1999;56(2):225–8.

112. Lee EA, Cho HI, Kim SS, Lee WY. Comparison of magnetic resonance imaging in subtypes of multiple system atrophy. Parkinsonism Relat Disord. 2004;10(6):363–8.

113. Ito S, Shirai W, Hattori T. Evaluating posterolateral linearization of the putaminal margin with magnetic resonance imaging to diagnose the Parkinson variant of multiple system atrophy. Mov Disord. 2007;22(4):578–81.

114. Kwon KY, Choi CG, Kim JS, Lee MC, Chung SJ. Diagnostic value of brain MRI and 18F-FDG PET in the differentiation of Parkinsonian-type multiple system atrophy from Parkinson's disease. Eur J Neurol. 2008;15(10):1043–9.

115. Ito S, Shirai W, Hattori T. Putaminal hyperintensity on T1-weighted MR imaging in patients with the Parkinson variant of multiple system atrophy. AJNR Am J Neuroradiol. 2009;30(4):689–92.

116. Lim TS, Lee PH, Kim HS, Yong SW. White matter hyperintensities in patients with multiple system atrophy. J Neurol. 2009;256(10):1663–70.

117. Sakurai K, Yamawaki T, Okita K, et al. Utility of the fluid-attenuated inversion recovery sequence in detecting a hyperintense putaminal rim in multiple system atrophy-parkinsonism: a preliminary study. Eur Neurol. 2011;66(1):42–6.

118. Kasahara S, Miki Y, Kanagaki M, et al. "Hot cross bun" sign in multiple system atrophy with predominant cerebellar ataxia: a comparison between proton density-weighted imaging and T2-weighted imaging. Eur J Radiol. 2012;81(10):2848–52.

119. Hauser TK, Luft A, Skalej M, et al. Visualization and quantification of disease progression in multiple system atrophy. Mov Disord. 2006;21(10):1674–81.

120. Kashihara K, Shinya T, Higaki F. Reduction of neuromelanin-positive nigral volume in patients with MSA, PSP and CBD. Intern Med. 2011;50(16):1683–7.

121. Shiga K, Yamada K, Yoshikawa K, et al. Local tissue anisotropy decreases in cerebellopetal fibers and pyramidal tract in multiple system atrophy. J Neurol. 2005;252(5):589–96.

122. Nilsson C, Markenroth Bloch K, Brockstedt S, et al. Tracking the neurodegeneration of parkinsonian disorders – a pilot study. Neuroradiology. 2007;49(2):111–19.

123. Arabia G, Morelli M, Paglionico S, et al. An magnetic resonance imaging T2*-weighted sequence at short echo time to detect putaminal hypointensity in Parkinsonisms. Mov Disord. 2010;25(16):2728–34.

Ataxia

Kathrin Reetz and Ferdinand Binkofski

Introduction

The term ataxia (from Greek α- [a negative prefix] + -τάξις [order] = "lack of order") stands for a neurological sign describing incoordination of voluntary muscle movements. Ataxia is a non-specific clinical condition resulting from a dysfunction of neural structures responsible for coordination of movements, for example the cerebellum causing cerebellar ataxia. The cerebellum is responsible for integrating a significant amount of neural information that is used to coordinate smoothly ongoing movements and to participate in motor planning. Although ataxia is not present with all cerebellar lesions, many conditions affecting the cerebellum do produce ataxia. Ataxia is characterized by irregular, uncoordinated movements manifesting as asthenia (lack of strength), asynergy (defective coordination), and delayed reaction time. Patients with cerebellar ataxia usually have difficulties in controlling the force, range, direction, velocity, and rhythm of muscle contractions. Besides the cerebellar syndrome, ataxia patients can also present with pigmentary retinopathy, extrapyramidal movement disorders, pyramidal signs, cortical symptoms (seizures, cognitive impairment, and/or behavioral symptoms), as well as peripheral neuropathy and disorders of other organs, for example the heart.

Cerebellar disorders can be divided into the more frequent sporadic forms and usually rare inherited diseases. Inherited ataxias include autosomal recessive cerebellar ataxias (detailed overview by [1], please see Table 14.1), autosomal dominant cerebellar ataxias (spinocerebellar ataxia) and episodic ataxias, and X-linked ataxias. This chapter will not focus on sporadic forms of ataxia, in which there is no family history and the genetic tests are negative, degenerative multiple system atrophy of the cerebellar type, which is covered in Chapter 13 of this book, and acute ataxias in which symptoms appear suddenly or in a few days often due to toxic, infectious, or nutritional deficiencies. The clinical diagnosis of subtypes of ataxias can be challenging due to phenotypic overlap of the genetic subtypes.

Autosomal recessive ataxias with known gene mutation

Friedreich's ataxia

Friedreich's ataxia (FRDA) is the most common of the genetically inherited ataxias with autosomal recessive transmission. The clinical hallmark symptoms at the average age of onset of 10 years are truncal and limb ataxia, scoliosis, limb weakness due to pyramidal involvement and sensorimotor axonal neuropathy, sensory loss due to posterior column involvement, dysarthria, and cardiomyopathy [2]. Additional clinical features may include diabetes mellitus, pes cavus, hypoacusia, and optic atrophy. FRDA is caused in more than 95% of cases by a homozygous triplet GAA expansion in the first intron of the frataxin gene (*FXN*, previously known as *FRDA, X25*) on chromosome 9q13, while the remaining patients are compound heterozygotes with a GAA expansion in the disease-causing range in one *FXN* allele and an inactivating point mutation in the other *FXN* allele [3, 4]. The homozygous and heterozygous GAA expansion result in severe dysfunction of frataxin [5, 6], which is a mitochondrial membrane protein involved in iron distribution, and lead to iron accumulation in mitochondria, primarily in cardiac muscle and in the cerebellar dentate nucleus. Characteristic neuropathological changes in FRDA include loss of neurons in the dorsal root ganglia; loss of sensory fibers in the

Magnetic Resonance Imaging in Movement Disorders, ed. Paul Tuite and Alain Dagher. Published by Cambridge University Press. © Cambridge University Press 2013.

Table 14.1. Autosomal recessive cerebellar ataxias*

Disease	Age at onset (years)	Clinical features	Laboratory findings	Brain MRI findings	Gene and protein
Cerebellar ataxia with pure sensory neuronopathy					
Friedreich's ataxia	Mean, 16; 7–25 in most cases, reported range, 2–60	Most frequent recessive ataxia, bilateral extensor plantar reflexes, scoliosis, square-wave jerks	GAA triplet repeat expansion in intron 1 of the *FXN* gene	No cerebellar atrophy, spinal cord atrophy	*FXN*, frataxin
Sensory axonal neuropathy with dysarthria and ophthalmoplegia	Range, 20–60	Ophthalmoparesis, dysarthria, ptosis, myoclonus	Variable elevation of serum lactic acid level	Variable cerebellar atrophy, cerebellar white matter changes, stroke-like lesions	*POLG*, polymerase gamma
Ataxia with vitamin E deficiency	Mean, 17; range, 2–50	Similar to Freidreich's ataxia, retinitis pigmentosa, variable head tremor	Significantly decreased serum vitamin E level[†]	Non-cerebellar atrophy, spinal cord atrophy	*TTPA*, α-tocopherol transfer protein
Abetalipoproteinemia	Birth	Vomiting, diarrhea, neonatal steatorrhea	Decreased serum levels of cholesterol, triglycerides, and vitamins A, D, E, and K; abetalipoproteinemia; acanthocytosis	No cerebellar atrophy	*MTP*, microsomal triglyceride transfer protein
Cerebellar ataxia with sensorimotor axonal neuropathy					
Ataxia telangiectasia	Range, 2–3; <5 in most cases	Telangiectasis; oculocephalic dissociation; susceptibility to infections and cancer; chorea, dystonia, or both	Elevated serum α-fetoprotein level, immunoglobulin deficiency, mosaic translocations (specific karyotype)[†]	Cerebellar atrophy	*ATM*, ataxia telangiectasia mutated
Ataxia with oculomotor apraxia type 1	Mean, 7; range, 1–20	Variable oculocephalic dissociation; chorea, dystonia, or both	Variable elevation of serum LDL cholesterol level and low serum albumin level	Cerebellar atrophy	*APTX*, aprataxin
Ataxia with ocular apraxia type 2	Mean, 15; range, 7–25	Variable oculocephalic dissociation; chorea, dystonia, or both	Elevated serum α-fetoprotein level[†]	Cerebellar atrophy	*SETX*, senataxin
Late-onset GM$_2$ gangliosidosis	Range, 15–45	Spasticity, weakness, dystonia, epilepsy, cognitive decline, psychosis, anterior horn involvement	Hexosaminidase A deficiency (late-onset Tay–Sachs disease), hexosaminidase A + B deficiency (Sandhoff's disease)	Cerebellar atrophy	*HEXA* (Tay–Sachs variant) or *HEXB* (Sandhoff's disease variant)

205

Table 14.1. *(cont.)*

Disease	Age at onset (years)	Clinical features	Laboratory findings	Brain MRI findings	Gene and protein
Congenital disorder of glycosylation type 1A	Birth	Mental retardation, retinitis pigmentosa, thoracic deformity, epilepsy	Serum transferrin isoelectric focusing	Cerebellar atrophy	*PMM2*, phospho-mannomutase
Autosonal recessive spastic ataxia of Charlevoix–Saguenay	Mean, 2; up to 12	Spastic paraparesis followed by spastic ataxia, demyelinating component of the neuropathy, hypertrophy of the myelinated fibers (of the fundus)		Anterior superior cerebellar atrophy, with variable T_2-weighted linear hypointensities in pons	*SACS*, sacsin
Refsum's disease	Range, 10–20	Retinitis pigmentosa, sensorineural deafness, demyelinating neuropathy	Elevated serum phytanic acid level[†]	No cerebellar atrophy	*PhyH*, phytanoyl-CoA hydroxylase and PEX7, PEX7
Cerebrotendinous xanthomatosis	Childhood	Spastic ataxia; mental retardation, dementia, or both; tendon xanthomas; chronic diarrhea; premature cataracts	Elevated serum cholestanol level[†]	Variable cerebellar atrophy, cerebellar or cerebral leukodystrophy	*CYP27*, sterol 27 hydroxylase
Cerebellar ataxia without neuropathy					
Autosomal recessive cerebellar ataxia type 1	Late onset; mean 32; range 17–46	Pure ataxia	Not applicable	Cerebellar atrophy	*SYNE1*, spectrin repeats-nuclear envelope 1
Autosomal recessive cerebellar ataxia type 2	Mean, 4; range, 1–11	Mental retardation, myoclonus, epilepsy, stroke-like condition, exercise intolerance	Variable elevation of serum lactic acid level and decreased coenzyme Q10 level	Cerebellar atrophy, stroke-like cerebral lesions	*ADCK3* (*CABC1*), aarf-domain containing kinase 3
Niemann–Pick type C disease	Range, 2–30	Vertical supranuclear ophthalmoplegia, splenomegaly, dystonia, cognitive disorder	Skin-biopsy findings (filipin staining)	Variable cerebellar or brain atrophy	*NPC1*, NPC1 and *NPC2*, NPC2

* Most congenital and inherited metabolic disorders are excluded. LDL denotes low-density lipoprotein.
† This biomarker is consistently altered (either increased or decreased) in the corresponding autosomal recessive cerebellar ataxia. GM₂, ganglioside monosialic type 2.
Obtained from Anheim *et al.* [1].

peripheral nerves; and degeneration of the posterior columns, spinocerebellar tracts, and corticospinal tracts of the spinal cord, dentate nucleus of the cerebellum, and myocardium [2, 7, 8].

Neuroimaging studies, mainly using magnetic resonance imaging (MRI), have revealed atrophy of the spinal cord in early stages of FRDA, followed by brainstem and cerebellar atrophy later in the course of the disease [9–12]. Voxel-based morphometry (VBM) has illustrated volume loss in the dentate region of the cerebellum, as well as in the dorsal medulla, inferomedial areas of the cerebellar hemispheres, and rostral vermis [13, 14]. The important role of the superior cerebellar peduncle, which connects the dentate nucleus as a relay center between the cortex and other brain structures, and its involvement in FRDA, has been shown using MRI [15], and has recently been further emphasized demonstrating the relationship of superior cerebellar peduncle changes to genetic and clinical features [16].

Neurodegenerative pathological processes can be characterized by increased water diffusivity, identifiable using diffusion-weighted imaging (DWI), or diffusion tensor imaging (DTI), as modification of brain tissue integrity, reducing the barriers that restrict the movement of water. A DWI study revealed higher mean diffusivity values in the medulla, inferior, middle, and superior cerebellar peduncles as well as optic radiations, cerebellar hemispheres, and vermis, which correlated with disease duration and severity, as measured by the International Cooperative Ataxia Rating Scale (ICARS) [17]. Integrity of the optic nerve in FRDA was investigated by measuring the apparent diffusion coefficient (ADC) of water, based on DWI [18]. The ADC values of optic radiations were increased and associated with genetic and clinical disease features, confirming that the visual system is involved in this mitochondrial disease [18]. Complementary to the DWI findings, DTI showed white matter fiber bundle atrophy in the central portion of the medulla oblongata, the dorsal upper pons, the superior cerebellar peduncles, the central portion of the midbrain, the medial portion of the right cerebral peduncle, the peridentate region, bilaterally, and the optic chiasm (Figure 14.1) [19]. Here, the severity of the neurological deficits correlated significantly with atrophy of the peridentate white matter, bilaterally, and that of the superior cerebellar peduncle decussation [19].

Little is known about the metabolic status of the brain in FRDA. High-field ^{1}H magnetic resonance spectroscopy (^{1}H MRS) is proposed as a powerful tool for the non-invasive characterization of biochemical alterations in the brain, because it allows the measurement of neurochemical profiles of several metabolites in localized brain regions in humans [20]. The few available MRS studies in FRDA mainly reported changes of metabolite ratios of N-acetylaspartate/creatine (NAA/Cr), choline/creatine (Cho/Cr), myo-inositol/creatine, and glutamate + glutamine/creatine [14, 21–24], supporting a perspective of distinct neurochemical patterns in FRDA.

Very few studies have examined cognitive function in FRDA. Slowed information processing is the major consistently reported feature, often leading to cognitive impairment; but mood disorders have also been described (see [25, 26] for review). Certain measures of cognitive function in FRDA can be confounded by the motor impairment, and therefore it is necessary to isolate cognitive function in tasks that require a motor response. Nevertheless, there is evidence of significant and potentially debilitating cognitive changes associated with FRDA [25, 27–29]. In more detail, a recent neuropsychological study in FRDA observed a pattern of impairment indicating executive and parietotemporal dysfunctions [29]. Based on neuropathological and neuroimaging studies in FRDA predominantly reporting only mild anomalies in the cerebral hemispheres, cognitive impairment in FRDA is thought to be associated with the interruption of the cerebrocerebellar circuits that have been proposed as the anatomical substrate of the cerebellar involvement in cognition [29]. A recent functional MRI (fMRI) study revealed that neurodegeneration in FRDA was associated with a mixed activation pattern of the brain. Hereby, a decreased activation in the primary motor cortex and cerebellum was linked to regional neuronal damage, whereas decreased activation of the thalamus and primary sensory cortex was related to a deafferentation phenomenon and, finally, the increased observed activation of the right parietal cortex and the striatum was interpreted as a possible compensatory strategy in FRDA [30].

Furthermore, impaired inhibition of prepotent motor tendencies in FRDA was demonstrated by the Simon interference task [31]. The slowing of response speed as a consequence of conflict is commonly known as the Simon effect [32]. FRDA subjects were disproportionally slower in processing

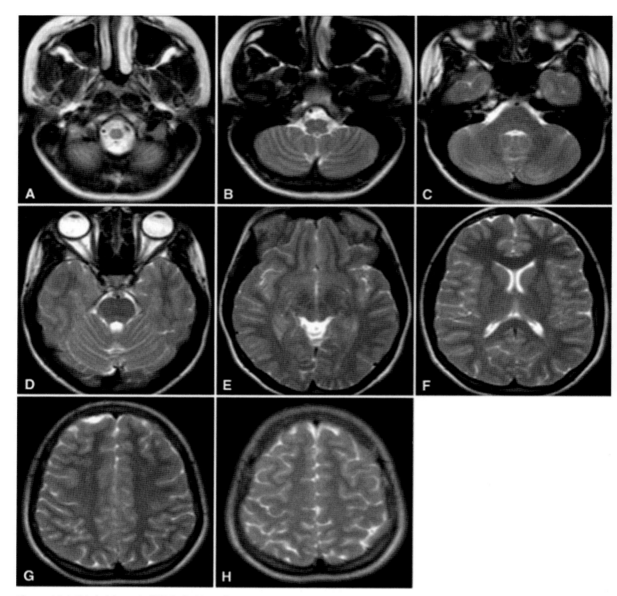

Figure 14.1 Friedreich ataxia (FRDA). (A–H) Axial T$_2$-weighted MR images in a 25-year-old woman with Friedreich ataxia (FRDA) show lack of diffuse or focal T$_2$ hyperintensity and subtle widening of the superior cerebellar sulci (D) and of the cerebrospinal fluid spaces surrounding the medulla (B). (Obtained from Pagani *et al.* [19].)

spatially incongruent stimuli requiring inhibition of a prepotent response. Therefore, it was proposed that such "dysmetria of thought" [33] results not simply from cerebellar compromise, but in large part also from deficits in cortico-ponto-cerebello-thalamo-cortical loops accessing critical cortical areas, in particular the frontoparietal circuitry [27].

Ataxia telangiectasia

Ataxia telangiectasia (A-T, Louis–Bar syndrome) is a rare autosomal recessive neurodegenerative disorder, caused by a defect in the *ATM* (ataxia telangiectasia mutated) gene [34], which is responsible for repairs in double-strand breaks in DNA. A-T results in progressive cerebellar degeneration affecting Purkinje cells, but also granule cells. However, cerebellar damage and loss of Purkinje and granule cells do not explain all of the neurological abnormalities in A-T. The effects of ATM deficiency on extracerebellar brain areas are therefore being actively investigated. A-T symptoms manifest mainly in early childhood and are characterized by cerebellar ataxia, choreoathetosis, impairment of the initiation of saccades (oculomotor apraxia) and oculocutaneous teleangiectasias, which result from widening of small vessels. Many patients are prone to infections of the respiratory tract (sinusitis, bronchitis, and pneumonia) and have an increased incidence of cancer (primarily, but not exclusively, lymphomas and leukemias). About two-thirds of patients with A-T have abnormalities of the immune system. The diagnosis of A-T is confirmed by specific laboratory abnormalities (elevated α-fetoprotein [AFP] levels, increased chromosomal breakage or cell death of white blood cells after exposure to X-rays, absence of ATM protein in white blood cells, or ATM mutations) [35].

The most prominent neuroimaging finding in A-T patients is cerebellar atrophy. This atrophy is dependent on age and on the stage of the disease [36]. Whereas the youngest patient in this study (2 years) had normal MRI results, early changes of atrophy were found in the next youngest patients (3–7 years) in the lateral cerebellum and superior vermis. The five patients who at the time of examination (over 9 years) were unable to walk all had diffuse atrophy involving both vermis and cerebellar hemispheres [36]. A combined clinical and MRI study on extracerebellar manifestations in A-T described marked hyperintense lesions in the cerebral white matter of T_2-weighted MR images in the most ataxic patients [37]. The six oldest patients suffered from spinal atrophy and two of them presented with extrapyramidal syndromes, one of which showed pathological findings in the basal ganglia. In a group of patients with normal IGF-1 (insulin growth factor 1, which is modulated by ATM) levels MRI showed cerebellar lesions in four patients, whereas spinal atrophy was found only in two. There was no involvement of the cerebral white matter or basal ganglia in this group suggesting that cerebral white matter involvement, spinal atrophy, and extrapyramidal symptoms are more often present in patients with pronounced deficiency of the growth hormone (GH)/IGF-1 axis accompanied by markedly reduced body weight and high ataxia scores [37]. Using ^{1}H MRS imaging it was demonstrated that A-T patients can be distinguished from controls by the profound loss of metabolites, such as NAA, Cho, and Cr, in the cerebellar vermis and to a lesser extent within the cerebellar hemispheres, but not in the basal ganglia [38]. There are very few functional imaging studies on A-T patients. A recent pilot fMRI study focused on the effects of betamethasone treatment on activation of the motor cortex during the performance of a pronation–supination task with the right hand [39]. In two tested patients the comparison of the measurement after steroid treatment with the baseline revealed a strong increase in activation in the motor areas [39]. The results should, however, be regarded with caution. It is not clear whether this increased activation of the motor areas results from increased motor performance or is a non-specific effect of corticosteroids. Taken together, all the presented imaging studies show clearly that the neuropathological changes in A-T start in the cerebellum and may spread to extracerebellar structures in the course of disease, which explains the complex clinical picture of A-T at the advanced stage.

Autosomal recessive ataxia with oculomotor apraxia type 1 and 2 (AOA1 and AOA2)

Ataxia with oculomotor apraxia type 1 (AOA1)

AOA1 is a rare, autosomal recessive disorder similar to A-T. It is caused by mutation in the gene (*APTX* gene) coding for the protein aprataxin. Aprataxin plays a role in the repair of single-stranded DNA. Some AOA1 patients have deficiency of co-enzyme Q10 in muscle, and many develop hypercholestolemia and hypoalbuminaemia. The dominant clinical features are cerebellar ataxia and oculomotor apraxia. The patients are unable to perform horizontal saccades and goal-directed eye movements. As a consequence they make jerky head movements towards intended targets in order to compensate for the oculomotor deficit. The clinical spectrum also includes chorea, polyneuropathy, and mental retardation. Individuals with AOA1 have a normal AFP level and normal measures of immune function. They may develop low serum levels of albumin after 10–15 years. The diagnosis can only be confirmed by genetic testing of the aprataxin gene. AOA1 usually

209

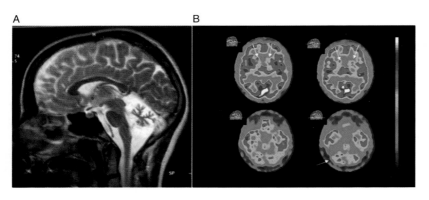

Figure 14.2 Ataxia with oculomotor apraxia type 1 (AOA1). (A) Brain MRI of an ataxia oculomotor apraxia type 1 (AOA1) patient. Sagittal T_2-weighted section showing severe cerebellar atrophy predominantly in the vermis. (B) Brain ECD-SPECT in another AOA1 patient. Arrows indicate cerebellar hypoperfusion in this patient associated with moderate bilateral hypoperfusion in the caudate nuclei. (Obtained from Le Ber *et al.* [40].)

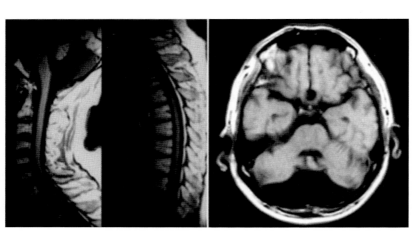

Figure 14.3 Ataxia with oculomotor apraxia type 2 (AOA2). MRI of the brain and spinal cord of a 57-year-old patient with ataxia oculomotor apraxia type 2 (AOA2) demonstrates a relatively spared spinal cord (left and central images) and a megacisterna magna and atrophy of the cerebellar hemispheres (right image). (Obtained from Asaka *et al.* [120].)

begins around the age of 7 years. The patients can reach adulthood, but are usually severely disabled.

In AOA1 cerebellar atrophy is the predominant neuroimaging feature, as demonstrated for example in a comprehensive study by Le Ber *et al.* [40]. Cerebellar atrophy was found on MRI in all eight investigated patients, predominantly in the vermis in most of them (62%) [40]. Additionally, cerebellar hypoperfusion was seen in three patients who underwent brain technetium-99m ethyl cysteinate dimer single-photon emission computed tomography (ECD-SPECT). In one of these patients, moderate bilateral hypoperfusion in the caudate nuclei was also seen (Figure 14.2) [40].

Ataxia with oculomotor apraxia type 2 (AOA2)

AOA2 is a rare autosomal recessive disorder caused by mutations in the senataxin gene (*SETX*). The protein senataxin plays a role in DNA repair and in the regulation of gene transcription.

The most prominent clinical symptoms are ataxia and polyneuropathy. The usual age of onset is around 15 years. Oculomotor apraxia is present in only half of affected individuals. Ocular telangiectasia does not develop. Therefore, the diagnosis AOA2 should also be considered in the absence of ocular symptoms. In AOA2, as in A-T but unlike in AOA1, all patients have an elevated serum AFP level. On the other hand, like AOA1 and unlike A-T, patients with AOA2 have normal markers of immune function. To distinguish AOA2 from A-T in vitro testing for susceptibility of lymphocytes to radiation can be performed. Genetic testing of the *SETX* gene can confirm the diagnosis.

Cerebellar atrophy is a consistent finding on MRI (96%), as shown in a study on a cohort of 90 AOA2 patients. No patient was lacking both peripheral neuropathy and cerebellar atrophy. Serial brain MRI in a group of AOA2 patients revealed severe cerebellar atrophy early in the course of the disease, suggesting that cerebellar involvement is present at the onset of symptoms of AOA2 [41]. In some patients the degree of cerebellar atrophy remained stable over the course of some 20 years (Figure 14.3).

Neuronal loss/dysfunction in the cerebellar vermis and hemispheres was indicated by lower total NAA levels than controls, and total NAA levels in the cerebellum strongly correlated with the FARS (Friedreich's Ataxia Rating Score) in a study using short-echo single-voxel ^{1}H MRS in nine patients with AOA2 [24]. The putative gliosis marker *myo*-inositol was higher than in controls in the vermis and pons. Lower glutamate in AOA2 than controls was observed in the vermis, indicating altered glutamatergic neurotransmission [24]. These spectroscopic findings hint at the complex pathophysiology of AOA2 and are of great potential value for monitoring disease progression and treatment.

Refsum's disease

Refsum's disease is another rare autosomal recessive disorder caused by mutations in the phytanoyl-CoA-hydroxylase gene. Phytanoyl-CoA-hydroxylase plays a crucial role in the α-oxidation of phytanic acid. The disease symptoms originate due to the accumulation of phytanic acid in tissue. Clinical features of Refsum's disease are progressive cerebellar ataxia, demyelinating sensorimotor neuropathy, retinal degeneration, inner ear deafness, cataract, night blindness, cardiac arrhythmias, and skin changes similar to ichthyosis. While the visual and auditory problems show a slow progression, acute exacerbations of the cardiac and neurological symptoms can occur. Those exacerbations are usually caused by low caloric intake, which causes a mobilization of phytanic acid from adipose tissue. The diagnosis can be confirmed by the detection of high serum levels of phytanic acid. Refsum's disease can be treated by a reduction of the dietary intake of phytanic acid, which can improve symptoms and prevent exacerbations. Patients should also have sufficient caloric intake, to prevent mobilization of phytanic acid from adipose tissue. With treatment the ataxia and polyneuropathy can improve; however, the progression of the visual and auditory deficits cannot be prevented.

Abnormal signal of the dentate nucleus is the most consistent MRI feature in infantile Refsum's disease [42]. MR images obtained at the time of diagnosis revealed patchy periventricular white matter hypointensities on T_2-weighted and fluid-attenuated inversion recovery (FLAIR) images [43]. The authors also found increased T_2 signal intensity in the cerebellar dentate nuclei in two patients with Refsum's disease. Follow-up MR imaging of the brain after more than 3 years in one patient showed further progression of the signal intensity changes in the periventricular white matter and dentate nuclei. In addition, there were new areas of abnormally increased T_2 and FLAIR signal intensity showing mild enhancement along the course of the cortical spinal tracts from the upper pons through the midbrain and into the internal capsules [43]. The neuroimaging findings mirror the clinical picture of Refsum's disease as a general progressive neurodegenerative disorder.

Ataxia with isolated vitamin E deficit (AVED)

AVED is an autosomal recessive inherited disorder, mostly found in North Africa and similar to FRDA, which is caused by mutations in the gene for α-tocopherol transporter protein. This protein is expressed in the liver and is responsible for the integration of vitamin E into very-low-density lipoproteins. The result is vitamin E deficiency, reflected in low serum levels. Since the absorption of vitamin E is not affected, AVED can be treated by oral intake of vitamin E. Differentiation of FRDA from acquired vitamin E deficiency (as might occur with micronutrient malabsorption) or AVED may prove challenging on clinical grounds.

Brain MRI is normal in most AVED cases. There are, however, reports of cerebellar atrophy in single cases. For example, a patient with AVED and mild cerebellar atrophy after 19 years of disease [44] and atrophy of cerebellar hemispheres in one of five patients investigated with computed tomography (CT) [45] have been reported.

Cerebrotendinous xanthomatosis (CTX)

CTX is an autosomal recessive inherited lipid storage disease caused by mutations of the gene *CYP27A1* coding for sterol 27-hydroxylase. In this rare disorder, sterol 27-hydroxylase is responsible for the decomposition of 7α-hydroxy-cholesterol to biliary acids. Additionally, cholesterol and 7α-hydroxy-cholesterol are increasingly metabolized to cholestanol. It is thought that the symptoms result from the accumulation of cholestanol in body tissue. CTX is a progressive multisystemic disease. The neurological symptoms consist of ataxia, pyramidal signs, cognitive deficits, epilepsy, and polyneuropathy. The patients also have chronic diarrhea, xanthomatous

211

swellings, and cataracts. Swelling of the tendons, which gives the disease its name in part, manifests in only 70% of patients. The diagnosis is confirmed by the identification of increased levels of cholestanol. CTX is treated by oral adminsitration of chenodeoxycholic acid. This can reduce the neurological symptoms, but it has no influence on cataracts and tendon swellings. Starting treatment in the presymptomatic stage can prevent the occurrence of symptoms.

A comprehensive neuroimaging study on 24 CTX patients found, apart from non-specific supratentorial atrophy and deep white matter changes, more typical hyperintense lesions on T_2-weighted images in the dentate nucleus (in 79% of patients), globus pallidus, substantia nigra, and inferior olive with extension into adjacent white matter as disease progressed [46]. In these locations, lipid crystal clefts and perivascular macrophages, neuronal loss, demyelination, fibrosis, and reactive astrocytosis were found on microscopic examination [46]. Hypointensity in the dentate nucleus on T_2-weighted images was sometimes found and was related to deposition of hemosiderin and calcifications. CT depicts fewer lesions, with hypointense appearance, except for calcifications, which are hyperintense. Spinal cord MR imaging revealed increased signal intensity in the lateral and dorsal columns on T_2-weighted images [46]. A multiparametric neuroimaging evaluation of CTX and its correlation with neuropsychological signs was performed using DTI, VBM analysis of T_1-weighted images, and SPECT in five CTX patients [47]. Patients had moderate mental retardation and performed worse than controls in all tested cognitive domains. Despite the extensive gray matter atrophy pattern, atrophy in the cerebellum, perisylvian regions, and parieto-occipital regions correlated with SPECT perfusion deficits. White matter atrophy located in the peridentate and left cerebral peduncle areas correlated with changes in diffusion measures, while axial and radial diffusivity patterns suggested both demyelinating and axonal changes. Changes in fractional anisotropy and mean diffusivity were correlated with VBM changes in the corpus callosum and corona radiata. Cognitive results correlated with fractional anisotropy changes. The study documents the complex pattern of decline in gray and white matter in CTX and indicates that disconnection of major fiber tracts that connect different cortical regions may contribute to cognitive impairment in this disease [47]. A recent functional dopaminergic

imaging study (^{123}I-FP-CIT SPECT) showed signs of presynaptic dopaminergic denervation in most CTX patients, while one patient had mildly reduced tracer uptake in the caudate [48]. This study confirmed a previous positron emission tomography (PET) finding of a presynaptic dysfunction of the nigrostriatal dopaminergic system in two CTX patients with parkinsonism [49].

As monitoring of the effects of chenodeoxycholic acid treatment brain SPECT with technetium-99m ethyl cysteate dimer was performed in a CTX patient to measure cerebral blood flow at onset and 2 years post-treatment [50]. Post-treatment SPECT showed better perfusion than pretreatment in frontal, parietal, and temporal cortices. This case illustrates the benefit of bile acid therapy for halting and even reversing neurological damage in this condition [50].

X-linked ataxias
Fragile X tremor/ataxia syndrome (FXTAS)

The fragile X syndrome is the most frequent form of a hereditary mental retardation in boys. It is an X-chromosomal inherited disease, which is caused by the expansion of a CGG repeat to more than 200 units (norm 6–44) in the 5'-region of the *FXTAS* gene. FXTAS has been described only recently in elderly male and very seldom in female carriers of a permutation of the *FXTAS* gene. Clinically, FXTAS manifests with progressive action tremor and cerebellar ataxia. Additionally, cognitive deficits, parkinsonian syndrome, polyneuropathy, and failure of the autonomic nervous system can occur.

MRI findings in FXTAS include global brain atrophy and white matter alterations manifested as increased T_2 signal intensity in the subcortical regions and in the middle cerebellar peduncles (MCPs) [51], consistent with a previous postmortem report of spongiosis in the deep cerebellar white matter [52]. A further characteristic finding in MRI scans of FXTAS patients is a hyperintense signal lateral to the dentate nucleus, extending to the MCPs [53]. The swelling of the MCPs is called the "MCP sign" and is relatively specific for FXTAS. However, it has also been reported in multiple system atrophy, acquired hepatocerebral degeneration, and other recessive ataxias. Increased T_2 signal intensity was also found symmetrically throughout the pons, appearing to reflect involvement of transverse pontine fibers and the corticospinal tract. Further, increased T_2 signal intensity of subependymal and deep white matter was demonstrated in the frontal and parietal lobes with mild to moderate cerebral cortical, cerebellar hemisphere, and vermis volume loss [54]. The characteristic findings are typically more severe in affected males than females [51]. Some asymptomatic carriers also show signs of atrophy, especially affecting the brainstem, whose volume was significantly smaller in unaffected male carriers than controls [55]. In a young woman with FXTAS, MRI of the brain showed diffuse cortical atrophy, while ^{1}H MRS revealed decreased levels of NAA in the cerebellum, basal ganglia, and pons [56], confirming the diffuse neurogenerative character of this disease.

Autosomal dominant spinocerebellar ataxias

Autosomal dominant spinocerebellar ataxias (SCAs) are a heterogeneous group of progressive neurodegenerative disorders, caused by diverse mutation types and complex pathogenesis, and clinically mainly characterized by cerebellar ataxia, resulting in unsteady gait, clumsiness, and dysarthria. The cerebellar syndrome is often associated with other neurological signs such as pyramidal or extrapyramidal signs, ophthalmoplegia, and cognitive impairment. Onset is generally during the third or fourth decade of life, but can occur in childhood or old age. Atrophy of the cerebellum and brainstem are most often the prominent imaging features, but other structures can be also affected, leading to a substantial range of phenotypes. The polyglutamine expansion SCAs share a mutational mechanism with other polyglutamine expansion diseases, such as Huntington's disease and spinal bulbar muscular atrophy. These disorders manifest above a threshold of CAG repeats that varies depending on the gene. Correlations between phenotype and genotype in the polyglutamine expansion SCAs have shown that differences in repeat size contribute to variation in disease progression and severity and to some of the clinical differences between patients. The most neuroimaging data are available for the subtypes SCA1, SCA2, SCA3, SCA6, and SCA17. Therefore in the following the chapter will focus on these. An overview for all SCAs is given in Table 14.2.

Spinocerebellar ataxia 1

SCA1 is clinically characterized by ataxia of gait, stance, and limbs; dysarthria; and oculomotor abnormalities (Table 14.2) [57]. The mutation causing SCA1 is a translated CAG repeat expansion in the coding gene for ataxin 1. SCA1 patients have one allele within the range of 40–81 repeats [58], whereas both normal and expanded CAG sequences may be interrupted by 1–3 CAT repeats. Normal repeat numbers in both copies of this gene are usually less than 36.

Clinically, along with the major symptoms of cerebellar ataxia and dysarthria, SCA1 patients can also develop highly variable non-cerebellar symptoms later in the disease, such as ophthalmoparesis and slow saccades, pyramidal signs, dysphagia, and – less commonly – amyotrophy, hyperkinesias, as well as sensory loss [59, 60]. In the first longitudinal natural history study over 2 years in SCA1, patients showed significant disease progression, with a decline in the ataxia score from the Scale for the Assessment and Rating of Ataxia (SARA) [61–63] and a measure of daily-life functional assessment (Unified Huntington Disease Rating Scale [UHDRS]) [64]. The observation of a faster disease progression in SCA1 compared to other SCAs is in line with the precedent baseline EUROSCA analysis [65] and a retrospective study on degenerative ataxias [66]. Onset is usually in the fourth decade. Anticipation has been observed in many SCA1 families. Median survival after onset of symptoms is 21 years. Postmortem examination revealed, at the macroscopic level, atrophy of the frontal, temporal, and parietal lobes, the cerebellum and its three peduncles, the brainstem, and the cranial nerves III, IV, and VI–XII and, on the light microscopic level, a severe degeneration in the cerebral cortex, basal forebrain, basal ganglia, thalamus, midbrain, pons, medulla oblongata, and cerebellum [67, 68].

Structural neuroimaging in SCA1 predominantly revealed atrophy in the brainstem, cerebellum, and basal ganglia (Figure 14.4) (e.g., [66, 69–71]).

Compared to other SCAs, the typical olivopontocerebellar atrophy was described as similar to but not as severe as in SCA2 [59, 71, 72] and more prominent than in SCA3 with respect to the cerebellar hemispheres [69]. A longitudinal MRI study, combining volumetry and VBM, revealed that pontine volume was the most sensitive measure of disease in SCA1,

Table 14.2. The spinocerebellar ataxias

SCA	Gene/locus	Mutation type	Key symptom in addition to cerebellar ataxia	Atrophy					
				Brainstem	Pons	Cerebellar hemispheres	Vermis	Basal ganglia	Cortical areas
1	ATXN1	CAG repeat	Dysphagia	++	++	++	++	+	+
2	ATXN2	CAG repeat	Oculomotor symptoms	++	+++	++	++		
3	ATXN3	CAG repeat	Dystonia, parkinsonism, neuropathy	++	+	+	++	+	
4	16q22.1	Unknown	Sensory neuropathy			+	+		
5	SPTBN2	Missense, n-frame deletion		−	−	++	++	−	−
6	CACNA1A	CAG repeat				++	+++		
7	ATXN7	CAG repeat	Visual loss		+++	++	++		
8	ATXN8OS	CTG repeat	Sensory neuropathy, spasticity	−	−	++	++		−
10	ATXN10	ATTCT repeat	Epilepsy			++	++		
11	TTBK-2	Frameshift				+	+		
12	PPP2R2B	CAG repeat		−	−	+	+	−	+
13	KCNC3	Point mutation	Mental retardation	+	+		+		
14	PRKCG	Missense, deletion	Myoclonus		(+)	++	++	−	−
15/16	ITPR1	Missense, frameshift		−	−	+	++		
17	TBP	CAG repeat	Dementia, psychiatric disorders			++	+	+	+
18	7q22−32	Unknown	Sensory neuropathy			+	+		(+)
19/22	KCND3	Unknown point mutation/insertion/deletion	Mental retardation			+	+		(+)
20*	11q12	260 KB duplication	Dysphonia, myoclonus			++	++		
21	7p21.3−p15.1	Unknown	Mental retardation			+	+		
23	PDYN	Missense	Sensory neuropathy, pyramidal signs			+	+		
25	2p21−2p13	Unknown	Sensory neuropathy	−	−	++	++		
26	19p13.3	Unknown		−	−	++	++		
27	FGF14	Point mutation	Dyskinesia, mental retardation	−	−	++	++	−	−

Table 14.2. (cont.)

SCA	Gene/ locus	Mutation type	Key symptom in addition to cerebellar ataxia	Atrophy					
				Brainstem	Pons	Cerebellar hemispheres	Vermis	Basal ganglia	Cortical areas
28	*AFG3L2*	Missense	Oculomotor symptoms	–	–	++	++		–
29	*ITPR1*	Missense mutation							
30	4q34.3–q35.1	Unknown							
31	*TK2, BEAN*	TGGAA repeat	Muscular hypotonia, auditory dysfunction						
32	7q32–q33	Unknown							
34	16p12.3–6p16.2	Unknown							
35	*TGM6*	Missense mutation							

ATXN, ataxin; SPTBN2, beta-III-spectrin; TTBK2, tau tubulin kinase 2; PPP2R2B, serine/threonine-protein phosphatase 2A; ITPR1, inositol triphosphate receptor type 1; TBP, TATA-box binding protein; PDYN, prodynorphin; FGF14, fibroblast growth factor 14; AFG3L2, ATPase family gene 3 like 2; TGM6, transglutaminase 6;–, no atrophy; (+), mild/inconsistently reported; +, mild atrophy; ++, moderate atrophy; +++, severe atrophy;. blank, not reported/unknown.
* Calcifications of dentate nucleus.

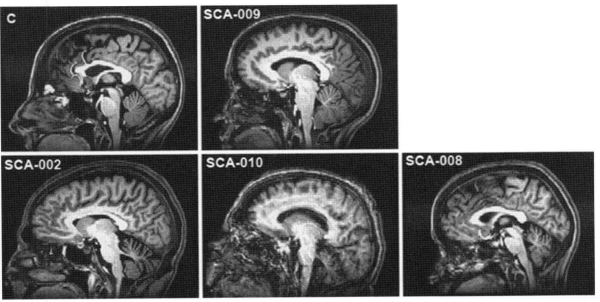

Figure 14.4 Cerebellar volume loss in spinocerebellar ataxia 1 (SCA1). Parasagittal sections depicting loss of cerebellar volumes as seen in magnetization-prepared rapid acquisition with gradient echo MRI. Images: c: Cerebellum section in a healthy control subject; SCA-009: presymptomatic individual with SCA1; and SCA-002, SCA-010, and SCA-008 are symptomatic SCA1 subjects. The cases are set according to severity of disease. Note that volume loss is not proportional to disease severity but rather to duration of illness. (Obtained from Solodkin *et al.* [76].)

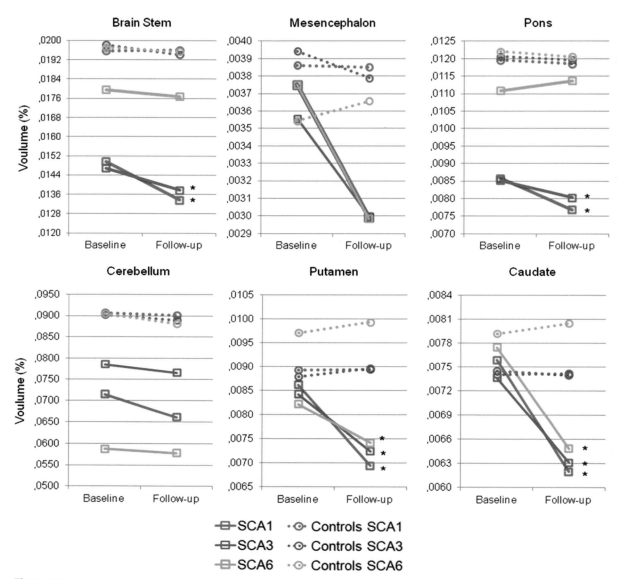

Figure 14.5 Longitudinal changes of brain volume in spinocerebellar ataxia (SCA) 1, 3 and 6. Volume of ROIs in each of the SCA genotypes (solid lines) and respective cross-sectional data of matched controls (round doted lines) at baseline and follow-up, showed increasing atrophy in the brainstem, cerebellum, and basal ganglia in all genotypes over time. Abbreviation: SCA, spinocerebellar ataxia. *Significant time effect for genotype. (Obtained from Reetz *et al.* [73].)

and that this was superior to the most sensitive clinical measure, SARA [73]. There was a mild correlation between CAG repeat length and volume loss of the bilateral cerebellum and the pons in SCA1 (Figure 14.5) [73].

Extending these neuroimaging findings and current neuropathological knowledge in SCA1, a recent

pathoanatomical study showed that brain damage in patients in the advanced clinical stages of SCA1 may go beyond the long-known macroscopic brain predilection sites (Figure 14.6) (for review see [74]) to involve the motor cerebello-thalamo-cortical and basal ganglia-thalamo-cortical circuits, the visual, auditory, somatosensory, oculomotor, vestibular,

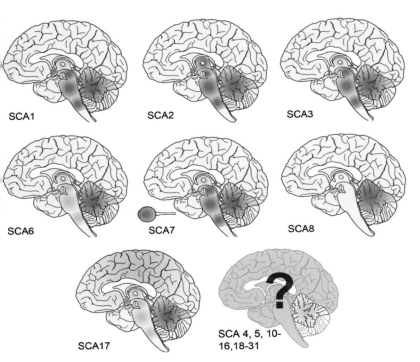

Figure 14.6 Distribution of neuronal loss in the brain of patients with spinocerebellar ataxias type 1 (SCA1), 2 (SCA2), 3 (SCA3), 6 (SCA6), 7 (SCA7), 8 (SCA8), and 17 (SCA17). Diagrammatic representation of midsagittal sections through the cerebrum, cerebellum, and brainstem of the human brain. The degree of neuronal loss in the cerebral cortex, basal forebrain, thalamus, cerebellum, and brainstem is indicated by red (severe) or light red (marked). (Obtained from Seidel *et al.* [74].)

ingestion-related, precerebellar, basal forebrain cholinergic, and midbrain dopaminergic systems [68]. This further emphasizes the idea that ongoing and extensive brain damage possibly explains the variable clinical phenotype in SCA1.

However, the brunt of the disease manifests as pontocerebellar atrophy, as shown by white matter assessment in a study using VBM, mean diffusivity, and Tract-Based Spatial Statistics (TBSS) in SCA1 [75]. To define the state of cerebellar connectivity, functional MRI and DTI were used, and revealed loss of intrinsic organization of cerebellar networks, which correlated with disease severity and duration in this disconnection syndrome [76].

MRS also demonstrates disease-related anomalies in NAA levels or the NAA/Cr ratio [23] in SCA1 [71]. Hereby, SCA1 patients presented with a decrease in the concentration of NAA in the pons and cerebellum.

Spinocerebellar ataxia 2

SCA2 is one of the most frequent SCAs worldwide, with a particularly high prevalence in the Holguin province of Cuba (Table 14.2). Its pathogenesis relies on a CAG repeat expansion in the disease gene ataxin-2 (*ATXN2*), which localizes to RNA-containing stress granules and associates with the endoplasmic reticulum/Golgi fraction [77]. Greater than 34 CAG repeats leads to full penetrance, while 32–34 repeats leads to incomplete penetrance [78, 79]. The age at onset is most commonly in the third to fourth decade, and is inversely correlated with the repeat length. The disease demonstrates anticipation and very long CAG expansions (>200) result in disease onset in infancy [57, 80]. The clinical picture of SCA2 includes ataxia, dysarthria, dysphagia, oculomotor dysfunction (slow saccades), rigidity, bradykinesia, somatosensory deficits as well as executive dysfunction and late cognitive decline [59, 80–85]. Neuropathological studies show widespread neuronal loss in SCA2 that severely affects the cerebral cortex, basal forebrain, basal ganglia, thalamus, midbrain, pons, medulla oblongata, and cerebellum (for review see [74]).

In vivo MRI neuroimaging reveals a marked atrophy of the cerebellum, pons, medulla oblongata, and spinal cord. Additionally, involvement of the parietal cortex and thalamus was reported (Figure 14.7) [86]. That some of these neurodegenerative findings can be linked to functional impairment was shown in a

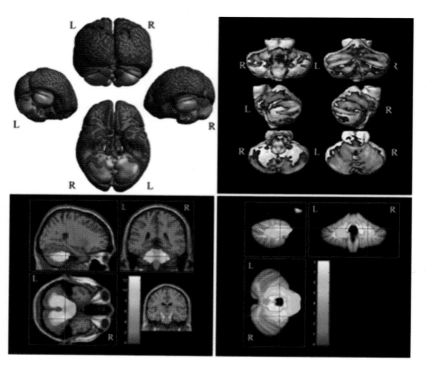

Figure 14.7 Voxel-based morphometry (VBM) comparison between controls and SCA2 patients. Upper left SCA2 versus controls gray matter (GM) comparison for DARTEL (algorithm for diffeomorphic image registration) normalized data, SPM maps projected onto a 3D rendering of the template created by DARTEL, upper right SCA2 versus controls GM comparison for spatially unbiased atlas template of the cerebellum and brainstem (SUIT) normalized data, SPM maps projected onto a 3D render of the SUIT template, lower left SCA2 versus controls white matter (WM) comparison for SUIT normalized data, SPM maps projected onto 3 orthogonal planes of the SUIT template, blue cross on the global maxima, lower right SCA2 versus controls WM comparison for DARTEL normalized data, projected onto 3 orthogonal planes of the Montreal Neurological Institute (MNI) Colin27 brain template, blue cross on the global maxima, detail of the corticospinal tracts involvement. For all the contrasts, the threshold was p < 0.001 uncorrected. (Obtained from D'Agata *et al.* [86].)

recent VBM study [86]. Using clinical and neuropsychological assessments this study linked impaired coordination to atrophy in the anterior cerebellum and executive impairment to atrophy in the posterior cerebellum.

Moreover, high-resolution volumetric MRI analysis in SCA2 showed that cerebellar and pontine volume loss specifically and closely correlate with functional staging scores [87]. Similar to SCA1, MRS revealed a decrease in the concentration of NAA in the pons and cerebellar hemispheres [71]. Using voxel-based ^{18}F-fluorodeoxyglucose (FDG) PET in SCA2, it was demonstrated that the glucose metabolic rate was significantly reduced in the cerebellum, pons, parahippocampal gyrus, and frontal cortex [88]. Compared to SCA3 and SCA6, cerebellar glucose metabolism was most severely compromised in SCA2 [88]. Another FDG-PET study showed reduced regional cerebral glucose metabolism in the brainstem and parietal cortex in SCA2 [89]. Given the clinical extrapyramidal symptoms and neurodegeneration in the basal ganglia and midbrain in SCA2 it is not surprising that investigation of the dopaminergic system using [^{11}C]d-threo-methylphenidate PET demonstrated reduced binding potential in the

striatum in SCA2, in a pattern that was distinct from Parkinson's disease [89].

Spinocerebellar ataxia 3

SCA3 is the most common SCA worldwide. Given the early onset in childhood or mid adulthood, the impact on the quality and length of life is severe (Table 14.2) [57]. The clinical phenotype in SCA3 is extremely heterogeneous. Besides cerebellar ataxia, familial parkinsonism, hereditary spastic paraplegia, hereditary neuropathy, restless-legs syndrome, and sleep disturbances, several non-specific symptoms have been reported, such as bulging eyes, faciolingual myokymia, and dystonia [57]. Longitudinal clinical data show that cerebellar ataxia-related symptoms, measured with SARA, and functional assessment of the UHDRS significantly deteriorated from baseline to follow-up over 2 years [90]. Related to other SCAs, the decline in SARA was less severe than in SCA1 but greater than in SCA6 [90].

Patterns of pontocerebellar atrophy in SCA3 have been reported in several neuroimaging studies [59, 69, 72, 91], which is well in line with postmortem macroscopic brain inspections, which also show pallor of the substantia nigra. Microscopic analyses reveal widespread neuronal loss in the cerebral cortex, basal ganglia, thalamus, midbrain, pons, medulla oblongata, and cerebellum (for review see [74]). Pontocerebellar atrophy as measured by MRI is similar to that in SCA1 [59, 72]. In addition, MRI reveals atrophy of the superior cerebellar peduncles, and the frontal and temporal lobes, as well as diminished transverse diameter of the pallidum [92]. The involvement of the basal ganglia in SCA3 has been further described in previous volumetric measurements in SCA3 but not in SCA1 and SCA2 [72]. A combined VBM and three-dimensional volumetric study revealed severe atrophy in total brainstem (consisting of midbrain, pons, and medulla), pons, medulla, total cerebellum, cerebellar hemispheres and cerebellar vermis, putamen, and caudate nucleus in SCA3 [69]. Also, a 2-year follow-up MRI study revealed that the most sensitive change was the striatal volume in SCA3 (Figure 14.5) [73]. Atrophy in the cerebellar hemispheres was less severe in SCA3 than in SCA1 or SCA6 [69].

Cerebral glucose metabolism measured with FDG-PET was decreased in the cerebellum, parahippocampal gyrus, and lentiform nucleus in SCA3 [88]. In contrast to SCA2, glucose metabolism in the lentiform nucleus and medulla was characteristically worse in SCA3 [88].

Spinocerebellar ataxia 6

SCA6 is primarily a cerebellar ataxia with relatively late onset, slow progression, and no significant impact on life expectancy (Table 14.2). Although SCA6 is mainly characterized by cerebellar ataxia, some cases present extracerebellar signs, such as mild peripheral neuropathy, brisk reflexes, pyramidal signs, bradykinesia, and dystonia [93] as well as oculomotor signs [65]. Moreover, a 2-year follow-up study in a larger cohort of SCA6 patients (n = 107) revealed two to three non-ataxia symptoms in this group [90], challenging the view of a purely cerebellar disorder. Neuroimaging studies report moderate to severe atrophy of the vermis, mild atrophy of the cerebellar hemispheres, and no atrophy of the MCPs, pons, or other structures of the posterior fossa [91, 93–95]. Furthermore, some studies document mild atrophy in the anteroposterior diameter of the pons and the diameter of the MCP [96], which nonetheless is never as severe as in SCA1 or SCA3. Notably, mild, diffuse atrophy of cortical areas has been reported in some SCA6 patients [93]. A cross-sectional volumetric and VBM study revealed atrophy in SCA6 predominantly in the cerebellum but also in total brainstem and pons (Figure 14.6) [69]. A 2-year longitudinal MRI study demonstrated that the most sensitive

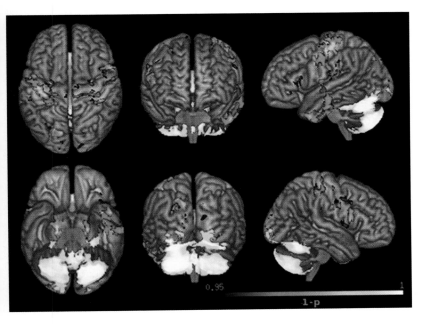

Figure 14.8 Spinocerebellar ataxia 7 (SCA 7) imaging. Three-dimensional image rendering on Montreal Neurological Institute (MNI) 152 template showing cortical regions with significant gray matter volume reductions (red–yellow, at a threshold of p < 0.05, corrected) in SCA7 patients when compared with a control group using VBM. (Obtained from Alcauter *et al.* [105].)

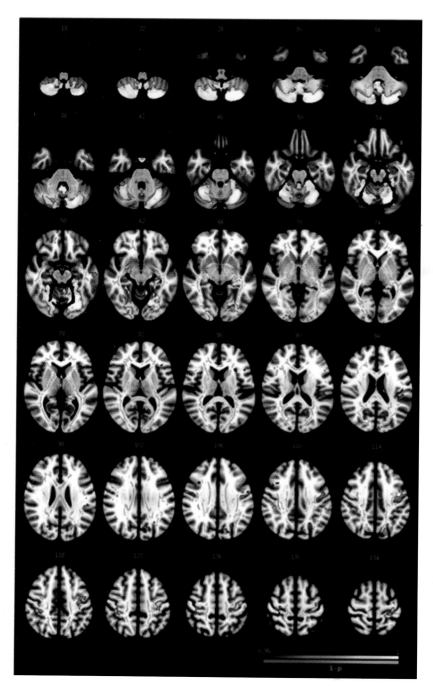

Figure 14.9 Spinocerebellar ataxia type 7 (SCA7) imaging. Axial sections showing areas with significant volume reduction of gray matter (red–yellow, threshold set at p < 0.05, corrected) obtained through VBM, and with a significant reduction in the fractional anisotropy (blue–green, at a threshold of p < 0.05, corrected) in SCA7 patients as compared with the control group. The results are projected on the MNI152 volume in the space of the Montreal Neurological Institute. Red labels indicate the z coordinate (in voxels), the left side of the image is the right side of the brain (radiological representation). (Obtained from Alcauter et al. [105].)

area to volume loss was the caudate; however, VBM showed the greatest gray matter loss in the cerebellum, thalamus, putamen, and pallidum (Figure 14.5) [73].

Spinocerebellar ataxia 7

SCA7 is an autosomal dominant inherited ataxia that differs from all others SCAs in having retinal degeneration as a consistent feature in addition to cerebellar

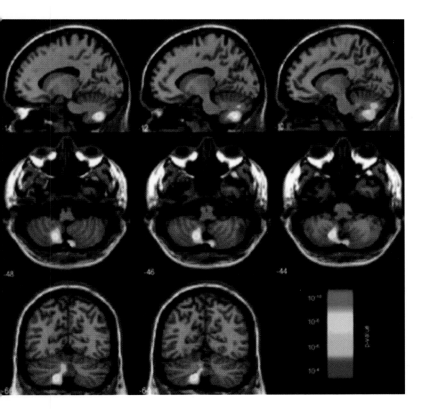

Figure 14.10 Voxel-based morphometry (VBM) of spinocerebellar ataxia 17 (SCA 17). Visual presentation of the VBM categorical comparison between the SCA17 patients and the controls in orthogonal sections (sagittal, coronal and axial view). The color bar represents the p values. (Obtained from Lasek *et al.* [115].) pFDR, positive false discovery rate.

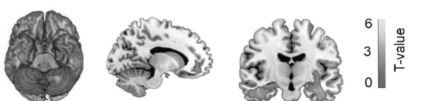

Figure 14.11 Longitudinal imaging in spinocerebellar ataxia 17 (SCA 17). Longitudinal findings contrasting the baseline and follow-up $(T_1 > T_2)$ assessments between SCA17 patients and healthy controls. Gray matter volume atrophy was found bilaterally in cerebellum, inferior frontal, and limbic structures such as parahippocampus. The overlay maps are superimposed and rendered on the SPM standard T_1-weighted template ($p < 0.05$). The color bar represents the T values. (Obtained from Reetz *et al.* [117].)

ataxia (Table 14.2). The causative gene mutation is a translated CAG repeat expansion in the gene encoding the ataxin 7 protein [97–99]. The normal range is 7–19 repeats, and the pathogenic alleles range from 37 to more than 300 repeats [97]. The ataxin 7 protein is crucial for retinal function. The clinical picture of SCA7 partly depends on the age of onset. Visual loss is due to a progressive atrophy of photoreceptor cells that results in macular degeneration often resulting in blindness in more advanced stages of the disease. Additional symptoms in SCA7 patients are progressive ataxia, dysarthria, dysphagia, and pyramidal and extrapyramidal signs. Tendon reflexes are usually absent. Clinical onset is usually in adulthood, with a mean age of about 30 years. As in other polyglutamine disorders, there is an inverse correlation between CAG repeat length and age of onset. Typically, the earlier the onset, the faster the disease progression. Lifespan is

221

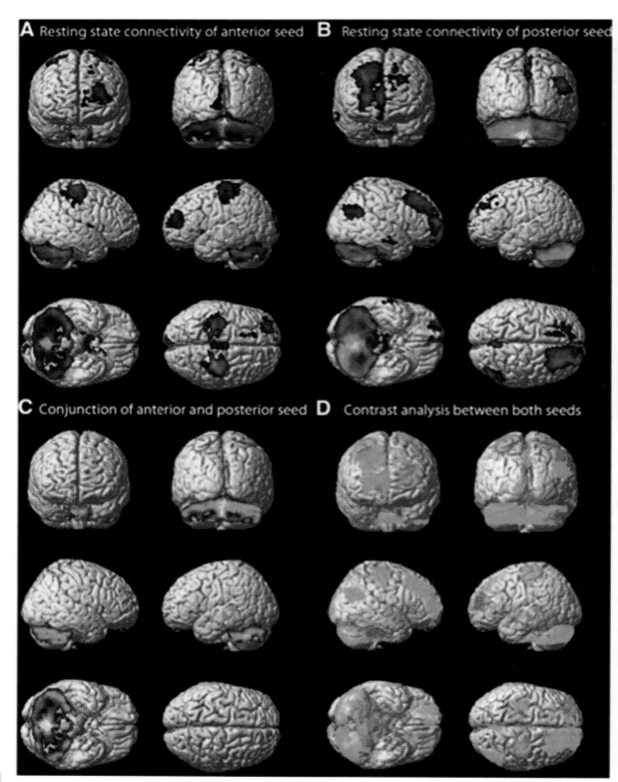

Figure 14.12 Function and connectivity in spinocerebellar ataxia 17 (SCA 17). Resting state connectivity. (A) Resting state connectivity with the anterior cerebellar cluster was observed mainly in lobules V–VII within the cerebellum extending to the striatum, pallidum, thalamus

often shortened and the cause of death is usually aspiration pneumonia due to dysphagia [100]. Postmortem macroscopic examinations disclose cerebellar and brainstem atrophy [101, 102]. Microscopy reveals widespread and severe neurodegeneration in the cerebral cortex, basal ganglia, thalamus, midbrain, pons, medulla oblongata, and cerebellum as well as significant retinal degeneration [99, 100, 102].

Accordingly, MRI studies have shown a diminished volume mainly in the cerebellum and pons [103, 104], while T_2 images have shown hyperintensities in transverse fibers at the pons. Overall, the most consistent finding in MRI studies is pontine atrophy. Compared to other SCAs, atrophy in the pons in SCA7 seems as severe as in SCA2, and more pronounced than in SCA3 and SCA6, whereas there is no difference in cerebellar atrophy between SCA7, SCA3, and SCA6 [103, 104]. A recent VBM and TBSS study demonstrated bilateral gray matter volume reductions in the cerebellar cortex and also in the pre- and postcentral gyrus, inferior and medial frontal cortex, inferior parietal cortex, parahippocampal gyrus, and occipital cortex (Figures 14.8 and 14.9) [105].

This study also showed diffuse reductions in fractional anisotropy in the cerebellar white matter, brainstem, cerebellar and cerebral peduncles, midbrain, anterior and posterior internal capsule, external/extreme capsule, corpus callosum, corona radiata, optical radiations, and the occipital, temporal, and frontal lobe white matter [105]. These results confirm previous evidence of widespread damage beyond the cerebellum and the pons in SCA7.

Spinocerebellar ataxia 17

SCA17 is caused by a polyglutamine expansion in the TATA-binding protein (TBP), a general transcription initiation factor [106, 107]. Aside from the clinical hallmark of cerebellar ataxia, the phenotypic spectrum of this disorder is highly variable and may comprise extrapyramidal motor symptoms [106, 108, 109] such as dystonia [109, 110] and chorea [111], as well as pyramidal signs such as spasticity [107, 110]. SCA17 may also manifest with epilepsy [112–114], and a broad spectrum of neuropsychiatric symptoms such as cognitive impairment, obsessive–compulsive personality disorder, and phobia [112, 113, 115]. Postmortem examinations of SCA17 patients demonstrate cerebellar but also widely distributed cortical and subcortical atrophy, as well as cerebellar and cerebral cell loss and gliosis [116]. MRI studies in SCA17 have revealed severe structural alterations in the cerebellum (Figure 14.10) [112, 115, 117].

It has been demonstrated that the extent of cerebellar neurodegeneration correlates with a variety of clinical motor features such as ataxia and extrapyramidal signs, but also to a broad spectrum of neuropsychiatric symptoms [115] and is negatively correlated with the CAG repeat size [118]. The motor-related neurodegeneration has been shown to be progressive in a longitudinal study (Figure 14.11) [117].

Recently, a task-based meta-analytic connectivity modeling (MACM) and task-free resting-state functional connectivity analysis showed differential functional connectivity of a cerebellar anterior and posterior cluster, obtained from a VBM analysis, in SCA17. This study highlights the manifold connections and anterior–posterior dichotomy of the human cerebellum, providing additional valuable information about disrupted cerebellar–cerebral connections and reflecting the brunt of motor and neuropsychiatric deficits in SCA17 (Figure 14.12) [119].

Caption for Figure 14.12 (*cont.*) and hippocampus. Cortically, significant correlations were mainly found in motor and sensorimotor regions (M1, PMC, SMA, SI), and further superior and middle frontal gyri, anterior cingulate cortex, and posterior insula. (B) For the posterior cluster significant resting state correlation was found mainly with posterior cerebellar lobules, with frontal gyri extending to mid-orbital and superior medial parts as well as the SMA in the frontal lobe. Further cortical clusters were located in parietal areas, the precuneus and middle temporal gyrus. (C) Conjunction analysis between both cerebellar seeds showed common connectivity only within the cerebellum, mainly in posterior lobules. (D) Contrasting the connectivity maps for the two clusters, the anterior cluster showed higher connectivity particularly with anterior cerebellar lobules, the thalamus, hippocampus, striatum, and motor as well as sensorimotor areas, frontal gyri, anterior cingulate, posterior insula, and parietal operculum (red blobs). The posterior cluster was more strongly correlated with posterior cerebellar lobules, orbital and medial regions of the frontal lobe, inferior and superior parietal areas, the precuneus, and middle temporal gyrus (green blobs). (Obtained from Reetz *et al.* [119].) SI = primary somatosensory cortex.

References

1. Anheim M, Tranchant C, Koenig M. The autosomal recessive cerebellar ataxias. *N Engl J Med.* 2012;**366**(7):636–46. Epub 2012/02/18.

2. Pandolfo M. Friedreich ataxia: the clinical picture. *J Neurol.* 2009;**256** Suppl 1:3–8. Epub 2009/04/11.

3. Pandolfo M. Friedreich ataxia: detection of GAA repeat expansions and frataxin point mutations. *Methods Mol Med.* 2006;**126**:197–216. Epub 2006/08/26.

4. Campuzano V, Montermini L, Molto MD, *et al.* Friedreich's ataxia: autosomal recessive disease caused by an intronic GAA triplet repeat expansion. *Science.* 1996;**271**(5254):1423–7. Epub 1996/03/08.

5. Pandolfo M. Frataxin deficiency and mitochondrial dysfunction. *Mitochondrion.* 2002;**2**(1–2):87–93. Epub 2005/08/27.

6. Durr A, Stevanin G, Cancel G, *et al.* Spinocerebellar ataxia 3 and Machado-Joseph disease: clinical, molecular, and neuropathological features. *Ann Neurol.* 1996;**39**(4):490–9. Epub 1996/04/01.

7. Pandolfo M. Friedreich ataxia. *Semin Pediatr Neurol.* 2003;**10**(3):163–72. Epub 2003/12/05.

8. Berciano J, Infante J, Mateo I, Combarros O. [Hereditary ataxias and paraplegias: a clinicogenetic review]. *Neurología.* 2002;**17**(1):40–51. Epub 2002/02/09.

9. Wullner U, Klockgether T, Petersen D, Naegele T, Dichgans J. Magnetic resonance imaging in hereditary and idiopathic ataxia. *Neurology.* 1993;**43**(2):318–25. Epub 1993/02/01.

10. Huang YP, Tuason MY, Wu T, Plaitakis A. MRI and CT features of cerebellar degeneration. *J Formos Med Assoc.* 1993;**92**(6):494–508. Epub 1993/06/01.

11. Ormerod IE, Harding AE, Miller DH, *et al.* Magnetic resonance imaging in degenerative ataxic disorders. *J Neurol Neurosurg Psychiatry.* 1994;**57**(1):51–7. Epub 1994/01/01.

12. De Michele G, Di Salle F, Filla A, *et al.* Magnetic resonance imaging in "typical" and "late onset" Friedreich's disease and early onset cerebellar ataxia with retained tendon reflexes. *Ital J Neurol Sci.* 1995;**16**(5):303–8. Epub 1995/06/01.

13. Della Nave R, Ginestroni A, Giannelli M, *et al.* Brain structural damage in Friedreich's ataxia. *J Neurol Neurosurg Psychiatry.* 2008;**79**(1):82–5. Epub 2007/07/20.

14. Franca MC, Jr., D'Abreu A, Yasuda CL, *et al.* A combined voxel-based morphometry and 1H-MRS study in patients with Friedreich's ataxia. *J Neurol.* 2009;**256**(7):1114–20. Epub 2009/03/13.

15. Della Nave R, Ginestroni A, Tessa C, *et al.* Brain white matter tracts degeneration in Friedreich ataxia. An in vivo MRI study using tract-based spatial statistics and voxel-based morphometry. *Neuroimage.* 2008;**40**(1):19–25. Epub 2008/01/30.

16. Akhlaghi H, Corben L, Georgiou-Karistianis N, *et al.* Superior cerebellar peduncle atrophy in Friedreich's ataxia correlates with disease symptoms. *Cerebellum.* 2011;**10**(1):81–7. Epub 2010/11/26.

17. Rizzo G, Tonon C, Valentino ML, *et al.* Brain diffusion-weighted imaging in Friedreich's ataxia. *Mov Disord.* 2011;**26**(4):705–12. Epub 2011/03/04.

18. Fortuna F, Barboni P, Liguori R, *et al.* Visual system involvement in patients with Friedreich's ataxia. *Brain.* 2009;**132**(Pt 1):116–23. Epub 2008/10/22.

19. Pagani E, Ginestroni A, Della Nave R, *et al.* Assessment of brain white matter fiber bundle atrophy in patients with Friedreich ataxia. *Radiology.* 2010;**255**(3):882–9. Epub 2010/05/27.

20. Tkac I, Oz G, Adriany G, Ugurbil K, Gruetter R. In vivo 1H NMR spectroscopy of the human brain at high magnetic fields: metabolite quantification at 4T vs. 7T. *Magn Reson Med.* 2009;**62**(4):868–79. Epub 2009/07/11.

21. Guerrini L, Belli G, Mazzoni L, *et al.* Impact of cerebrospinal fluid contamination on brain metabolites evaluation with 1H-MR spectroscopy: a single voxel study of the cerebellar vermis in patients with degenerative ataxias. *J Magn Reson Imaging.* 2009;**30**(1):11–17. Epub 2009/06/27.

22. Mascalchi M, Cosottini M, Lolli F, *et al.* Proton MR spectroscopy of the cerebellum and pons in patients with degenerative ataxia. *Radiology.* 2002;**223**(2):371–8. Epub 2002/05/09.

23. Viau M, Marchand L, Bard C, Boulanger Y. (1)H magnetic resonance spectroscopy of autosomal ataxias. *Brain Res.* 2005;**1049**(2):191–202. Epub 2005/06/21.

24. Iltis I, Hutter D, Bushara KO, *et al.* (1)H MR spectroscopy in Friedreich's ataxia and ataxia with oculomotor apraxia type 2. *Brain Res.* 2010;**1358**:200–10. Epub 2010/08/18.

25. Corben LA, Georgiou-Karistianis N, Fahey MC, *et al.* Towards an understanding of cognitive function in Friedreich ataxia. *Brain Res Bull.* 2006;**70**(3):197–202. Epub 2006/07/25.

26. Mantovan MC, Martinuzzi A, Squarzanti F, *et al.* Exploring mental status in Friedreich's

ataxia: a combined neuropsychological, behavioral and neuroimaging study. *Eur J Neurol.* 2006;**13**(8):827–35. Epub 2006/08/02.

27. Corben LA, Delatycki MB, Bradshaw JL, *et al.* Impairment in motor reprogramming in Friedreich ataxia reflecting possible cerebellar dysfunction. *J Neurol.* 2010;**257**(5):782–91. Epub 2009/12/04.

28. Fielding J, Corben L, Cremer P, *et al.* Disruption to higher order processes in Friedreich ataxia. *Neuropsychologia.* 2010; **48**(1):235–42. Epub 2009/09/22.

29. Nieto A, Correia R, de Nobrega E, *et al.* Cognition in Friedreich ataxia. *Cerebellum.* 2012;**11**(4): 834–44. Epub 2012/02/22.

30. Ginestroni A, Diciotti S, Cecchi P, *et al.* Neurodegeneration in Friedreich's ataxia is associated with a mixed activation pattern of the brain. A fMRI study. *Hum Brain Mapp.* 2012;**33**(8):1780–91. Epub 2011/06/16.

31. Corben LA, Akhlaghi H, Georgiou-Karistianis N, *et al.* Impaired inhibition of prepotent motor tendencies in Friedreich ataxia demonstrated by the Simon interference task. *Brain Cogn.* 2011;**76**(1):140–5. Epub 2011/03/01.

32. Simon JR, Rudell AP. Auditory S-R compatibility: the effect of an irrelevant cue on information processing. *J Appl Psychol.* 1967;**51**(3):300–4. Epub 1967/06/01.

33. Schmahmann JD. Disorders of the cerebellum: ataxia, dysmetria of thought, and the cerebellar cognitive affective syndrome. *J Neuropsychiatry Clin Neurosci.* 2004;**16**(3):367–78. Epub 2004/09/21.

34. Savitsky K, Bar-Shira A, Gilad S, *et al.* A single ataxia telangiectasia gene with a product similar to PI-3 kinase. *Science.*

1995;**268**(5218):1749–53. Epub 1995/06/23.

35. Sun X, Becker-Catania SG, Chun HH, *et al.* Early diagnosis of ataxia-telangiectasia using radiosensitivity testing. *J Pediatr.* 2002;**140**(6):724–31. Epub 2002/06/20.

36. Tavani F, Zimmerman RA, Berry GT, *et al.* Ataxia-telangiectasia: the pattern of cerebellar atrophy on MRI. *Neuroradiology.* 2003;**45**(5): 315–19. Epub 2003/05/13.

37. Kieslich M, Hoche F, Reichenbach J, *et al.* Extracerebellar MRI-lesions in ataxia telangiectasia go along with deficiency of the GH/IGF-1 axis, markedly reduced body weight, high ataxia scores and advanced age. *Cerebellum.* 2010;**9**(2):190–7. Epub 2009/11/10.

38. Lin DD, Crawford TO, Lederman HM, Barker PB. Proton MR spectroscopic imaging in ataxia-telangiectasia. *Neuropediatrics.* 2006;**37**(4): 241–6. Epub 2006/12/21.

39. Quarantelli M, Giardino G, Prinster A, *et al.* Steroid treatment in ataxia-telangiectasia induces alterations of functional magnetic resonance imaging during prono-supination task. *Eur J Paediatr Neurol.* 2012;**17**(2):135–40. Epub 2012/07/06.

40. Le Ber I, Moreira MC, Rivaud-Pechoux S, *et al.* Cerebellar ataxia with oculomotor apraxia type 1: clinical and genetic studies. *Brain.* 2003;**126**(Pt 12):2761–72. Epub 2003/09/25.

41. Anheim M, Monga B, Fleury M, *et al.* Ataxia with oculomotor apraxia type 2: clinical, biological and genotype/phenotype correlation study of a cohort of 90 patients. *Brain.* 2009;**132**(Pt 10):2688–98. Epub 2009/08/22.

42. Dubois J, Sebag G, Argyropoulou M, Brunelle F. MR findings in infantile Refsum disease: case report of two family

members. *AJNR Am J Neuroradiol.* 1991;**12**(6): 1159–60. Epub 1991/11/01.

43. Choksi V, Hoeffner E, Karaarslan E, Yalcinkaya C, Cakirer S. Infantile refsum disease: case report. *AJNR Am J Neuroradiol.* 2003;**24**(10): 2082–4. Epub 2003/11/20.

44. Anheim M, Fleury M, Monga B, *et al.* Epidemiological, clinical, paraclinical and molecular study of a cohort of 102 patients affected with autosomal recessive progressive cerebellar ataxia from Alsace, Eastern France: implications for clinical management. *Neurogenetics.* 2010;**11**(1):1–12. Epub 2009/05/15.

45. Benomar A, Yahyaoui M, Meggouh F, *et al.* Clinical comparison between AVED patients with 744 del A mutation and Friedreich ataxia with GAA expansion in 15 Moroccan families. *J Neurol Sci.* 2002;**198**(1–2):25–9. Epub 2002/06/01.

46. Barkhof F, Verrips A, Wesseling P, *et al.* Cerebrotendinous xanthomatosis: the spectrum of imaging findings and the correlation with neuropathologic findings. *Radiology.* 2000;**217**(3):869–76. Epub 2000/12/09.

47. Chang CC, Lui CC, Wang JJ, *et al.* Multi-parametric neuroimaging evaluation of cerebrotendinous xanthomatosis and its correlation with neuropsychological presentations. *BMC Neurol.* 2010;**10**:59. Epub 2010/07/07.

48. Mignarri A, Falcini M, Vella A, *et al.* Parkinsonism as neurological presentation of late-onset cerebrotendinous xanthomatosis. *Parkinsonism Relat Disord.* 2012;**18**(1):99–101. Epub 2011/07/19.

49. Ohno T, Kobayashi S, Hayashi M, Sakurai M, Kanazawa I. Diphenylpyraline-responsive

parkinsonism in cerebrotendinous xanthomatosis: long-term follow up of three patients. *J Neurol Sci.* 2001;**182**(2):95–7. Epub 2001/01/04.

50. Selva-O'Callaghan A, Bardes I, Jacas C, *et al.* SPECT imaging for brain improvement quantification in a patient with cerebrotendinous xanthomatosis. *Clin Nucl Med.* 2011;**36**(1):38–9. Epub 2010/12/16.

51. Adams JS, Adams PE, Nguyen D, *et al.* Volumetric brain changes in females with fragile X-associated tremor/ataxia syndrome (FXTAS). *Neurology.* 2007;**69**(9): 851–9. Epub 2007/08/29.

52. Greco CM, Hagerman RJ, Tassone F, *et al.* Neuronal intranuclear inclusions in a new cerebellar tremor/ataxia syndrome among fragile X carriers. *Brain.* 2002;**125**(Pt 8):1760–71. Epub 2002/07/24.

53. Jacquemont S, Hagerman RJ, Leehey M, *et al.* Fragile X premutation tremor/ataxia syndrome: molecular, clinical, and neuroimaging correlates. *Am J Hum Genet.* 2003;**72**(4):869–78. Epub 2003/03/15.

54. Jacquemont S, Orrico A, Galli L, *et al.* Spastic paraparesis, cerebellar ataxia, and intention tremor: a severe variant of FXTAS? *J Med Genet.* 2005;**42**(2): e14. Epub 2005/02/04.

55. Cohen S, Masyn K, Adams J, *et al.* Molecular and imaging correlates of the fragile X-associated tremor/ataxia syndrome. *Neurology.* 2006;**67**(8):1426–31. Epub 2006/10/25.

56. Sarac H, Henigsberg N, Markeljevic J, *et al.* Fragile X-premutation tremor/ataxia syndrome (FXTAS) in a young woman: clinical, genetics, MRI and 1H-MR spectroscopy correlates. *Coll Antropol.* 2011;**35** Suppl 1:327–32. Epub 2011/06/09.

57. Schols L, Bauer P, Schmidt T, Schulte T, Riess O. Autosomal dominant cerebellar ataxias: clinical features, genetics, and pathogenesis. *Lancet Neurol.* 2004;**3**(5):291–304.

58. Orr HT, Chung MY, Banfi S, *et al.* Expansion of an unstable trinucleotide CAG repeat in spinocerebellar ataxia type 1. *Nat Genet.* 1993;**4**(3):221–6. Epub 1993/07/01.

59. Bürk K, Abele M, Fetter M, *et al.* Autosomal dominant cerebellar ataxia type I clinical features and MRI in families with SCA1, SCA2 and SCA3. *Brain.* 1996;**119**(Pt 5): 1497–505. Epub 1996/10/01.

60. Dubourg O, Durr A, Cancel G, *et al.* Analysis of the SCA1 CAG repeat in a large number of families with dominant ataxia: clinical and molecular correlations. *Ann Neurol.* 1995;**37**(2):176–80. Epub 1995/02/01.

61. Schmitz-Hubsch T, du Montcel ST, Baliko L, *et al.* Scale for the assessment and rating of ataxia: development of a new clinical scale. *Neurology.* 2006;**66**(11):1717–20. Epub 2006/06/14.

62. Schmitz-Hubsch T, Fimmers R, Rakowicz M, *et al.* Responsiveness of different rating instruments in spinocerebellar ataxia patients. *Neurology.* 2010;**74**(8):678–84. Epub 2010/02/24.

63. Weyer A, Abele M, Schmitz-Hubsch T, *et al.* Reliability and validity of the scale for the assessment and rating of ataxia: a study in 64 ataxia patients. *Mov Disord.* 2007;**22**(11):1633–7. Epub 2007/05/23.

64. Unified Huntington's Disease Rating Scale: reliability and consistency. Huntington Study Group. *Mov Disord.* 1996;**11**(2):136–42. Epub 1996/03/01.

65. Schmitz-Hubsch T, Coudert M, Bauer P, *et al.* Spinocerebellar ataxia types 1, 2, 3, and 6: disease severity and nonataxia symptoms.
Neurology. 2008;**71**(13):982–9. Epub 2008/08/08.

66. Klockgether T, Ludtke R, Kramer B, *et al.* The natural history of degenerative ataxia: a retrospective study in 466 patients. *Brain.* 1998;**121**(Pt 4): 589–600. Epub 1998/05/13.

67. Gilman S, Sima AA, Junck L, *et al.* Spinocerebellar ataxia type 1 with multiple system degeneration and glial cytoplasmic inclusions. *Ann Neurol.* 1996;**39**(2):241–55. Epub 1996/02/01.

68. Rüb U, Bürk K, Timmann D, *et al.* Spinocerebellar ataxia type 1 (SCA1): new pathoanatomical and clinico-pathological insights. *Neuropathol Appl Neurobiol.* 2012;**38**(7):665–80. Epub 2012/02/09.

69. Schulz JB, Borkert J, Wolf S, *et al.* Visualization, quantification and correlation of brain atrophy with clinical symptoms in spinocerebellar ataxia types 1, 3 and 6. *Neuroimage.* 2010;**49**(1):158–68. Epub 2009/07/28.

70. Ginestroni A, Della Nave R, Tessa C, *et al.* Brain structural damage in spinocerebellar ataxia type 1: a VBM study. *J Neurol.* 2008;**255**(8):1153–8. Epub 2008/04/29.

71. Guerrini L, Lolli F, Ginestroni A, *et al.* Brainstem neurodegeneration correlates with clinical dysfunction in SCA1 but not in SCA2. A quantitative volumetric, diffusion and proton spectroscopy MR study. *Brain.* 2004;**127**(Pt 8):1785–95.

72. Klockgether T, Skalej M, Wedekind D, *et al.* Autosomal dominant cerebellar ataxia type I. MRI-based volumetry of posterior fossa structures and basal ganglia in spinocerebellar ataxia types 1, 2 and 3. *Brain.* 1998;**121**(Pt 9):1687–93.

73. Reetz K, Costa A, Mirzazade S, *et al.* Genotype specific patterns of atrophy progression are more

sensitive than clinical decline in SCA1, SCA3 and SCA6. *Brain.* 2013;**136**(Pt 3):905–17.

74. Seidel K, Siswanto S, Brunt ER, *et al.* Brain pathology of spinocerebellar ataxias. *Acta Neuropathol.* 2012;**124**(1):1–21. Epub 2012/06/12.

75. Della Nave R, Ginestroni A, Tessa C, *et al.* Brain white matter damage in SCA1 and SCA2. An in vivo study using voxel-based morphometry, histogram analysis of mean diffusivity and tract-based spatial statistics. *Neuroimage.* 2008;**43**(1):10–19. Epub 2008/08/02.

76. Solodkin A, Peri E, Chen EE, Ben-Jacob E, Gomez CM. Loss of intrinsic organization of cerebellar networks in spinocerebellar ataxia type 1: correlates with disease severity and duration. *Cerebellum.* 2011;**10**(2):218–32. Epub 2010/10/05.

77. Lastres-Becker I, Rüb U, Auburger G. Spinocerebellar ataxia 2 (SCA2). *Cerebellum.* 2008;**7**(2):115–24. Epub 2008/04/18.

78. Cancel G, Durr A, Didierjean O, *et al.* Molecular and clinical correlations in spinocerebellar ataxia 2: a study of 32 families. *Hum Mol Genet.* 1997;**6**(5):709–15. Epub 1997/05/01.

79. Hernandez A, Magarino C, Gispert S, *et al.* Genetic mapping of the spinocerebellar ataxia 2 (SCA2) locus on chromosome 12q23-q24.1. *Genomics.* 1995;**25**(2):433–5. Epub 1995/01/20.

80. Schols L, Gispert S, Vorgerd M, *et al.* Spinocerebellar ataxia type 2. Genotype and phenotype in German kindreds. *Arch Neurol.* 1997;**54**(9):1073–80. Epub 1997/10/06.

81. Bürk K, Globas C, Bosch S, *et al.* Cognitive deficits in spinocerebellar ataxia type 1, 2, and 3. *J Neurol.* 2003;**250**(2):207–11.

82. Bürk K, Fetter M, Abele M, *et al.* Autosomal dominant cerebellar ataxia type I: oculomotor abnormalities in families with SCA1, SCA2, and SCA3. *J Neurol.* 1999;**246**(9):789–97. Epub 1999/10/20.

83. Durr A, Smadja D, Cancel G, *et al.* Autosomal dominant cerebellar ataxia type I in Martinique (French West Indies). Clinical and neuropathological analysis of 53 patients from three unrelated SCA2 families. *Brain.* 1995;**118**(Pt 6):1573–81. Epub 1995/12/01.

84. Klinke I, Minnerop M, Schmitz-Hubsch T, *et al.* Neuropsychological features of patients with spinocerebellar ataxia (SCA) types 1, 2, 3, and 6. *Cerebellum.* 2010;**9**(3):433–42. Epub 2010/05/27.

85. Le Pira F, Zappala G, Saponara R, *et al.* Cognitive findings in spinocerebellar ataxia type 2: relationship to genetic and clinical variables. *J Neurol Sci.* 2002;**201**(1–2):53–7. Epub 2002/08/07.

86. D'Agata F, Caroppo P, Boghi A, *et al.* Linking coordinative and executive dysfunctions to atrophy in spinocerebellar ataxia 2 patients. *Brain Struct Funct.* 2011;**216**:275–88.

87. Ying SH, Choi SI, Perlman SL, *et al.* Pontine and cerebellar atrophy correlate with clinical disability in SCA2. *Neurology.* 2006;**66**(3):424–6. Epub 2006/02/16.

88. Wang PS, Liu RS, Yang BH, Soong BW. Regional patterns of cerebral glucose metabolism in spinocerebellar ataxia type 2, 3 and 6: a voxel-based FDG-positron emission tomography analysis. *J Neurol.* 2007;**254**(7):838–45. Epub 2007/05/01.

89. Wullner U, Reimold M, Abele M, *et al.* Dopamine transporter positron emission tomography in spinocerebellar ataxias type 1, 2, 3, and 6. *Arch Neurol.*

2005;**62**(8):1280–5. Epub 2005/08/10.

90. Jacobi H, Bauer P, Giunti P, *et al.* The natural history of spinocerebellar ataxia type 1, 2, 3, and 6: a 2-year follow-up study. *Neurology.* 2011;**77**(11):1035–41. Epub 2011/08/13.

91. Lukas C, Schols L, Bellenberg B, *et al.* Dissociation of grey and white matter reduction in spinocerebellar ataxia type 3 and 6: a voxel-based morphometry study. *Neurosci Lett.* 2006;**408**(3):230–5. Epub 2006/09/29.

92. Murata Y, Yamaguchi S, Kawakami H, *et al.* Characteristic magnetic resonance imaging findings in Machado-Joseph disease. *Arch Neurol.* 1998;**55**(1):33–7. Epub 1998/01/27.

93. Schols L, Kruger R, Amoiridis G, *et al.* Spinocerebellar ataxia type 6: genotype and phenotype in German kindreds. *J Neurol Neurosurg Psychiatry.* 1998;**64**(1):67–73. Epub 1998/01/22.

94. Satoh JI, Tokumoto H, Yukitake M, *et al.* Spinocerebellar ataxia type 6: MRI of three Japanese patients. *Neuroradiology.* 1998;**40**(4):222–7. Epub 1998/05/21.

95. Butteriss D, Chinnery P, Birchall D. Radiological characterization of spinocerebellar ataxia type 6. *Br J Radiol.* 2005;**78**(932):694–6. Epub 2005/07/28.

96. Murata Y, Kawakami H, Yamaguchi S, *et al.* Characteristic magnetic resonance imaging findings in spinocerebellar ataxia 6. *Arch Neurol.* 1998;**55**(10):1348–52. Epub 1998/10/21.

97. David G, Abbas N, Stevanin G, *et al.* Cloning of the SCA7 gene reveals a highly unstable CAG repeat expansion. *Nat Genet.* 1997;**17**(1):65–70. Epub 1997/09/01.

98. Lebre AS, Brice A. Spinocerebellar ataxia 7 (SCA7). *Cytogenet*

227

Genome Res. 2003;**100**(1–4): 154–63. Epub 2003/10/04.

99. Michalik A, Martin JJ, Van Broeckhoven C. Spinocerebellar ataxia type 7 associated with pigmentary retinal dystrophy. *Eur J Hum Genet.* 2004;**12**(1):2–15. Epub 2003/10/23.

100. Rüb U, Brunt ER, Petrasch-Parwez E, *et al.* Degeneration of ingestion-related brainstem nuclei in spinocerebellar ataxia type 2, 3, 6 and 7. *Neuropathol Appl Neurobiol.* 2006;**32**(6):635–49. Epub 2006/11/07.

101. David G, Durr A, Stevanin G, *et al.* Molecular and clinical correlations in autosomal dominant cerebellar ataxia with progressive macular dystrophy (SCA7). *Hum Mol Genet.* 1998;**7**(2):165–70. Epub 1998/03/21.

102. Rüb U, Brunt ER, Gierga K, *et al.* Spinocerebellar ataxia type 7 (SCA7): first report of a systematic neuropathological study of the brain of a patient with a very short expanded CAG-repeat. *Brain Pathol.* 2005;**15**(4):287–95. Epub 2006/01/05.

103. Dohlinger S, Hauser TK, Borkert J, Luft AR, Schulz JB. Magnetic resonance imaging in spinocerebellar ataxias. *Cerebellum.* 2008;**7**(2):204–14. Epub 2008/04/18.

104. Bang OY, Huh K, Lee PH, Kim HJ. Clinical and neuroradiological features of patients with spinocerebellar ataxias from Korean kindreds. *Arch Neurol.* 2003;**60**(11): 1566–74. Epub 2003/11/19.

105. Alcauter S, Barrios FA, Diaz R, Fernandez-Ruiz J. Gray and white matter alterations in spinocerebellar ataxia type 7: an in vivo DTI and VBM study.

106. Nakamura K, Jeong SY, Uchihara T, *et al.* SCA17, a novel autosomal dominant cerebellar ataxia caused by an expanded polyglutamine in TATA-binding protein. *Hum Mol Genet.* 2001;**10**(14):1441–8.

107. Koide R, Kobayashi S, Shimohata T, *et al.* A neurological disease caused by an expanded CAG trinucleotide repeat in the TATA-binding protein gene: a new polyglutamine disease? *Hum Mol Genet.* 1999;**8**(11):2047–53.

108. Zuhlke C, Hellenbroich Y, Dalski A, *et al.* Different types of repeat expansion in the TATA-binding protein gene are associated with a new form of inherited ataxia. *Eur J Hum Genet.* 2001;**9**(3):160–4. Epub 2001/04/21.

109. Hernandez D, Hanson M, Singleton A, *et al.* Mutation at the SCA17 locus is not a common cause of parkinsonism. *Parkinsonism Relat Disord.* 2003;**9**(6):317–20.

110. Hagenah JM, Zuhlke C, Hellenbroich Y, Heide W, Klein C. Focal dystonia as a presenting sign of spinocerebellar ataxia 17. *Mov Disord.* 2004;**19**(2):217–20.

111. Toyoshima Y, Yamada M, Onodera O, *et al.* SCA17 homozygote showing Huntington's disease-like phenotype. *Ann Neurol.* 2004;**55**(2):281–6.

112. Rolfs A, Koeppen AH, Bauer I, *et al.* Clinical features and neuropathology of autosomal dominant spinocerebellar ataxia (SCA17). *Ann Neurol.* 2003;**54**(3):367–75.

113. Maltecca F, Filla A, Castaldo I, *et al.* Intergenerational instability

and marked anticipation in SCA-17. *Neurology.* 2003;**61**(10):1441–3.

114. De Michele G, Maltecca F, Carella M, *et al.* Dementia, ataxia extrapyramidal features, and epilepsy: phenotype spectrum in two Italian families with spinocerebellar ataxia type 17. *Neurol Sci.* 2003;**24**(3):166–7.

115. Lasek K, Lencer R, Gaser C, *et al.* Morphological basis for the spectrum of clinical deficits in spinocerebellar ataxia 17 (SCA17). *Brain.* 2006;**129**(Pt 9):2341–52.

116. Bruni AC, Takahashi-Fujigasaki J, Maltecca F, *et al.* Behavioral disorder, dementia, ataxia, and rigidity in a large family with TATA box-binding protein mutation. *Arch Neurol.* 2004;**61**(8):1314–20.

117. Reetz K, Lencer R, Hagenah JM, *et al.* Structural changes associated with progression of motor deficits in spinocerebellar ataxia 17. *Cerebellum.* 2010;**9**(2):210–17. Epub 2009/12/18.

118. Reetz K, Kleiman A, Klein C, *et al.* CAG repeats determine brain atrophy in spinocerebellar ataxia 17: a VBM study. *PLoS One.* 2011;**6**(1):e15125. Epub 2011/02/12.

119. Reetz K, Dogan I, Rolfs A, *et al.* Investigating function and connectivity of morphometric findings – exemplified on cerebellar atrophy in spinocerebellar ataxia 17 (SCA17). *Neuroimage.* 2012;**62**(3):1354–66. Epub 2012/06/05.

120. Asaka T, Yokoji H, Ito J, Yamaguchi K, Matsushima A. Autosomal recessive ataxia with peripheral neuropathy and elevated AFP: novel mutations in SETX. *Neurology.* 2006;**66**(10):1580–1. Epub 2006/05/24.

Chapter 15

Magnetic resonance spectroscopy in Parkinson's disease

Uzay E. Emir and Gülin Öz

Introduction

Parkinson's disease (PD) is a progressive neurodegenerative disorder that usually appears after the age of 50 and occurs in all ethnic groups [1]. The major pathological marker of PD is the degeneration of nigrostriatal dopaminergic neurons, which leads to a reduction in dopamine (DA) content within the striatum [2]. While loss of the nigrostriatal dopaminergic neurons represents a hallmark of PD, the pathology in PD extends beyond these neurons. Recent evidence indicates that caudal brainstem structures are involved in PD pathology even before the nigrostriatal pathology [3]. Several processes have been proposed to underlie neurodegeneration in PD, including mitochondrial dysfunction [4] and iron-related oxidative stress [5]. Although there have been many advances in understanding the pathophysiology of PD, the diagnosis of PD still largely relies on the clinical judgment of a neurologist. Misdiagnoses could compromise therapeutic decisions. Hence, the development of biomarkers to confirm diagnosis and to monitor progression and response to therapeutic interventions is of critical importance to clinical practice. Neuroimaging techniques have much to offer for an objective and potentially more accurate in vivo means to assess the brain structure, physiology, chemistry, and function in PD.

Non-invasive magnetic resonance spectroscopy (MRS) techniques can be utilized for the evaluation of brain physiology, chemistry, and function in neurodegenerative disorders since they provide unique information on chemical composition of the brain tissue. Using MRS at 7T it is possible to measure the signals from up to 17 metabolites [6] that are reflective of different pathophysiological processes of PD. Thus, this method has the potential to improve the understanding of the etiology, progression, and the response to therapy in PD. In this chapter we will review MRS studies that were used to investigate neurochemical alterations in PD.

Magnetic resonance spectroscopy

MRS is a non-invasive technique that can be used to quantify compounds or metabolites that are present in high concentrations in a single voxel or multiple voxels within tissues. The technique is based on the same physical principles as MRI; however, the MRS measurement results in a spectrum where metabolite nuclei resonate at characteristic frequencies depending on their chemical and physical vicinity in a molecule. The surroundings change the local magnetic field experienced by the nuclei (nuclear shielding) and thus their resonance frequency. MRS has been demonstrated in vivo for different nuclei, including ^1H, ^{31}P, ^{13}C, ^{15}N, ^{19}F, and ^{23}Na. However, clinical applications are mostly limited to ^1H and ^{31}P isotopes. Therefore, this chapter will focus on the use of ^1H and ^{31}P nuclei for MRS.

Briefly, in MRS, the nuclei of interest (e.g., ^1H, ^{31}P) are placed in a strong external magnetic field and the volume of interest is excited using broadband excitation radiofrequency (RF) pulses. Subsequently, the response to the excitation RF pulses is recorded and Fourier transformed to obtain a spectrum consisting of peaks at specific resonant frequencies (Figure 15.1). The signal intensity (amplitude on the y-axis) and linewidth provide the "area" which can be used to quantitate the amount of the observed chemical. The technical background of this approach has been described in detail [7].

The most widely used MRS approach is ^1H MRS since it can be executed with standard MR equipment and offers a large sensitivity advantage over other

Magnetic Resonance Imaging in Movement Disorders, ed. Paul Tuite and Alain Dagher. Published by Cambridge University Press. © Cambridge University Press 2013.

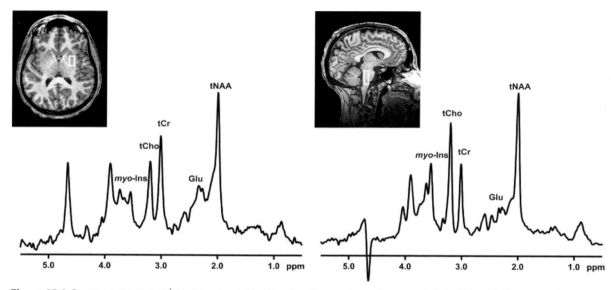

Figure 15.1 Representative in vivo ^{1}H MR spectra obtained in a healthy volunteer with a modified SEMI-LASER [59] sequence (TR = 5 s, TE = 28 ms) at 3T (Siemens Tim Trio) from the posterior putamen and pons. The positions of the voxels are shown on T_1-weighted images. These regions were chosen based on a recent ^{1}H MRS study that indicated significant GABA elevation in the putamen and pons [15]. Processing: Reconstruction of single scan free induction decays (FIDs) from phased array data, frequency and phase correction of FID arrays, FID summation, correction for residual eddy current effects, Gaussian multiplication (σ = 0.15 s), Fourier transform (FT), zero-order phase correction. tNAA, total *N*-acetylaspartate; tCho, total choline; tCr, total creatine; *myo*-Ins, *myo*-inositol; Glu, glutamate.

nuclei, by having not only the highest gyromagnetic ratio γ of non-radioactive nuclei, but also a high natural abundance. ^{1}H MRS allows detection of a variety of metabolites, including *N*-acetylaspartate (NAA) as a marker of neuronal loss/dysfunction, creatine (Cr) as a marker for deficits in energy metabolism, choline (Cho) as a marker for cell membrane turnover, and glutamate (Glu) and γ-aminobutyric acid (GABA), the primary excitatory and inhibitory neurotransmitters, respectively. Although not as commonly utilized as ^{1}H MRS, ^{31}P MRS can be performed if appropriate RF coils, amplifiers, and electronics are available. ^{31}P MRS evaluates high-energy phosphate compounds (HEPs), which reflect intracellular energy metabolism, such as adenosine triphosphate (ATP), phosphocreatine (PCr), and inorganic phosphate (P$_i$). The detection of these metabolites has been valuable in understanding the neuropathology or biochemical abnormalities in PD, as well as in evaluating disease progression and response to therapeutic interventions.

In the following sections we will review clinically relevant and MRS-detectable metabolites and illustrate potential applications in PD. Furthermore, if applicable, we will provide examples from translational research as they relate to the pathophysiology of PD.

N-acetylaspartate

The most prominent proton metabolite signal in the central nervous system, resonating at 2.02 ppm, originates from the *N*-acetyl group of NAA, with usually unresolved contribution from *N*-acetylaspartylglutamate (NAAG) at 2.04 ppm (except at high fields) [7]. Together with NAAG, it is often referred to as "total NAA" (tNAA). Total NAA concentration in the human brain is in the range of 8–14 μmol/g under normal conditions [6]. NAA is widely regarded as a marker of neuronal viability, synaptic health, and metabolism since it has several functions such as myelin synthesis, cell-specific signaling, and maintenance of the intracellular osmotic balance by removing large amounts of metabolic water generated by neuronal glucose metabolism [8]. Thus, it is reasonable to expect alterations in tNAA concentration in neurodegenerative conditions. Any changes in tNAA concentration, either as an absolute concentration or as a ratio between tNAA and total Cr (tNAA/tCr) or total Cho (tNAA/tCho), have proven diagnostically important. For instance, in cerebral artery stroke with massive neuronal loss, NAA was decreased [9]. NAA also appears to reflect mitochondrial health, and studies using mitochondrial respiratory chain inhibitors revealed that reductions in NAA correlated with impaired oxidative phosphorylation [10].

Using MRS, decreased NAA/Cr and NAA/Cho ratios have been reported in different brain regions in PD. Specifically, NAA/Cr was significantly lower in the pre-supplementary motor area [11], the temporoparietal cortex [12], and the motor cortex [13] of patients with PD relative to controls. While neuronal loss of the nigrostriatal dopaminergic neurons is well known in PD, demonstration of supportive findings using NAA levels or its ratios in the basal ganglia have been mixed. For instance, early ^{1}H MRS studies at 1.5T reported a lower NAA/Cho ratio from the putamen contralateral to the more severely affected side in PD compared to controls [14]. However, more recent studies at a higher field did not reveal significant reductions in NAA or its ratios in the basal ganglia of patients with early to moderate PD [15, 16].

On the other hand, animal models of PD have tended to show more consistent differences in NAA levels than those observed in patients. Animal model studies have primarily employed the 1-methyl-4-phenyl-1,2,3,6-tetrahydropyridine (MPTP) model, a neurotoxin that leads to loss of dopaminergic neurons in the substantia nigra, resulting in parkinsonian features. Lower NAA levels were observed in the striatum or substantia nigra of mouse [17], rat [18], and primate [19] MPTP models, suggesting neuronal loss and mitochondrial dysfunction.

Creatine and phosphocreatine

The Cr signals (3.03 and 3.93 ppm), which are composite peaks consisting of the methyl and methylene protons of Cr and PCr [7], are usually considered a marker of energy metabolism as Cr and PCr preserve constant ATP levels through the Cr kinase reaction [20]. Because the sum of the concentrations of Cr and PCr was suggested to be relatively constant in the human brain (6–10 μmol/g in gray matter) [7], tCr is often used as an internal reference signal. However, tCr level should be used with caution as an internal concentration reference since it might change with disease, complicating the interpretation of changes in ratios relative to tCr [21].

Most ^{1}H MRS studies in PD used tCr as an internal reference assuming that tCr was present at a constant level [11, 13, 22, 23]. Studies that quantified tCr in PD found no significant difference in patients versus controls [15, 24] except for one study, which reported lower tCr in patients with bilateral PD symptoms of at least moderate severity relative to healthy controls [25].

On the other hand, a significant depletion of PCr in the putamen and midbrain of patients with PD was detected using ^{31}P MRS [26]. This reduction in PCr indicates mitochondrial dysfunction and oxidative damage, which are presumed contributing factors to the pathogenesis of PD.

Choline-containing compounds

Cho is a major constituent of the phospholipid metabolism of cell membranes and is involved in membrane synthesis and degradation [7]. The peak for Cho-containing compounds occurs at 3.21 ppm. The total MRS observable Cho concentration in the human brain is approximately 1–2 μmol/g [7]. This signal includes contributions from overlapping resonances of glycerophosphocholine, phosphocholine, and phosphatidylcholine and to a small extent acetylcholine; thus, together they are often referred to as "total Cho" (tCho). tCho shows quite strong regional variations in the brain, usually with higher tCho concentration in regions such as the thalamus, hypothalamus, insular cortex, and pons [27]. Increased tCho appears in areas with increased cell membrane breakdown, such as tumors [28].

Both increases and decreases in tCho have been reported in PD using ^{1}H MRS. Lower tCho was reported in several cortical areas of patients with PD, such as the motor [13] and temporoparietal cortex [12]. On the other hand, in one study of patients with PD, an increase in tCho/tCr was shown in a voxel containing the putamen and globus pallidus [22]. Other studies concerning human PD with ^{1}H MRS did not, however, report significant differences in tCho [15, 24].

Only a few ^{1}H MRS animal model studies have reported tCho abnormalities in PD. In a study on MPTP-treated monkeys, striatal tissue exhibited increased tCho/tCr ratio for up to 2 years after MPTP administration [19]. However, in rats treated with 6-hydroxydopamine (6-OHDA) for intraparenchymal neurochemical lesioning of the nigrostriatal pathway, a lower tCho/tCr ratio was reported in the striatum of the ipsilateral hemisphere [29].

myo-Inositol

myo-Inositol (myo-Ins) is almost exclusively located in glial cells and is therefore considered a glial marker [30]. It also has an established role in osmoregulation [31]. The three moieties of myo-Ins resonate at 3.27, 3.56, and 4.05 ppm. myo-Ins is one of the larger signals in short echo time spectra, with a concentration of 5–10 µmol/g [7]. One of the isomers of myo-Ins, scyllo-inositol, has substantially lower concentrations in the brain (less than 1 µmol/g) and is hard to detect by MRS [7]. Elevated myo-Ins levels were found in several neurological disorders, including Alzheimer's disease [32] and spinocerebellar ataxias [21].

Most of the ^{1}H MRS studies in humans and animal models did not show a significant difference in myo-Ins levels between subjects with PD and controls. However, a recent study reported higher myo-Ins levels in the basal ganglia of two parkinsonian patients with PINK1 mutations as compared to findings seen in controls [33].

Glutamate and glutamine

Glu is the most abundant amino acid and has a variety of metabolic roles in addition to being the key neurotransmitter of excitatory signaling in the brain [34]. Glu is not only a precursor for GABA, glutamine (Gln), and glutathione (GSH); but also represents a link between the tricarboxylic acid cycle and amino acid synthesis [34]. It has an average concentration of 6–13 µmol/g with significant differences between gray and white matter. Glu has two methylene groups and a methine group that are strongly coupled, which gives rise to a complicated spectral pattern spread between 2.0 and 3.8 ppm, resulting in low intensities of individual peaks despite its relative abundance [7]. Gln is synthesized from Glu by Gln synthetase in glia at a concentration of 2–4 µmol/g and converted back to Glu by glutaminase in neurons, completing the Glu–Gln cycle [34]. Since Gln and Glu are coupled through the Glu–Gln cycle, it has been suggested that alterations of their levels in neurological diseases indicate impaired neurotransmission and Glu–Gln cycling. For instance, reciprocal alterations in Glu and Gln concentrations were reported in spinocerebellar ataxias [21].

It has been shown that degeneration of dopamine nigral neurons is followed by striatal dopaminergic denervation, which increases the activity of the glutamatergic projections from the subthalamic nucleus to the basal ganglia [35]. These altered glutamatergic projections appear to have an impact on the pathophysiology of PD by altering the normal functioning of basal ganglia circuitry [35]. Thus, monitoring the glutamatergic system may help to better understand PD.

It was not possible to report Glu and Gln concentrations separately in early ^{1}H MRS studies of PD performed at low magnetic fields (1.5T) due to the complicated spectral patterns of Glu and Gln and their substantial overlap with each other. Recent advances in MRI, particularly with the use of higher magnetic fields (3T and above), have allowed for independent quantification of both Glu and Gln thanks to increased resolution and sensitivity. One recent study reported reduced Glu/tCr ratios in the anterior cingulate gyrus of patients with PD [23], whereas studies of the basal ganglia in PD showed no differences in Glu or Gln [15, 16, 24].

Although anatomical studies in 6-OHDA-lesioned rats and MPTP-treated primates revealed adaptive changes at cortico-striatal synapses suggestive of hyperactivity at these glutamatergic synapses, only a few ^{1}H MRS studies have reported altered glutamatergic tone in animal models of PD. Specifically, one group showed increased concentration of both Glu and Gln in the striatum of MPTP-treated mice [36].

γ-aminobutyric acid

GABA is the most abundant inhibitory neurotransmitter in the central nervous system and has a cortical concentration of circa 1 µmol/g [7]. GABA has three different multiplets corresponding to three methylene groups [7]. Two triplet resonances appear at 3.01 ppm and 2.28 ppm, while the GABA quintet is centered at 1.89 ppm [37]. All three resonances of GABA overlap with other, more intense signals arising, for example, from the more abundant metabolites of NAA at 2 ppm, Cr at 3 ppm, and Glu and Gln at 2.3 ppm. Since the GABAergic system accounts for almost half of synaptic activity in the human brain, monitoring GABA concentration becomes important in evaluating various neurological disorders and the effect of therapies. Alterations in brain GABA concentrations and in GABAergic pathways are implicated in the pathophysiology of a number of neurological and psychiatric disorders such as epilepsy [38] and depression [39].

Various techniques have been introduced to extract reliable GABA concentrations from spectra with overlapping resonant peaks. It is possible to isolate the GABA peak from other overlapping resonances in the spectrum by applying one of a series of spectral editing methods [40]. Alternatively, transferring overlapped and hidden information into a second frequency dimension in two-dimensional MRS can alleviate overlap between signals [41]. The third approach is to move to higher field strength, since the relative width of multiplets (in ppm) scales inversely with field strength [15].

Dopaminergic nigrostriatal neurons are under tonic feedback control via nigrostriatal pathways that use GABA as their neurotransmitter and abnormalities of these GABAergic systems have been described in PD [42]. Postmortem studies of individuals with advanced disease demonstrated elevated striatal GABA levels, particularly in the putamen [43]. An inverse correlation between GABA and DA was observed in the putamen in this postmortem work; suggesting that the striatal GABA elevation was associated with dopaminergic terminal loss in PD. Hence, in vivo monitoring of GABA concentration with MRS in PD might provide a measure of disease severity. There are only a few studies of ^{1}H MRS which reported GABA concentrations in PD. In a study of the substantia nigra at 4T no statistically significant differences were detected in GABA levels [24]. One recent study reported elevated GABA levels in the pons and putamen of patients with mild to moderate PD at 7T [15].

In line with the postmortem and MRS findings in the putamen in humans [15, 43], a significant increase in GABA concentration was also shown in the striatum of the MPTP-treated mouse model of PD [36]. One recent study in lesioned (6-OHDA) and genetic rat models has reported an increased striatal GABA level [44].

Glutathione and ascorbate

Ascorbate (Asc, vitamin C) and reduced GSH are the most concentrated chemical antioxidants in the central nervous system with average concentrations of around 1–3 μmol/g [45]. The Asc peaks appear as a doublet at 4.49 ppm and multiplets at 4.00 ppm and 3.73 ppm, whereas GSH peaks appear as a singlet at 3.77 ppm, multiplets at 2.15 and 2.55 ppm, and doublet of doublets at 2.93, 2.98, and 4.56 ppm [37]. Asc

and GSH are scavengers of free radicals formed from the interaction of iron and hydrogen peroxide, and play a major role in cellular detoxification [45].

Both Asc and GSH are MRS-detectable antioxidants. However, similar to GABA, there are technical challenges associated with detection of these low concentration metabolites since Asc and GSH resonances are not resolved from overlapping resonances with conventional MRS [7]. They can be detected using selective editing techniques [46]. In addition, direct detection of GSH and Asc is possible at short echo times at high fields thanks to the gain in sensitivity and spectral resolution [6].

Because of their high metabolic rate, the basal ganglia are at high risk of free radical injury mediated by excessive formation of hydrogen peroxide, superoxide anions, and hydroxyl radicals, especially in the event of reductions in antioxidant concentrations [47]. On this point, significantly lower GSH content was demonstrated in pooled samples of tissue from the putamen, globus pallidus, substantia nigra, nucleus basalis of Meynert, amygdaloid nucleus, and frontal cortex of PD brains [48]. Thus, having a non-invasive measure of cerebral GSH is desirable and could help to understand PD and responses to treatment better. Only a few studies have reported GSH and Asc concentrations in PD and detected no significant differences with disease [15, 24].

Lactate

Lactate (Lac) is an intermediate product of energy metabolism. Lac is normally present at a low concentration of circa 0.5–1 μmol/g [7]. It appears as a doublet at 1.33 ppm with 7 Hz splitting and a multiplet at 4.10 ppm. Increased energy consumption or decreased oxygen availability shifts catabolism from the mitochondrial oxidative pathway to anaerobic glycolysis, leading to Lac accumulation [49]. Decreased complex I activity, indicative of respiratory chain defects in mitochondria, has been demonstrated in the postmortem substantia nigra of people with PD [50]. Thus, one would expect to find elevated Lac levels in this area with in vivo MRS. However, there are technical challenges associated with detection of Lac with MRS due to overlapping lipid resonances, originating from either the brain or the scalp. Several approaches can be used to distinguish Lac from lipids, including the use of spectral editing techniques and the use of an echo time of approximately 140 ms

233

where the Lac resonance is inverted [7]. Although the Lac doublet can be masked by lipid resonances, it is detectable at short echo times at high fields as long as clean localization is achieved and lipid resonances from outside the region of interest are sufficiently suppressed [6].

Increased Lac content in PD has been reported in the occipital cortex using ^{1}H MRS [51], providing further support for a defect in brain energy metabolism. However, a subsequent study raised the possibility that the increased tissue Lac may have been due to contamination from ventricular cerebrospinal fluid as elevated Lac has been reported in the right posterior horn of the lateral ventricle in patients with PD [52].

Animal model studies also showed elevated basal ganglia Lac levels using ^{1}H MRS. Specifically, elevated Lac levels were observed in the presence of normal levels of NAA in MPTP-treated mice [53]. Similar results were reported in MPTP rat [18] and primate [19] models.

Adenosine triphosphate

ATP is a nucleotide consisting of adenine, ribose sugar, and three phosphate groups. It is the major source of usable chemical energy in metabolism. The brain has a high energy demand, which is provided by the cellular energy metabolism through ATP production. Since HEP metabolites such as ATP and PCr are measurable by in vivo ^{31}P MRS, this technique is suitable for investigating mitochondrial dysfunction in PD. For instance, in a recent ^{31}P MRS study, a bilateral reduction of HEPs was reported in the putamen and midbrain of early and advanced patients with PD [26]. In another study, HEPs were monitored in the visual cortex of patients with PD and controls at rest and during and after visual activation. The alterations in HEPs showed the same pattern in patients with PD and controls at rest and during visual stimulation; however, HEPs fell significantly in the recovery period following visual stimulation only in patients with PD, suggesting the presence of mitochondrial dysfunction [54].

Potential sources of variability in MRS studies

Although MRS may provide valuable insights into PD, published results may be conflicting due to technical differences such as different voxel sizes, field strengths, pulse sequences used, and variable spectral quality achieved. Regarding spectral quality, broad linewidths in many PD studies can be the result of several factors, including failure of the shimming methodology, the presence of iron in the tissue, or simply tissue–air magnetic susceptibility differences. The caudate nucleus, globus pallidus, putamen, and substantia nigra are known regions that display field inhomogeneity due to high tissue iron levels. These structures are of high interest for PD, and typically result in broader intrinsic linewidths in MR spectra than other brain regions, which may contribute to the variability of the reported MRS results. MRS can particularly benefit from substantial gains in signal-to-noise ratio (SNR) and spectral resolution at high fields, enabling the quantification of numerous metabolites from small volumes of interest with minimal partial volume effects [6]. Apart from utilization of MRS at ultra-high field, there are also practical concerns for achievable spectral quality with MRS techniques on clinical platforms, which contribute to the uncertainties in the literature. Namely, vendor-provided MRS packages on clinical scanners may not be fully optimized, resulting in, for example, baseline distortions, unwanted echoes, and poor water suppression. Thus, in order to generate more reliable findings, MRS methods need to be optimized by a physicist in order to assist the MRI operator in obtaining optimal data on clinical platforms. Figure 15.1 demonstrates that high spectral quality (marked by high spectral resolution, SNR, and efficient water and unwanted coherence suppression) can be obtained with standard 3T clinical MRI equipment. Automation and standardization of such optimized, advanced MRS technology on widely available clinical platforms is expected to minimize the variability between findings in PD at different sites and studies.

Conclusions and future directions

By providing concentrations of a profile of neurochemicals, MRS may improve our understanding of pathogenic mechanisms of PD and could be helpful in longitudinal monitoring of disease progression and determining the response to therapeutic interventions. In addition, in vivo MRS of animal models has proven to be an invaluable method for non-invasive monitoring of brain neurochemistry in longitudinal therapeutics and pathology studies [29, 36, 44].

While not reviewed in detail in this chapter, MRS is also expected to have a role in the differential diagnosis of parkinsonian disorders. Namely, clinically distinguishing idiopathic PD from atypical parkinsonian disorders, for example progressive supranuclear palsy (PSP), multiple system atrophy (MSA), and corticobasal degeneration (CBD), can be difficulty in early stages since signs and symptoms overlap between conditions, which may lead to misdiagnoses [55]. The MRS literature has consistently demonstrated that patients with PSP, MSA, and CBD display more prominent neurochemical alterations than patients with idiopathic PD [56, 57], and in the future these findings may be utilized as a means to separate PD from atypical parkinsonian conditions.

Finally, current trends suggest that multimodal imaging approaches to neurodegenerative diseases are likely to be more fruitful than a single modality such as MRS. For instance, the combination of the structural (e.g., diffusion tensor imaging), functional (e.g.,

functional MRI), molecular (e.g., positron emission tomography), and neurochemical (e.g., MRS) imaging may provide a more comprehensive understanding of PD. As for animal studies, combining MRS with the novel methodology of light-activated optogenetic probes (opto-MRS) may enhance our understanding of stimulation, inhibition, or manipulation of biochemical events within PD-related brain regions of PD models [58].

Acknowledgements

The preparation of this chapter was supported by the National Institute of Neurological Disorders and Stroke (NINDS) grant R01 NS070815. The Center for MR Research is supported by National Center for Research Resources (NCRR) biotechnology research resource grant P41 RR008079, National Institute of Biomedical Imaging and Bioengineering (NIBIB) grant P41 EB015894, and Neuroscience Center Core Blueprint Award P30 NS057091 and P30 NS076408.

References

1. Lang AE, Lozano AM. Parkinson's disease. Second of two parts. *N Engl J Med*. 1998;**339**(16): 1130–43.

2. Obeso JA, Rodriguez-Oroz MC, Goetz CG, et al. Missing pieces in the Parkinson's disease puzzle. *Nat Med*. 2010;**16**(6):653–61.

3. Braak H, Del Tredici K, Rüb U, et al. Staging of brain pathology related to sporadic Parkinson's disease. *Neurobiol Aging*. 2003;**24**(2):197–211.

4. Bueler H. Impaired mitochondrial dynamics and function in the pathogenesis of Parkinson's disease. *Exp Neurol*. 2009;**218**(2):235–46.

5. Gerlach M, Ben-Shachar D, Riederer P, Youdim MB. Altered brain metabolism of iron as a cause of neurodegenerative diseases? *J Neurochem*. 1994;**63**(3):793–807.

6. Emir UE, Auerbach EJ, Van De Moortele PF, et al. Regional neurochemical profiles in the human brain measured by (1)H MRS at 7 T using local B(1)

shimming. *NMR Biomed*. 2012;**25**(1):152–60.

7. Graaf RAD. *In Vivo NMR Spectroscopy: Principles and Techniques*. New York: John Wiley & Sons; 2002.

8. Moffett JR, Ross B, Arun P, Madhavarao CN, Namboodiri AM. N-Acetylaspartate in the CNS: from neurodiagnostics to neurobiology. *Prog Neurobiol*. 2007;**81**(2):89–131.

9. Barker PB, Gillard JH, van Zijl PC, et al. Acute stroke: evaluation with serial proton MR spectroscopic imaging. *Radiology*. 1994;**192**(3):723–32.

10. Dautry C, Vaufrey F, Brouillet E, et al. Early N-acetylaspartate depletion is a marker of neuronal dysfunction in rats and primates chronically treated with the mitochondrial toxin 3-nitropropionic acid. *J Cereb Blood Flow Metab*. 2000;**20**(5):789–99.

11. Camicioli RM, Hanstock CC, Bouchard TP, et al. Magnetic resonance spectroscopic evidence for presupplementary motor area neuronal dysfunction in

Parkinson's disease. *Mov Disord*. 2007;**22**(3):382–6.

12. Taylor-Robinson SD, Turjanski N, Bhattacharya S, et al. A proton magnetic resonance spectroscopy study of the striatum and cerebral cortex in Parkinson's disease. *Metab Brain Dis*. 1999;**14**(1):45–55.

13. Lucetti C, Del Dotto P, Gambaccini G, et al. Influences of dopaminergic treatment on motor cortex in Parkinson disease: a MRI/MRS study. *Mov Disord*. 2007;**22**(15):2170–5.

14. Ellis CM, Lemmens G, Williams SC, et al. Changes in putamen N-acetylaspartate and choline ratios in untreated and levodopa-treated Parkinson's disease: a proton magnetic resonance spectroscopy study. *Neurology*. 1997;**49**(2):438–44.

15. Emir UE, Tuite PJ, Oz G. Elevated pontine and putamenal GABA levels in mild-moderate Parkinson disease detected by 7 tesla proton MRS. *PLoS One*. 2012;**7**(1):e30918.

16. Kickler N, Krack P, Fraix V, et al. Glutamate measurement in

Parkinson's disease using MRS at 3 T field strength. *NMR Biomed.* 2007;**20**(8):757–62.

17. Boska MD, Lewis TB, Destache CJ, *et al.* Quantitative 1H magnetic resonance spectroscopic imaging determines therapeutic immunization efficacy in an animal model of Parkinson's disease. *J Neurosci.* 2005;**25**(7):1691–700.

18. Jenkins BG, Brouillet E, Chen YC, *et al.* Non-invasive neurochemical analysis of focal excitotoxic lesions in models of neurodegenerative illness using spectroscopic imaging. *J Cereb Blood Flow Metab.* 1996;**16**(3):450–61.

19. Brownell AL, Jenkins BG, Elmaleh DR, *et al.* Combined PET/MRS brain studies show dynamic and long-term physiological changes in a primate model of Parkinson disease. *Nat Med.* 1998;**4**(11):1308–12.

20. Bessman SP, Geiger PJ. Transport of energy in muscle: the phosphorylcreatine shuttle. *Science.* 1981;**211**(4481):448–52.

21. Oz G, Iltis I, Hutter D, *et al.* Distinct neurochemical profiles of spinocerebellar ataxias 1, 2, 6, and cerebellar multiple system atrophy. *Cerebellum.* 2011;**10**(2):208–17.

22. Clarke CE, Lowry M. Basal ganglia metabolite concentrations in idiopathic Parkinson's disease and multiple system atrophy measured by proton magnetic resonance spectroscopy. *Eur J Neurol.* 2000;**7**(6):661–5.

23. Griffith HR, den Hollander JA, Okonkwo OC, *et al.* Brain metabolism differs in Alzheimer's disease and Parkinson's disease dementia. *Alzheimers Dement.* 2008;**4**(6):421–7.

24. Oz G, Terpstra M, Tkac I, *et al.* Proton MRS of the unilateral substantia nigra in the human brain at 4 tesla: detection of high GABA concentrations.

Magn Reson Med. 2006; **55**(2):296–301.

25. O'Neill J, Schuff N, Marks WJ, Jr., *et al.* Quantitative 1H magnetic resonance spectroscopy and MRI of Parkinson's disease. *Mov Disord.* 2002;**17**(5):917–27.

26. Hattingen E, Magerkurth J, Pilatus U, *et al.* Phosphorus and proton magnetic resonance spectroscopy demonstrates mitochondrial dysfunction in early and advanced Parkinson's disease. *Brain.* 2009; **132**(Pt 12):3285–97.

27. Baker EH, Basso G, Barker PB, *et al.* Regional apparent metabolite concentrations in young adult brain measured by (1)H MR spectroscopy at 3 Tesla. *J Magn Reson Imaging.* 2008;**27**(3):489–99.

28. Aboagye EO, Bhujwalla ZM. Malignant transformation alters membrane choline phospholipid metabolism of human mammary epithelial cells. *Cancer Res.* 1999;**59**(1):80–4.

29. Kickler N, Lacombe E, Chassain C, *et al.* Assessment of metabolic changes in the striatum of a rat model of parkinsonism: an in vivo (1)H MRS study. *NMR Biomed.* 2009;**22**(2):207–12.

30. Brand A, Richter-Landsberg C, Leibfritz D. Multinuclear NMR studies on the energy metabolism of glial and neuronal cells. *Dev Neurosci.* 1993;**15**(3–5):289–98.

31. Thurston JH, Sherman WR, Hauhart RE, Kloepper RF. myo-inositol: a newly identified nonnitrogenous osmoregulatory molecule in mammalian brain. *Pediatr Res.* 1989; **26**(5):482–5.

32. Kantarci K. 1H magnetic resonance spectroscopy in dementia. *Br J Radiol.* 2007;**80** Spec No 2:S146–52.

33. Prestel J, Gempel K, Hauser TK, *et al.* Clinical and molecular characterisation of a Parkinson family with a novel PINK1

mutation. *J Neurol.* 2008;**255**(5):643–8.

34. Oz G, Okar D, Henry P-G. Glutamate-glutamine cycle and anaplerosis. In: Choi I-Y, Gruetter R, editors. *Neural Metabolism In Vivo.* New York: Springer US; 2012. 921–46.

35. Blandini F, Greenamyre JT, Nappi G. The role of glutamate in the pathophysiology of Parkinson's disease. *Funct Neurol.* 1996;**11**(1):3–15.

36. Chassain C, Bielicki G, Keller C, Renou JP, Durif F. Metabolic changes detected in vivo by 1H MRS in the MPTP-intoxicated mouse. *NMR Biomed.* 2010;**23**(6):547–53.

37. Govindaraju V, Young K, Maudsley AA. Proton NMR chemical shifts and coupling constants for brain metabolites. *NMR Biomed.* 2000;**13**(3):129–53.

38. Doelken MT, Hammen T, Bogner W, *et al.* Alterations of intracerebral gamma-aminobutyric acid (GABA) levels by titration with levetiracetam in patients with focal epilepsies. *Epilepsia.* 2010;**51**(8):1477–82.

39. Hasler G, van der Veen JW, Tumonis T, *et al.* Reduced prefrontal glutamate/glutamine and gamma-aminobutyric acid levels in major depression determined using proton magnetic resonance spectroscopy. *Arch Gen Psychiatry.* 2007; **64**(2):193–200.

40. Mescher M, Merkle H, Kirsch J, Garwood M, Gruetter R. Simultaneous in vivo spectral editing and water suppression. *NMR Biomed.* 1998;**11**(6): 266–72.

41. Wang ZJ, Bergqvist C, Hunter JV, *et al.* In vivo measurement of brain metabolites using two-dimensional double-quantum MR spectroscopy – exploration of GABA levels in a ketogenic diet. *Magn Reson Med.* 2003;**49**(4):615–19.

42. Tepper JM, Lee CR. GABAergic control of substantia nigra dopaminergic neurons. *Prog Brain Res.* 2007;**160**:189–208.

43. Kish SJ, Rajput A, Gilbert J, *et al.* Elevated gamma-aminobutyric acid level in striatal but not extrastriatal brain regions in Parkinson's disease: correlation with striatal dopamine loss. *Ann Neurol.* 1986;**20**(1):26–31.

44. Coune P, Craveiro M, Gaugler M, *et al.* An in vivo ultrahigh field 14.1 T (1) H-MRS study on 6-OHDA and alpha-synuclein-based rat models of Parkinson's disease: GABA as an early disease marker. *NMR Biomed.* 2013;**26**(1):43–50.

45. Rice ME, Russo-Menna I. Differential compartmentalization of brain ascorbate and glutathione between neurons and glia. *Neuroscience.* 1998;**82**(4): 1213–23.

46. Terpstra M, Marjanska M, Henry PG, Tkac I, Gruetter R. Detection of an antioxidant profile in the human brain in vivo via double editing with MEGA-PRESS. *Magn Reson Med.* 2006; **56**(6):1192–9.

47. Thomas B, Beal MF. Mitochondrial therapies for Parkinson's disease. *Mov Disord.* 2010;**25** Suppl 1:S155–60.

48. Riederer P, Sofic E, Rausch WD, *et al.* Transition metals, ferritin, glutathione, and ascorbic acid in parkinsonian brains. *J Neurochem.* 1989;**52**(2):515–20.

49. Veech RL. The metabolism of lactate. *NMR Biomed.* 1991;**4**(2):53–8.

50. Janetzky B, Hauck S, Youdim MB, *et al.* Unaltered aconitase activity, but decreased complex I activity in substantia nigra pars compacta of patients with Parkinson's disease. *Neurosci Lett.* 1994;**169**(1–2):126–8.

51. Bowen BC, Block RE, Sanchez-Ramos J, *et al.* Proton MR spectroscopy of the brain in 14 patients with Parkinson disease. *AJNR Am J Neuroradiol.* 1995;**16**(1):61–8.

52. Henchcliffe C, Shungu DC, Mao X, *et al.* Multinuclear magnetic resonance spectroscopy for in vivo assessment of mitochondrial dysfunction in Parkinson's disease. *Ann N Y Acad Sci.* 2008;**1147**:206–20.

53. Koga K, Mori A, Ohashi S, *et al.* H MRS identifies lactate rise in the striatum of MPTP-treated C57BL/ 6 mice. *Eur J Neurosci.* 2006;**23**(4):1077–81.

54. Rango M, Bonifati C, Bresolin N. Parkinson's disease and brain mitochondrial dysfunction: a functional phosphorus magnetic resonance spectroscopy study. *J Cereb Blood Flow Metab.* 2006;**26**(2):283–90.

55. Poewe W, Wenning G. The differential diagnosis of Parkinson's disease. *Eur J Neurol.* 2002;**9** Suppl 3:23–30.

56. Davie CA, Wenning GK, Barker GJ, *et al.* Differentiation of multiple system atrophy from idiopathic Parkinson's disease using proton magnetic resonance spectroscopy. *Ann Neurol.* 1995;**37**(2):204–10.

57. Watanabe H, Fukatsu H, Katsuno M, *et al.* Multiple regional 1H-MR spectroscopy in multiple system atrophy: NAA/Cr reduction in pontine base as a valuable diagnostic marker. *J Neurol Neurosurg Psychiatry.* 2004;**75**(1):103–9.

58. Kravitz AV, Freeze BS, Parker PR, *et al.* Regulation of parkinsonian motor behaviours by optogenetic control of basal ganglia circuitry. *Nature.* 2010;**466**(7306):622–6.

59. Oz G, Tkac I. Short-echo, single-shot, full-intensity proton magnetic resonance spectroscopy for neurochemical profiling at 4 T: validation in the cerebellum and brainstem. *Magn Reson Med.* 2011;**65**(4):901–10.

Chapter

16

The image of essential tremor: current neuroimaging and clues to disease localization, pathogenesis, and diagnosis

Hiral Shah and Elan D. Louis

Introduction

Essential tremor (ET) is among the most common movement disorders; prevalence estimates range from 0.4% (all ages) to 21.7% among those greater than 95 years of age [1]. Despite this high prevalence, its pathophysiology is not well understood. Previously thought to be benign and monosymptomatic, ET is increasingly recognized as a more complex entity with both motor and non-motor features. New insights into ET in recent years have prompted a renewed interest in its clinical features and pathophysiology. The primary motor finding of ET is kinetic tremor of the arms, but tremor in the arms may additionally be present during sustained arm extension (i.e., postural tremor), at rest, or with intention; tremors may also involve cranial structures (neck, jaw, voice) [2]. Mild problems with force and timing of motion (e.g., mild dysmetria or ataxia) [3] are also common. Non-motor features include anxiety, depressive symptoms and depression, personality features, cognitive impairment, and even dementia [4].

Research over the past 5–10 years has begun to coalesce on several elemental questions. These are as follows: (1) Does the disease process originate in the cerebellum or a cerebellar motor loop system, or does it originate in the brainstem? (2) Is ET neurodegenerative? (3) Can one use neuroimaging as a diagnostic tool to distinguish ET from Parkinson's disease (PD)? This chapter will set out to address each of these three emerging questions; the emphasis will be on the review of available neuroimaging data, inclusive of magnetic resonance imaging (MRI) as well as other modalities. To complement postmortem (i.e., pathological) studies, MRI and other imaging methods offer a valuable non-invasive approach for understanding in vivo functional anatomy and metabolic abnormalities in disease. Though the underlying pathophysiology of ET is not well understood, there are two current alternative hypotheses: (1) aberrant activity of primary cerebellar–thalamic pathways with impaired central inhibition and/or γ-aminobutyric acid (GABA) dysfunction in tremorigenesis, and (2) the presence of a central pacemaker, possibly in the brainstem, that drives abnormal downstream cerebellar–thalamic pathway activity. In the past, routine neuroimaging in ET was thought to be unremarkable, but more recent advances in the field now exploit a broad array of neuroimaging techniques, including MRI, for studying ET.

Question 1: Does the disease process originate in the cerebellum or a cerebellar motor loop system, or does it originate in the brainstem?

Introduction

There is growing consensus that ET is a disease primarily of cerebellar or cerebellar systems dysfunction. This view is based upon lesion data as well as postmortem and clinical data, among other evidence. When little was known about the pathophysiology of ET, inferences were made from lesion studies that pointed to the central (i.e., central nervous system) origin of the ET. Lesions of the ipsilateral cerebellum [5] as well as the contralateral pyramidal tract [6], and the ventral intermediate nucleus (VIM) of the thalamus [7] terminated the tremor of ET. Additionally, intraoperative recordings during stereotactic surgery in patients with ET revealed neuronal bursts in the

Magnetic Resonance Imaging in Movement Disorders, ed. Paul Tuite and Alain Dagher. Published by Cambridge University Press. © Cambridge University Press 2013.

thalamus [8]. Initial neuroimaging work, beginning in the early 1990s, used positron emission tomography (PET) and ^{1}H magnetic resonance spectroscopic imaging (MRSI), and focused on the identification, distribution, and laterality of changes seen in the brains of ET patients. In one of these reports, investigators used resting PET imaging, and described hypermetabolism in the thalami, bilateral medulla, and, to some extent, in the cerebellar hemispheres in eight ET patients versus ten normal controls [9]. Although there are many bilateral brainstem nuclei, one possibility is that the observed hypermetabolism was originating in the inferior olivary nucleus; the resolution of the imaging method did not allow this hypothesis to be addressed directly. Nonetheless, the findings of thalamic, medullary, and cerebellar involvement were posited to represent an abnormal olivary-cerebello-thalamic circuit. This circuit theory was further supported by data from a toxin-based animal model of tremor produced by treatment with harmaline and harmine. The core event in this toxin-based tremor seems to be the involvement of the inferior olivary nucleus and its climbing fiber connections to the cerebellum [10]. In this toxin-based model, unit recordings in the cat demonstrate that harmine has a direct effect on the inferior olive [10]. Previous investigators have found that the inferior olivary nucleus can fire synchronously at a rate of 10 Hz [11], and this firing is enhanced by harmine, which results in a rhythmic firing that is synchronous with tremor [12], and can be abolished with lesioning of the inferior olive [13], leading some to postulate that this is the structure responsible for the production of tremor in ET. One question, though, is whether pathomechanistic claims derived from animal studies of a toxin-based, lesional model of non-specific tremor can be extrapolated to the human disease ET.

Though animal model evidence seems to point to the inferior olivary nucleus as a possible tremor generator, with the cerebellum and its output pathways as the passive recipients, the panoply of subsequent evidence points away from this notion. Human postmortem studies are limited, but have demonstrated clear structural pathological changes in the cerebellum of many ET cases, including Purkinje cell changes (axonal swellings [torpedoes], dendritic swellings, Purkinje cell loss), basket cell changes (hypertrophy of basket cell processes), and glial changes (gliosis) [14], all in the setting of normal

inferior olivary nuclei, pointing to a possible principal role of the cerebellum in this disease entity. Hence, at the moment, the current question remains: Does the disease process in ET originate in the cerebellum or does it originate in the brainstem? Below, we review the relevant neuroimaging evidence supporting each view.

The disease process in ET originates in the cerebellum: neuroimaging evidence

The first reports in the imaging literature that implicated the cerebellum as having a primary role in ET were PET studies in the early 1990s [15–18]. Briefly, PET allows for an indirect measurement of neural activation via changes in cerebral blood flow. In an initial PET study in 1990 [15] conducted with inhaled $C^{15}O_2$, cerebral blood flow was assessed in two conditions (first at rest and then during sustained arm extension) in two groups (four ET cases and four controls). The main case–control difference was as follows: in ET cases, there was an increase in bilateral cerebellar blood flow during arm extension; this was not the observation in controls [15]. Three years later, the investigators completed a follow-up $C^{15}O_2$ PET study with additional subjects (11 ET cases and 8 controls); this study showed that at rest, ET cases had increased blood flow in both cerebellar hemispheres when compared with controls [16]. Further, in ET cases, additional activation of the cerebellar hemispheres occurred with postural tremor. Most interesting was that the contralateral cerebellar activation, associated with postural tremor among ET subjects, was determined to be pathological; voluntary movements in control subjects mainly resulted in isolated activation of the cerebellar vermis and ipsilateral cerebellar hemisphere [16]. A $H_2^{15}O$ PET study by the same group (seven ET cases and six controls) 1 year later revealed abnormal cerebellar, red nuclear, and thalamic activity [17]. Unlike their prior studies, they included the medulla in their fields of view, so that they could attempt to assess the role of the inferior olivary nuclei in ET. At rest, cerebellar blood flow was bilaterally increased in the seven ET cases versus six controls but olivary activation did not differ between the two groups. In ET, there was a further increase in bilateral cerebellar blood flow during arm extension (i.e., in the presence of postural tremor), but no involvement of the inferior olives [17, 18].

Given the clinical observation that ethanol has a therapeutic effect on the tremor in ET, in 1996, a group of investigators examined brain metabolic changes ($H_2{}^{15}O$) with ethanol ingestion in six ET cases with ethanol-responsive tremor and six controls. Ethanol ingestion led to bilateral decreases of cerebellar blood flow (in both cases and controls) and increases of blood flow in the inferior olivary nuclei (only in cases). The authors suggested that ethanol-induced tremor suppression in ET might be mediated by a reduction in cerebellar synaptic activity resulting in an increase in afferent input to the inferior olivary nuclei [19].

The first reports utilizing MRI techniques in ET were conducted with ^{1}H MRSI. An initial study (2002) of metabolic changes in 20 patients with ET and 11 controls demonstrated an approximately 20% reduction of the neuronal marker N-acetylaspartate (NAA) (expressed as a ratio to total creatine, tCr) in the cerebellar hemispheres of cases versus controls; a follow-up study by that group in 2004 revealed a relative symmetry to these metabolic changes in ET, mirroring the relatively symmetric nature of the tremor in patients [20, 21]. There was an inverse association between cerebellar cortical NAA/tCr and dominant arm tremor severity (r = −0.59, p = 0.02) [20]. Similarly, another group later reported low NAA/Cr in the cerebellar hemispheres in ten ET patients compared to ten controls, again implicating the cerebellum for the pathological abnormality [22].

In 1997, a functional MRI (fMRI) study examined cerebral activation patterns associated with unilateral postural tremor in 12 ET cases, comparing them to 15 controls. Involuntary postural tremor in ET patients was associated with a significantly larger extent of activation in the cerebellar hemispheres and red nucleus compared with mimicked tremor in the control group [23].

The disease process in ET originates in the brainstem: neuroimaging evidence

Though the majority of evidence seems to point to the central and primary involvement of the cerebellum in ET, there is some contrary evidence that should be considered. As noted above, in an early ^{18}F-fluorodeoxyglucose study of eight ET cases and ten controls, the former showed a 71% increase in resting glucose hypermetabolism in the medulla, 10–12% in the thalami, and 3–14% in the cerebellar cortices. The latter difference, though, was not significant [9]. The authors hypothesized that the inferior olivary nuclei were responsible for the changes seen in the medulla.

Summary

The majority of neuroimaging evidence is in favor of a central role of cerebellar involvement in the pathobiology of ET. Not only is there metabolic activation of bilateral cerebellar hemispheres both at rest and with action with several PET studies, but MRS studies point to metabolic dysfunction and possible neuronal death in the cerebellar hemispheres. fMRI also reveals excessive activation in the cerebellar hemispheres in ET. Clinicopathological data are also supporting this hypothesis. The primary evidence in support of the alternative, olivary, hypothesis, comes from animal studies, and investigators have appropriately begun to question the validity of comparisons between ET, a human disease state, and a toxin-induced animal model of non-specific action tremor, especially given differences in clinical findings between the human disease state and the toxin-induced tremor (limb tremor versus more generalized tremor). Likely the cerebellum is at the center of a larger network that is involved in the pathogenesis of ET. The connections that this structure makes via the thalamus to the motor cortex, frontal lobe, spinal cord, midbrain, and medulla are likely to be important in the propagation and expression of tremor in ET.

Question 2: Is ET neurodegenerative?
Introduction

ET has also recently been hypothesized to be a neurodegenerative disease [24, 25]. Clinically, this concept seems plausible given the observed insidious and progressive nature of the clinical symptoms and signs, as well as the exponential increase in tremor prevalence with advanced age [14]. Postmortem data have documented degenerative changes, which were principally found in the cerebellum. Specifically, studies in ET have found pathological evidence of degeneration (reductions in the number of Purkinje cells) as well as other structural changes, including increased number of Purkinje cell axonal swellings ("torpedoes"), increased number of displaced or heterotopic Purkinje cells, and hypertrophy of basket cell processes ("hairy baskets") [24, 26–28]. Of note, pathological findings have been found to be somewhat heterogeneous, with an increase in the numbers of brainstem Lewy bodies and intranuclear inclusions in some studies [28]. And even beyond pathological findings, epidemiological studies indicate increased odds and risks of other degenerative conditions (Alzheimer's disease and PD) among those with ET [29], suggesting a possible common degenerative pathway.

Given the extensive evidence of cerebellar involvement in ET, and possible neurodegeneration, many have focused on this structure and searched for neuroimaging evidence of a neurodegenerative process, that is, evidence of atrophy or neuronal loss. MRI is the technique of choice to address these questions and examine quantitative measures of volume loss. Pathological changes in the brain may ultimately result in cell loss, which is detected as atrophy by structural MRI [30]. Voxel-based morphometry (VBM) is a technique typically used to study gray matter volume changes by utilizing T_1-weighted scans and performing statistical analysis across all voxels to detect volume differences between tissue regions. Magnetic resonance diffusion tensor imaging (DTI) also allows the examiner to look at tissue microstructure. DTI sequences provide quantitative measures of white matter structure using fractional anisotropy (FA), a measure of directionality, and mean diffusivity (MD), which both correlate with data on microstructure. Reductions of FA and increases in MD are complementary to reduction in fiber density or abnormal fiber integrity [31], which could be markers of fiber tract degeneration.

ET is neurodegenerative: neuroimaging evidence

The first reports utilizing MR techniques were conducted with ^{1}H MRS. As already mentioned, initial studies of patients with ET demonstrated a reduction of NAA to tCR ratio in the cerebellar hemispheres, implying a loss of neuronal integrity [20–22] and an underlying degenerative process. In 2008, a VBM study in Italy (50 ET cases and 32 controls) used 1.5T MRI and divided ET cases into those with arm tremor versus those with head tremor. Patients with arm tremor showed a trend towards cerebellar vermal gray matter volume loss compared with controls. Cerebellar volume and vermal area were reduced in the ET cases with head tremor compared with controls [32]. Studies of volume loss in ET have not focused solely on the cerebellum. In fact, investigators

have observed changes in both the gray and white matter of the cerebellum as well as cerebral hemispheres. Widespread changes have been observed and characterized. A VBM study in Spain in 2009 used 3T MRI (19 ET cases and 20 controls), and the investigators reported widespread changes in the white and gray matter. Specifically, there were white matter changes in the cerebellum, medulla, parietal lobe, and limbic lobe as well as gray matter changes in the cerebellum, parietal lobes, frontal lobe, and insula. This work corroborated prior findings and supported the notion of the structural involvement of the cerebello-thalamo-cortical network in ET [33]. A VBM study in India in 2010 used 3T MRI (20 ET cases and 17 controls), showing that ET cases had widespread areas of atrophy both in the cerebellar and the cerebral gray matter [34]. A DTI study in Germany (14 ET cases and 20 controls) found evidence of localized pathology in cerebellar circuits and more general alterations in white matter tracts throughout the brain, indicating that the integrity of neuronal fibers in ET was impaired [31].

ET is not neurodegenerative: neuroimaging evidence

Though many studies have found metabolic and structural changes that suggest loss of neuronal and/or fiber tract integrity in ET, there have been limited studies that have found no abnormalities among ET patients. One VBM study, using 1.5T MRI, found no decrease in cerebellar gray matter volume in ET [35]. As noted above, DWI may act as a surrogate for neuronal and axonal damage as well as neurodegeneration. One group studied ten patients with ET and found no abnormality on DWI when compared to ten controls, and specifically examined structures previously thought to be altered in ET subjects (pons, middle cerebellar peduncles, cerebral white matter, dentate nucleus, red nucleus, thalamus, caudate, putamen, pallidum, frontal, and precentral white matter) [36].

Summary

The majority though not all neuroimaging evidence, derived from MRSI, VBM, and DTI studies, points to changes in neuronal integrity and neuronal loss in ET, supporting the notion that ET is a neurodegenerative process. These imaging data are further supported by postmortem, clinical, and epidemiological data, as reviewed above. Yet there exists heterogeneity of findings across studies; given widespread localization of findings across brain regions, this should be the focus of continued study and investigation.

Question 3: Can one use neuroimaging as a diagnostic tool to distinguish ET from PD?

Introduction

Although the clinical features of ET and PD are often fairly distinctive, the presence of a range of different types of tremor in each disease remains a continued source of diagnostic difficulty for clinical neurologists. Indeed, several studies have shown that approximately 30% of "ET" cases do not have ET but have other diagnoses, with PD being common among these. Clinicians have also observed a tendency of ET patients to develop PD [37]. Neuroimagers have thus sought to identify methods to distinguish between the two diseases.

Neuroimaging may be used as a diagnostic tool to distinguish ET from PD

From an imaging perspective, the diagnosis of PD relies upon the identification of a deficit in presynaptic striatal dopamine. The key distinction is that there is a clear dopamine deficit in the nigrostriatal pathway in PD in contrast to ET. Even in early PD, dopamine transporter (DAT) availability is probably the most sensitive measurable parameter of pathological change; this is due to early downregulation of DAT activity. Cuberas-Borros and colleagues used ^{123}I-FP-CIT, a cocaine analog that attaches to presynaptic DATs, single-photo emission computed tomography (SPECT) and compared PD cases to ET cases, demonstrating significant differences, especially in putaminal uptake. These findings support the principle of the relatively preserved nigrostriatal dopaminergic system among patients with ET [38]. Studies examining presynaptic DATs have shown that there are significant qualitative differences in the uptake in the caudate and putamen in patients with PD when compared to ET. PET studies examining the DAT via the radioligand [^{11}C]d-threomethylphendiate as well as [11-C]FE-CIT found that ET cases did not exhibit altered DAT availability when compared to control subjects [39, 40]. A study

of eight familial ET cases also observed that they had normal striatal 18F-dopa uptake [41]. In comparison to healthy controls or patients with PD, ET cases demonstrated no abnormality in striatal [^{123}I]β-CIT binding ratios, indicating normal function of the dopa-decarboxylase enzyme and normal uptake and metabolism of dopa [42, 43].

In a 2008 study of 32 ET cases, 47 PD cases, and 31 controls using ^{123}I-ioflupane SPECT [44], striatal DAT function binding differed in ET cases and PD cases. First, PD cases but not ET cases differed from controls with respect to the asymmetry index (defined as ^{123}I-ioflupane binding asymmetry in putamen, caudate, and stratium: [ipsilateral – contralateral]/[ipsilateral + contralateral]). Thus, the asymmetry index was higher in PD cases than controls. Second, PD cases but not ET cases differed from controls with respect to the putamen–caudate index (defined as the relationship between ^{123}I-ioflupane binding in the putamen and caudate, both ipsilateral and contralateral: [putamen – caudate]/[putamen + caudate]). Thus, the index was higher in PD cases than controls. Also, dopamine deficiency was observed to be in a pattern involving the entire striatum in ET patients; this was in contrast to the pattern observed in PD (i.e., predominant involvement of the posterior putamen) [44].

Neuroimaging may not be used as a diagnostic tool to distinguish ET from PD

There are also data to suggest that there is some dysfunction in dopamine transport or uptake in some ET cases. These data "muddy the water." The radioligand ^{99m}Tc-TRODAT-1 was used in a study that attempted to differentiate 27 early PD and 12 ET cases [45]. A cutoff point was determined as the value for the contralateral striatal uptake that best separated PD cases from ET cases; using that cutoff point, the sensitivity and specificity for differentiating PD from ET were 96.4% and 91.7%, respectively. Thus, while there was reasonable separation, there was also some overlap, and this cutoff point has not been reproduced.

Indeed, in the 2008 study discussed previously [44], while the investigators showed PD versus control differences using ^{123}I-Ioflupane SPECT, they found that striatal DAT binding was lower in ET cases compared to controls, though higher than in PD cases. These results may be interpreted in several ways; first, there may be a presynaptic dopaminergic deficit in some ET cases or, alternatively, ET cases with DAT binding abnormalities might be developing early PD [44]. In an additional study by the same investigators using ^{123}I-ioflupane SPECT, a discriminant analysis clustered 70% of the ET cases in a distinct group with abnormal values in the caudate nucleus contralateral to the most affected body side [46].

Isolated action tremor is typically a representation of ET; however, it can be seen as the first clinical feature of PD. Using ^{123}I-FP-CIT SPECT, Coria *et al.* set out to determine if there was any evidence of dopaminergic denervation (i.e., preclinical evidence of PD) in individuals with isolated action tremor [47]. Interestingly, among 167 patients with isolated action tremor, 114 (68.3%) were found to have reduced striatal uptake, with the remaining 53 (31.7%) having normal striatal uptake. Of those with reduced uptake, 86.8% had mild reduction in uptake (DAT-SPECT Visual Rating Scale: grades I and II), and 91.2% had asymmetrical uptake (typical of PD). Asymmetric tremor and late onset of tremor (after 50 years of age) were predictive of reduced striatal uptake [47].

Summary

Though much evidence exists that the status of striatal dopamine and dopamine transport is relatively normal among ET subjects when compared to PD patients, recent evidence suggests that there might be an intermediate level of abnormality in the striatum in some ET cases, which is between that seen in healthy controls and PD cases. One suspects that these studies have identified patients with preclinical PD, although this remains to be determined.

Summary and future directions

In summary, MRI, PET, and SPECT evidence supports the notion that the cerebellum is likely at the center of the pathophysiology of ET. It certainly is part of a larger network including the thalamus, motor cortex, and frontal lobe explaining many of the clinical features of the disease. There is sufficient evidence of neuronal loss in both gray and white matter, suggesting underlying degeneration. These imaging findings are bolstered by postmortem, clinical, and epidemiological evidence. In addition, pure ET cases likely have a different underlying pathology and absence of dopaminergic denervation compared to PD cases, therefore providing a useful biomarker to differentiate ET subjects from healthy controls and PD subjects.

Ultimately, to understand the pathophysiology underlying ET, further pathological studies and correlation with imaging need to be conducted. Imaging provides a more accessible, non-invasive, real-time examination of the metabolic and structural changes in patients with ET. As further genetic studies are done and genetic targets are identified, possible other sources for study may include the identification of a more sensitive and specific biomarker. Prospective and follow-up studies that examine volume loss over time or axonal loss over time may help to answer the question of whether ET is a neurodegenerative disease. Additional study is warranted to examine substructures that have been identified in prior studies. For example, insular changes seen by Benito-Leon *et al.* that could point to a pathological cause of non-motor symptoms in ET patients should be examined further [33].

Acknowledgements

Elan D. Louis receives research support from the National Institutes of Health: NINDS #R01 NS042859 (principal investigator), NINDS #R01 NS39422 (principal investigator), NINDS #R01 NS073872 (principal investigator), NINDS #T32 NS07153–24 (principal investigator), NINDS #R21 NS077094 (co-investigator), and NINDS #R01 NS36630 (co-investigator), as well as the Parkinson's Disease Foundation (principal investigator), the Arlene Bronstein Essential Tremor Research Fund (Columbia University), and the Claire O'Neil Essential Tremor Research Fund (Columbia University).

References

1. Louis ED, Ferreira JJ. How common is the most common adult movement disorder? Update on the worldwide prevalence of essential tremor. *Mov Disord.* 2010;**25**(5):534–41.

2. Louis ED, Frucht SJ, Rios E. Intention tremor in essential tremor: prevalence and association with disease duration. *Mov Disord.* 2009; **24**(4):626–7.

3. Singer C, Sanchez-Ramos J, Weiner WJ. Gait abnormality in

essential tremor. *Mov Disord.* 1994;**9**(2):193–6.

4. Troster AI, Woods SP, Fields JA, *et al.* Neuropsychological deficits in essential tremor: an expression of cerebello-thalamo-cortical pathophysiology? *Eur J Neurol.* 2002;**9**(2):143–51.

5. Dupuis MJ, Delwaide PJ, Boucquey D, Gonsette RE. Homolateral disappearance of essential tremor after cerebellar stroke. *Mov Disord.* 1989;**4**(2):183–7.

6. Young RR. Essential familial tremor. In: Vinken PJ. Bruyn GW, Klawans HL, editors. *Handbook of Clinical Neurology.* Vol. 49. Amsterdam: Elsevier; 1986. 565–81.

7. Hirai T, Miyazaki M, Nakajima H, Shibazaki T, Ohye C. The correlation between tremor characteristics and the predicted volume of effective lesions in stereotaxic nucleus ventralis intermedius thalamotomy. *Brain.* 1983;**106**(Pt 4):1001–18.

8. Narabayashi H. Stereotaxic Vim thalamotomy for treatment of tremor. *Eur Neurol.* 1989; **29** Suppl 1:29–32.

9. Hallett M, Dubinsky RM. Glucose metabolism in the brain of patients with essential tremor. *J Neurol Sci.* 1993;**114**(1):45–8.

10. Longo VG, Massotti M. Effect of tremorigenic agents on the cerebellum: a review of biochemical and electrophysiological data. *Int Rev Neurobiol.* 1985;**26**:315–29.

11. Llinas RR. Electrophysiological properties of the olivocerebellar system. *Exp Brain Res Ser.* 1989;**17**:201–8.

12. Llinas RR. Rebound excitation as the physiological basis for tremor: a biophysical study of the oscillatory properties of mammalian central nervous system in vitro. In: Findley LJ, Capildeo R, editors. *Movement Disorders: Tremor.* New York:

Oxford University Press; 1984. 165–82.

13. Lamarre Y. Tremorgenic mechanisms in primates. In: Meldrum BS, Marsden CD, editors. *Primate Models of Neurologic Disorders.* New York: Raven Press; 1975. 23–34.

14. Louis ED. Essential tremors: a family of neurodegenerative disorders? *Arch Neurol.* 2009;**66**(10):1202–8.

15. Colebatch JG, Findley LJ, Frackowiak RS, Marsden CD, Brooks DJ. Preliminary report: activation of the cerebellum in essential tremor. *Lancet.* 1990;**336**(8722):1028–30.

16. Jenkins IH, Bain PG, Colebatch JG, *et al.* A positron emission tomography study of essential tremor: evidence for overactivity of cerebellar connections. *Ann Neurol.* 1993;**34**(1):82–90.

17. Wills AJ, Jenkins IH, Thompson PD, Findley LJ, Brooks DJ. Red nuclear and cerebellar but no olivary activation associated with essential tremor: a positron emission tomographic study. *Ann Neurol.* 1994;**36**(4):636–42.

18. Wills AJ, Jenkins IH, Thompson PD, Findley LJ, Brooks DJ. A positron emission tomography study of cerebral activation associated with essential and writing tremor. *Arch Neurol.* 1995;**52**(3):299–305.

19. Boecker H, Wills AJ, Ceballos-Baumann A, *et al.* The effect of ethanol on alcohol-responsive essential tremor: a positron emission tomography study. *Ann Neurol.* 1996;**39**(5):650–8.

20. Louis ED, Shungu DC, Chan S, *et al.* Metabolic abnormality in the cerebellum in patients with essential tremor: a proton magnetic resonance spectroscopic imaging study. *Neurosci Lett.* 2002;**333**(1):17–20.

21. Louis ED, Shungu DC, Mao X, Chan S, Jurewicz EC. Cerebellar metabolic symmetry in essential

tremor studied with 1H magnetic resonance spectroscopic imaging: implications for disease pathology. *Mov Disord.* 2004;**19**(6):672–7.

22. Pagan FL, Butman JA, Dambrosia JM, Hallett M. Evaluation of essential tremor with multi-voxel magnetic resonance spectroscopy. *Neurology.* 2003;**60**(8):1344–7.

23. Bucher SF, Seelos KC, Dodel RC, Reiser M, Oertel WH. Activation mapping in essential tremor with functional magnetic resonance imaging. *Ann Neurol.* 1997;**41**(1):32–40.

24. Louis ED. Essential tremor: evolving clinicopathological concepts in an era of intensive post-mortem enquiry. *Lancet Neurol.* 2010;**9**(6):613–22.

25. Benito-Leon J. Essential tremor: one of the most common neurodegenerative diseases? *Neuroepidemiology.* 2011;**36**(2):77–8.

26. Kuo SH, Erickson-Davis C, Gillman A, *et al.* Increased number of heterotopic Purkinje cells in essential tremor. *J Neurol Neurosurg Psychiatry.* 2011;**82**(9):1038–40.

27. Erickson-Davis CR, Faust PL, Vonsattel JP, *et al.* "Hairy baskets" associated with degenerative Purkinje cell changes in essential tremor. *J Neuropathol Exp Neurol.* 2010;**69**(3):262–71.

28. Louis ED, Erickson-Davis C, Pahwa R, *et al.* Essential tremor with ubiquitinated Purkinje cell intranuclear inclusions. *Acta Neuropathol.* 2010;**119**(3):375–7.

29. LaRoia H, Louis ED. Association between essential tremor and other neurodegenerative diseases: what is the epidemiological evidence? *Neuroepidemiology.* 2011;**37**(1):1–10.

30. Whitwell JL. Voxel-based morphometry: an automated technique for assessing structural changes in the brain. *J Neurosci.* 2009;**29**(31):9661–4.

31. Klein JC, Lorenz B, Kang JS, et al. Diffusion tensor imaging of white matter involvement in essential tremor. *Hum Brain Mapp*. 2011;**32**(6):896–904.

32. Quattrone A, Cerasa A, Messina D, et al. Essential head tremor is associated with cerebellar vermis atrophy: a volumetric and voxel-based morphometry MR imaging study. *AJNR Am J Neuroradiol*. 2008;**29**(9):1692–7.

33. Benito-Leon J, Alvarez-Linera J, Hernandez-Tamames JA, et al. Brain structural changes in essential tremor: voxel-based morphometry at 3-Tesla. *J Neurol Sci*. 2009;**287**(1–2):138–42.

34. Bagepally BS. Decrease in cerebral and cerebellar gray matter in essential tremor: A voxel-based morphometric analysis under 3T MRI. *J Neuroimaging*. 2010;**XX**: 1–4.

35. Daniels C, Peller M, Wolff S, et al. Voxel-based morphometry shows no decreases in cerebellar gray matter volume in essential tremor. *Neurology*. 2006;**67**(8):1452–6.

36. Martinelli P, Rizzo G, Manners D, et al. Diffusion-weighted imaging study of patients with essential tremor. *Mov Disord*. 2007;**22**(8):1182–5.

37. Minen MT, Louis ED. Emergence of Parkinson's disease in essential tremor: a study of the clinical correlates in 53 patients. *Mov Disord*. 2008;**23**(11):1602–5.

38. Cuberas-Borros G, Lorenzo-Bosquet C, Aguade-Bruix S, et al. Quantitative evaluation of striatal I-123-FP-CIT uptake in essential tremor and parkinsonism. *Clin Nucl Med*. 2011;**36**(11):991–6.

39. Antonini A, Moresco RM, Gobbo C, et al. The status of dopamine nerve terminals in Parkinson's disease and essential tremor: a PET study with the tracer [11-C]FE-CIT. *Neurol Sci*. 2001;**22**(1):47–8.

40. Breit S, Reimold M, Reischl G, Klockgether T, Wullner U. [(11)C]d-threo-methylphenidate PET in patients with Parkinson's disease and essential tremor. *J Neural Transm*. 2006;**113**(2):187–93.

41. Brooks DJ, Playford ED, Ibanez V, et al. Isolated tremor and disruption of the nigrostriatal dopaminergic system: an 18F-dopa PET study. *Neurology*. 1992;**42**(8):1554–60.

42. Benamer TS, Patterson J, Grosset DG, et al. Accurate differentiation of parkinsonism and essential tremor using visual assessment of [123I]-FP-CIT SPECT imaging: the [123I]-FP-CIT study group. *Mov Disord*. 2000;**15**(3):503–10.

43. Asenbaum S, Pirker W, Angelberger P, et al. [123I]beta-CIT and SPECT in essential tremor and Parkinson's disease. *J Neural Transm*. 1998;**105**(10–12):1213–28.

44. Isaias IU, Canesi M, Benti R, et al. Striatal dopamine transporter abnormalities in patients with essential tremor. *Nucl Med Commun*. 2008;**29**(4):349–53.

45. Wang J, Jiang YP, Liu XD, et al. 99mTc-TRODAT-1 SPECT study in early Parkinson's disease and essential tremor. *Acta Neurol Scand*. 2005;**112**(6):380–5.

46. Isaias IU, Marotta G, Hirano S, et al. Imaging essential tremor. *Mov Disord*. 2010;**25**(6):679–86.

47. Coria F, Gimenez-Garcia M, Samaranch L, et al. Nigrostriatal dopaminergic function in subjects with isolated action tremor. *Parkinsonism Relat Disord*. 2012;**18**(1):49–53.

Clinical applications

Michael Samuel and Jozef Jarosz

Introduction

Magnetic resonance imaging (MRI) is central to clinical practice and neurology constitutes a large proportion of clinical MRI scanning time in most hospitals. In movement disorders specifically, there are few other diagnostic tests, unlike, for example, neurological inflammatory disease, neuropathy, or myology in which cerebrospinal fluid examination, neurophysiology, or histology can confirm diagnosis. In movement disorders, MRI is principally an adjunct to clinical examination to support or refute a diagnosis. In some scenarios, it can also be used to assess disease progression or therapy, but these instances are rarer. To maximize the clinical application, this chapter will use exclusively 1.5 Tesla images since 1.5 Tesla scanners are most often employed in routine clinical practice worldwide. Variations in scanner hardware, processing, lower and higher magnetic field strengths, and commercial differences are outside the scope of this chapter, as are variations in images as the infant brain develops and matures.

This chapter will focus on how MRI can be used to add weight to clinical diagnosis for adult movement disorders. First, it is assumed that readers have familiarity with the clinical features of the disorders as we concentrate predominantly on MRI features here. Second, for convenience, and in line with clinical presentation of the illnesses, we discuss MRI findings in relation to types of clinical presentations, rather than on a disease-by-disease basis. It is common for cases of movement disorders to present clinically with more than one movement disorder phenotype, but for practical reasons, we present here the main clinical disorder associated with each figure. Standard clinical sequences will be described. Accepted abbreviations are used throughout and include: T_1, T_2, T_2^*, fluid-attenuated inversion recovery (FLAIR), diffusion-weighted imaging (DWI), and apparent diffusion coefficient (ADC). Some more advanced structural imaging techniques, such as volumetry, segmentation, and diffusion tensor imaging, have to date not reached routine clinical practice and so are excluded from this chapter.

Common normal and non-specific abnormalities

Some MRI features and minor abnormalities may co-exist in patients presenting with movement disorders. They are included here for awareness that they may not be pathological and should not prevent other detailed diagnostic tests for diagnoses. These include non-specific atrophy, small vessel vascular disease within the basal ganglia or white matter, simple cysts, large perivascular spaces, and dilated ventricles, as in Figure 17.1. Vascular findings and ventricular dilation can be associated with parkinsonism, isolated gait failure, or the triad of dementia, incontinence, and gait difficulty. The distinction between global atrophy and normal pressure hydrocephalus can be difficult, but in the latter the ventricular dilation is disproportionate to the degree of sulcal widening. Where doubt exists, a trial of cerebrospinal fluid removal can be attempted to see if the symptoms improve rapidly, but transiently.

Normal and abnormal metal deposition affecting the basal ganglia
Calcium: physiological versus pathological calcification of the basal ganglia

Calcium normally appears dark on T_2 MRI, although there are variations, appearing as mixed signal on both T_1 and T_2, or high signal on T_1 (Figures 17.2 and 17.3).

Magnetic Resonance Imaging in Movement Disorders, ed. Paul Tuite and Alain Dagher. Published by Cambridge University Press. © Cambridge University Press 2013.

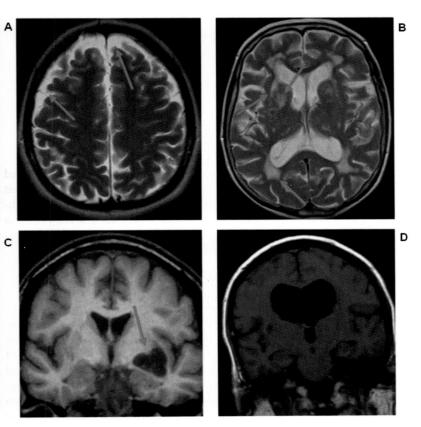

Figure 17.1 Common non-specific and/or asymptomatic abnormalities. (A) T_2 non-specific frontal atrophy, (B) T_2 bilateral basal ganglia, deep white matter, and periventricular small vessel disease, (C) T_1 left basal ganglia giant perivascular space, and (D) ventricular dilation, can be asymptomatic but can also be seen in normal pressure hydrocephalus.

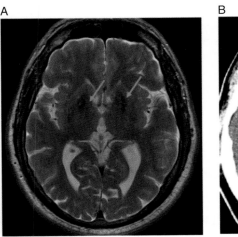
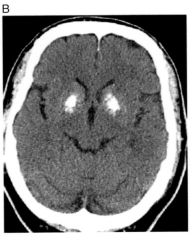

Figure 17.2 Physiological asymptomatic calcification of the basal ganglia on (A) T_2 MRI and (B) computed tomography (CT).

When searching for calcium metabolic disorders, computed tomography (CT) is more sensitive. Figure 17.2 shows modest asymptomatic calcification and can be compared with Figure 17.3 of Fahr syndrome, which can present with parkinsonism, a mixed movement disorder, cognitive or psychiatric disturbance. Calcification of the basal ganglia, particularly the striatum and pallidum, can also be seen in hypoparathyroidism, allied calcium disorders, familial and infantile cases, and with other structural

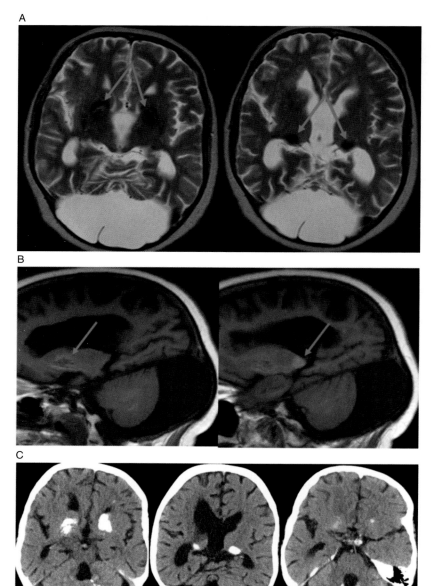

Figure 17.3 (A) Calcium deposition on T_2 MRI in Fahr syndrome. Mixed signal in the basal ganglia but low signal in the posterior thalamus. Dandy Walker abnormality is also present. (B) Same patient, T_1 MRI. Calcium deposition is seen as mixed signal in the basal ganglia but high signal in the posterior thalamus. Dandy Walker abnormality is also present. (C) Same patient, with analogous sections on plain CT, showing more obvious abnormality, including calcification of the dentate nucleus, which was less noticeable on MRI.

abnormalities, for example microcephaly, or Dandy Walker syndrome (Figure 17.3).

Iron: physiological versus pathological iron deposition within the basal ganglia

Iron deposition in the globus pallidus, red nucleus, substantia nigra, and dentate nucleus occurs in childhood and early adult life as a normal finding. It is visible as hypointensity on T_2 images, usually between the ages of 10 and 25 [1]. Hence, it can be similar to the MRI appearance of calcium in some instances, but CT will usually distinguish these readily as iron shows no abnormal signal on CT. Physiological iron deposition becomes more pronounced with age and it can be difficult to be certain of the significance of subtle signal change. As a general rule,

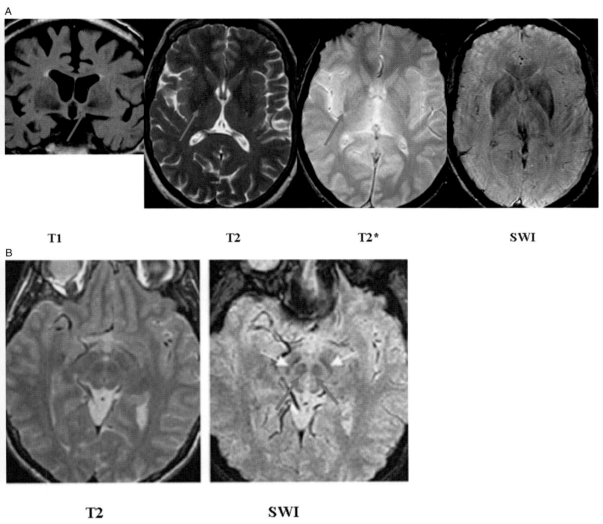

Figure 17.4 (A) Basal ganglia normal physiological iron deposition in the striatum. This is a non-specific finding and can be seen as a normal variant. (B) SWI of smaller basal ganglia structures. Compared with routine T_2 images of the subthalamic nucleus (white arrows) and the red nucleus (red arrows), SWI shows more contrast in these structures. (With permission from O'Gorman *et al.* [2].)

it should be classified as physiological unless clearly very abnormal and in the correct clinical setting. New techniques, such as susceptibility-weighted imaging (SWI), may help to improve specificity (Figures 17.4A and 17.4B). In this method, the phase change associated with the magnetic susceptibility of iron can provide an additional source of MR image contrast, and so it is most appropriate to apply it to structures normally higher in iron content, such as the basal ganglia. While only recently becoming routinely available for clinical use, it can be used to better define normal basal ganglia anatomy for

neurosurgery, for example localization of small target nuclei in deep brain stimulation [2].

Pathological iron deposition occurs in a variety of "iron disorders," also called neuronal brain iron accumulation (NBIA) syndromes. These usually start in childhood. Patients may, however, re-present in adulthood requesting more modern investigations. Presentations are usually with dystonia/parkinsonism/cognitive changes along with a family history, although the latter may not be easily detectable in the autosomal recessive disorders. Current terminology is changing rapidly as new genetic tests become

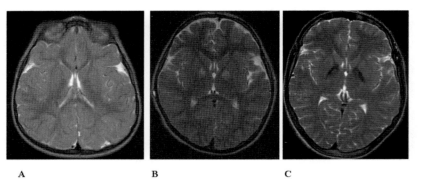

A   B   C

Figure 17.5 High central pallidal signal on T_2 (which can develop over time) suggests PKAN. Usually, this is surrounded by hypointense pallidal signal, but this can be variable. (A) T_2 MRI of PKAN at age 1 year and 8 months, the basal ganglia appear normal. (B) T_2 MRI of the same patient at age 5 years 10 months. High signal centrally in pallida. (C) T_2 MRI of a different patient but more typical example – "eye of the tiger." (Courtesy of Dr. Jean-Pierre Lin, Evelina Children's Hospital, London.)

available for clinical diagnoses. These disorders include pantothenate kinase-associated neurodegeneration (PKAN), phospholipase A2-associated neurodegeneration (PLAN) (also called PLA2G6-associated neurodegeneration), fatty acid hydroxylase-associated neurodegeneration (FAHN), mitochondrial protein-associated neurodegeneration (MPAN), Kufor–Rakeb disease, aceruloplasminemia, and neuroferritinopathy [3]. Diagnosis has been reported to be directed by the character, location, and associated abnormalities identified on routine brain MRI. For example, PKAN is reported to be associated with the T_2 "eye of the tiger" sign, while PLAN is not associated with central high signal in the pallida. Neuroferritinopathy is reported to be associated with dentate iron deposition and pallidal cavitation [4]. Figures 17.5 and 17.6 show variations amongst these disorders. The diagnostic accuracy of imaging alone remains an area of study as it should be noted that some MRI abnormalities can develop over time (Figures 17.5A and 17.5B). The correlation between signal abnormality, disease duration, phenotype, and severity is currently not known.

Copper

Copper deposition occurs in the basal ganglia, amongst other areas, in Wilson's disease, manifesting on T_2 MRI as putaminal, pallidal, thalamic, and internal capsule hyperintensity. Additional MRI abnormalities can include the "face of the giant panda" in the midbrain (high T_2 signal in the tegmentum with normal red nuclei signal) and "face of the panda cub" in the pons (low signal of central tegmental tracts with high signal around the aqueductal opening to the fourth ventricle) as in Figure 17.7 [5]. These signal abnormalities may resolve with

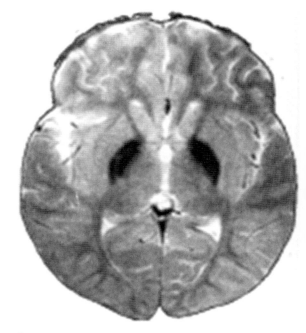

Figure 17.6 Other iron deposition disorders, without central high T_2 signal. PLAN, see text. (With permission from McNeill et al. [4].)

improved symptoms with treatment although there are patients for whom MRI and clinical time courses are not concordant [6].

Hepatic disorders and manganese

The non-wilsonian form of acquired hepatolenticular syndrome has typical imaging features of high T_1 pallidal and nigral signal, as in Figure 17.8. In particular, other MRI sequences are typically normal. Other causes of this unusual high T_1 pallidal signal are relatively rare and can usually be distinguished

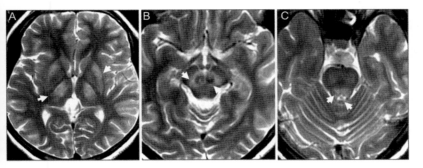

Figure 17.7 T$_2$-weighted axial MRI demonstrates: (A) Symmetric hyperintense signals in the putamen, posterior internal capsule, and thalami (arrows). (B) "Face of the giant panda" in midbrain with high signal in tegmentum and normal red nuclei (arrows). (C) "Face of the panda cub" in pons with hypointensity of central tegmental tracts with hyperintensity of aqueductal opening to fourth ventricle (arrows). (With permission from Shivakumar *et al.* [5].)

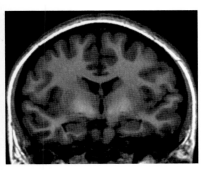

Figure 17.8 Acquired hepatolenticular syndrome from liver cirrhosis. Note high T$_1$ pallidal signal. Similar appearances can be seen in other disorders (see text).

from acquired hepatolenticular syndrome on clinical grounds. These include Wilson's disease, recent hyperglycemia, hypoxia, carbon monoxide injury, calcification of the basal ganglia, NBIA, neurofibromatosis, and micro-hemorrhages. Clinical features of acquired hepatolenticular syndrome include parkinsonism, dystonia, unsteadiness, and cognitive slowing, in the presence of porto-systemic shunting. The most common form of shunting is that related to cirrhosis of the liver, which may be cryptogenic at the time of the movement disorder presentation. The MRI appearances are so suggestive of hepatic disorders in the appropriate setting that we and others [7] have seen examples in which the liver pathology was first identified after liver investigations were initiated based on the abnormal T$_1$ pallidal signal on brain MRI. There does not appear to be a correlation between the severity of the movement disorder and the severity of the liver disease, nor its duration. Neither is there a correlation between movement disorder severity and MRI abnormality. The similarity of the MRI appearances to manganese toxicity

from inhalation of fumes during welding or manganese mining, or the injection of recreational drugs high in manganese, or manganese-rich parenteral nutrition suggests that in these conditions, one common factor is the deposition of manganese in the basal ganglia, particularly the pallida, which constitute the postsynaptic dopaminergic pathways of the basal ganglia–thalamo-cortical circuits. This location of signal abnormality is thought to underlie the usual lack of response that such patients have to levodopa for treatment of their parkinsonism. For a review of acquired hepatolenticular syndrome, see [8]. Very recently, a new manganese-related disorder of dystonia, associated with mutations in the *SLC30A10* gene, has been described [9].

Other rare disorders involving heavy metals

Other rare heavy metal-associated disorders may cause movement disorders not by direct accumulation in the brain, but by affecting enzymatic pathways involved in basal ganglia metabolism. The basal ganglia seem to be one of the most susceptible brain regions to hypoxia or failure of energy metabolism. Molybdenum is one such heavy metal, and genetic deficiency of molybdenum cofactor leads to infantile severe movement disorders and cognitive decline. Diagnosis is by finding high urinary sulfite, high serum xanthine and hypoxanthine, followed by genetic testing. The basal ganglia appearances can be non-specific [10] and progressive [11], (Figure 17.9). Symmetrical T$_2$ high signal abnormality within the cerebellar deep nuclei, reduced white matter bulk, and thinning of the corpus callosum have been described in a patient with late presentation [12]. One clue to the diagnosis of this condition is ocular lens dislocation.

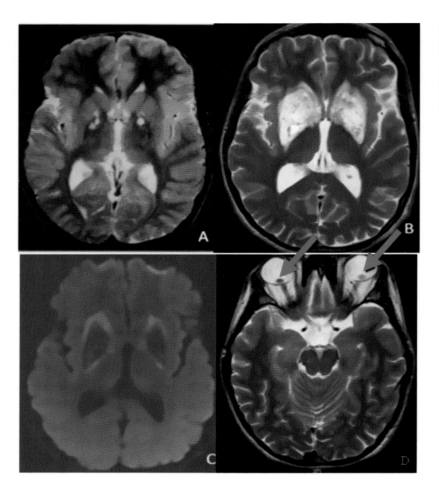

Figure 17.9 A, early and B, late basal ganglia features of molybdenum co-factor deficiency. C. DWI showing free diffusion centrally and intermediate diffusion peripherally around the areas of signal abnormality. D. Note the ocular lens dislocations (arrows). (With permission from Alkufri *et al.* [11].)

Extrapyramidal disorders

These disorders include parkinsonism, chorea, ballism, myoclonus of cerebral origin, and dystonia. The brain MRI can be normal in all. The following are typical examples of how the abnormal brain MRI, when present, can be helpful in reaching a diagnosis in the appropriate clinical setting, with sensitivity of approximately 70% [13]. There are no specific abnormalities associated with the movement disorders of myoclonus, akathisia, tics, and drug-induced movement disorders and rarely are there abnormalities which are more specific for tremor and ataxia.

Parkinsonism

In idiopathic Parkinson's disease, including young-onset and genetically determined Parkinson's disease, MRI is typically normal. In dementia with Lewy bodies and patients with Parkinson's disease dementia, non-specific atrophy may be seen. Vascular parkinsonism is associated with either vascular disease within the basal ganglia or deep white matter small vessel disease, as in Figure 17.1B, and parkinsonism associated with hydrocephalus as in Figure 17.1D.

MRI can be helpful in the differentiation of parkinson-plus disorders from idiopathic Parkinson's disease. When axial features, postural instability, frontal signs, cognitive changes, and supranuclear palsy may co-exist, the presence of midbrain atrophy, best seen sagitally as the "hummingbird" sign [14] and axially as dilation of the cisterns around the superior colliculus, suggests a diagnosis of progressive supranuclear palsy as in Figure 17.10.

When pontocerebellar atrophy is seen on MRI in the presence of clinical features of parkinsonism, then multiple system atrophy can be suspected, although

A

B

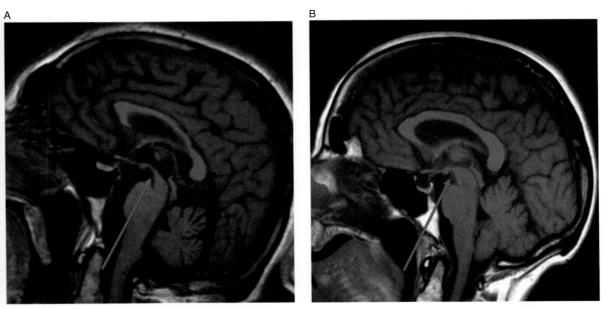

Figure 17.10 Thinning of the upper brainstem, seen on T$_1$ sagittal MRI (the "hummingbird" sign) and/or midbrain atrophy suggest progressive supranuclear palsy. Non-specific cortical atrophy may co-exist. (A) Supranuclear palsy at presentation age 69 years. (B) For comparison, normal brainstem at 69 years.

the radiological atrophy is not typically gross. A sign which supports a diagnosis of multiple system atrophy is the pontine "hot cross bun" sign on T$_2$ or proton density MRI [15], although this can also be seen in the genetic spinocerebellar ataxias (SCA2, 3, 7, and 8) [16] and other conditions. We have seen a similar appearance in a case of progressive multifocal leukoencephalopathy and in Wolfram syndrome. Additional signs suggestive of multiple system atrophy include high signal in the middle cerebellar peduncles on T$_2$, and posterior putaminal atrophy manifesting as dark posterior putamen with a high signal lateral rim on T$_2$ (Figures 17.11A–E). Parkinsonism, in the presence of a family history of descendants with learning difficulties or the combination of ataxia with cognitive changes, can suggest a diagnosis of fragile X permutation tremor/ataxia syndrome, in which MRI shows global atrophy, cerebellar T$_2$ hyperintensity around the dentate nucleus, and middle cerebellar T$_2$ high signal [17]. Note that the directionality of diffusion which is inherent of the DWI technique can produce an apparent "hot cross bun" sign, which is a false positive (Figure 17.12).

Asymmetrical parkinsonism, cortical signs, alien limb, myoclonus, and cognitive changes suggest a diagnosis of corticobasal degeneration/syndrome.

MRI may be normal but the diagnosis can be supported by posterior frontal asymmetrical focal atrophy contralateral to the parkinsonism/dystonia as in Figure 17.13.

Chorea

Choreic disorders can usually be identified by the presence or absence of other features. MRI can be normal in the presence of chorea. In Huntington's disease, T$_1$ MRI can show non-specific atrophy but caudate atrophy, seen best on T$_1$ coronal images, can be seen late in the illness as in Figure 17.14. Vascular generalized chorea can be identified by vascular disease in the basal ganglia or deep white matter. Post-infective chorea is reported rarely to be associated with gadolinium-enhanced basal ganglia abnormality [18] although it is often normal, as is chorea related to medication or chorea gravidarum. When hemichorea exists, a specific search should be made for small infarcts or hemorrhages in the region of the contralateral subthalamic nucleus, as in Figure 17.15A. When bilateral chorea/ballism commences abruptly, vascular lesions can be responsible but may be outside the subthalamic region and may involve the sub cortical white matter, as in Figure 17.15B, or

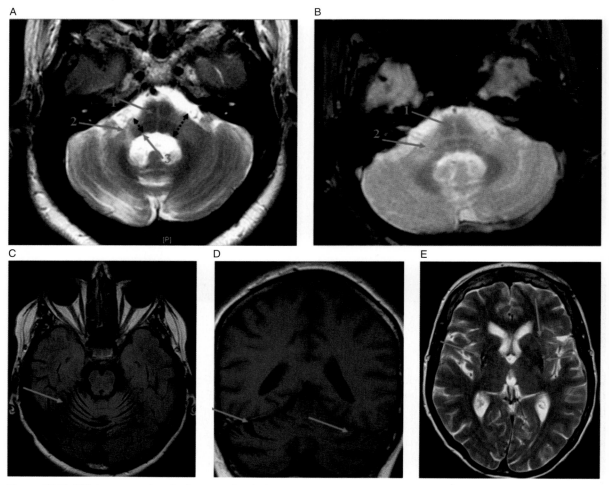

Figure 17.11 MRI signs supportive of a diagnosis of multiple system atrophy. (A) With and (B) without middle cerebellar peduncle atrophy. (A) T$_2$ MRI. 1. "Hot cross bun," 2. Middle cerebellar peduncle hyperintensity, 3. Right middle cerebellar peduncle atrophy, compare black arrow right and left. (B) Proton density MRI. 1. "Hot cross bun," 2. Middle cerebellar peduncle hyperintensity without middle cerebellar peduncle atrophy. (C) T$_1$ axial and (D) T$_1$ coronal images of cerebellar atrophy. (E) T$_2$ posterior putaminal atrophy, putaminal hypointensity, and putaminal lateral rim of hyperintensity.

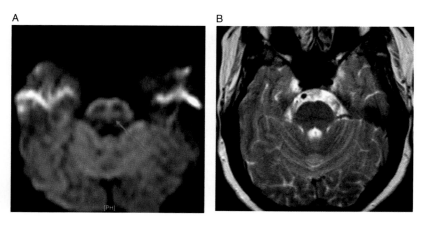

Figure 17.12 Apparent "hot cross bun" sign in DWI. This is a false positive and is normal. It is due to the technique. (A) DWI false-positive "hot cross bun." (B) T$_2$ – no "hot cross bun."

A

B

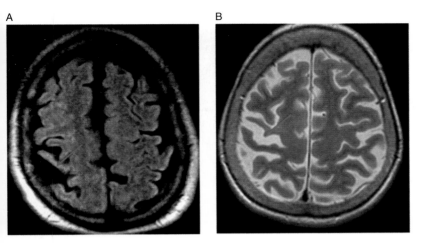

Figure 17.13 Asymmetrical right posterior frontal focal atrophy in corticobasal degeneration/syndrome. (A) Axial FLAIR MRI. (B) Axial T_2. Marked atrophy of the right precentral gyrus and widening of right peri-Rolandic sulci.

A

B

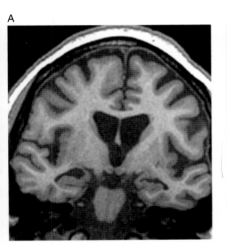
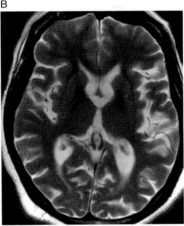

Figure 17.14 Huntington's disease with pronounced atrophy of the heads of the caudate nuclei; seen better on coronal T_1 (A) than on axial T_2 (B) MRI.

lentiform nuclei [19]. HIV infection should be considered. Global atrophy may co-exist.

Dystonia

Primary dystonias, for example idiopathic cervical dystonia, have normal MRI imaging. Some secondary dystonias can have abnormal imaging relating to the etiology, for example vascular, hypoxic, metabolic, or structural lesions. The term "hereditary" or "genetic" dystonia continues to be difficult to classify as some of these dystonias can be grouped into primary or secondary. Some, for example DYT1, 5, and 11, have normal imaging. Other hereditary conditions, for

example NBIA, have abnormal MRI, as above, and the term "hereditary–degenerative" has sometimes been applied. The use of MRI in the diagnosis of dystonia is mainly to look for lesions which if found would point away from a diagnosis of primary dystonias.

Figure 17.16 shows some examples of MRI abnormalities of secondary dystonia. Figure 17.16 shows (A) hypoxic focal lesions specifically in the posterior putamen, (B) diffuse hypoxic injury to the white matter, (C) hypoxic structurally small left putamen with normal signal, (D and E) putaminal necrosis from Leigh's disease, (F–H) glutaric acidemia type 1 showing (F) dentate hyperintensity, (G) putaminal

255

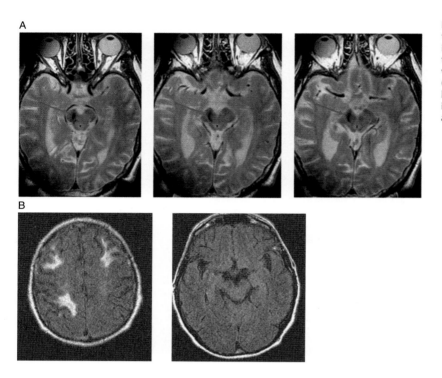

Figure 17.15 (A) Hemichorea. Serial thin sections of brainstem showing infarction/hemosiderin in the region of the right subthalamic nucleus in a patient with left hemichorea and some dystonia. (B) Bilateral chorea/ballism. Vascular lesions outside the subthalamic nucleus, in this case multiple cortical watershed areas.

mixed intensity lesions, and (H) diffuse marked white matter T_2 hyperintensity, and (I) hyperglycemia with left striatal hyperintensity, best seen on T_1 MRI. Hyperglycemia can cause chorea additionally.

Ataxia

Hereditary

When ataxia is present, MRI can help if abnormalities of the cerebellar cortex, hemispheres, cerebellar nuclei, or cerebellar connections are identified, but it should be noted that not all ataxias are cerebellar in origin, and even if the ataxia is severe and due to cerebellar dysfunction, MRI can be normal. The paraneoplastic disorders typically have normal brain MRI. Slowly progressive genetic spinocerebellar ataxias have marked global cerebellar atrophy. Midsagittal sections can visually overestimate cerebellar atrophy and coronal or axial T_1 or FLAIR are more influential. Figure 17.17 shows typical isolated cerebellar atrophy, which is a non-specific finding. The degree of atrophy in the posterior fossa outweighs the supratentorial atrophy. MRI findings cannot distinguish the spinocerebellar ataxias.

Progressive ataxia with palatal tremor (PAPT) can have many causes [20]. This syndrome is characterized by palatal tremor on clinical examination and inferior olivary hypertrophy on T_2 or proton density MRI (Figure 17.18). The olivary hypertrophy can be transient, becoming less notable on proton density or T_2 MRI despite persistence of palatal tremor.

The combination of unilateral or bilateral olivary hypertrophy with spinal cord and brainstem atrophy suggests adult-onset Alexander disease, as in Figure 17.19 [21]. The adult form of this autosomal dominant disorder is distinct from the infantile and juvenile forms both clinically and radiologically [22]. In the adult form, the cerebral white matter need not show major abnormalities as is more typical in the other leukodystrophies.

Unilateral cerebellar lesions are usually easy to identify on MRI. When associated with disruption of the cerebellar peduncles, red nucleus, or thalamus, unilateral olivary hypertrophy can suggest the syndrome of symptomatic palatal tremor, as in Figure 17.20.

A variety of movement disorders are associated with mutations in the polymerase gamma (*POLG*)

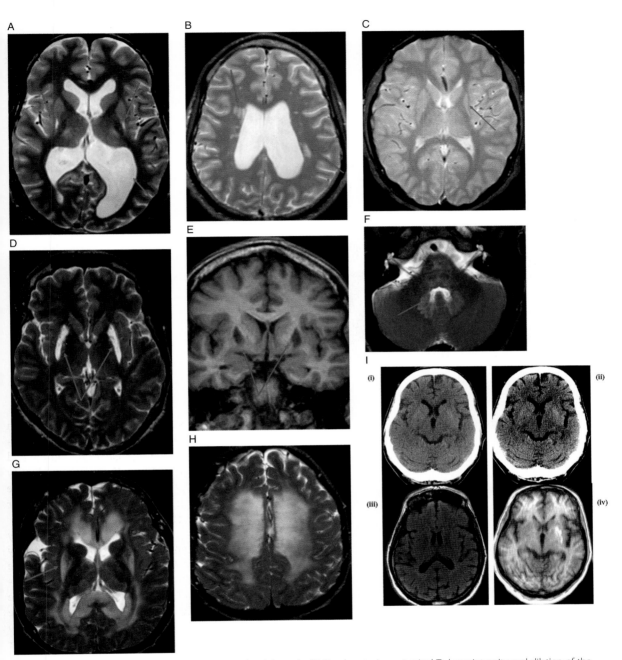

Figure 17.16 Hypoxic brain injury leading to generalized dystonia. (A) Focal posterior putaminal T_2 hyperintensity and dilation of the posterior ventricles. (B) T_2 diffuse deep white matter hyperintensity. (C) T_2 MRI of focal hypoxic brain injury leading to small left putamen in right hemidystonia with normal signal. (D and E) Leigh's disease. (D) T_2 putaminal necrosis. (E) T_1 putaminal necrosis. (F, G ,and H) Glutaric acidemia type I. See text. (Courtesy of Dr. Jean-Pierre Lin, Evelina Children's Hospital, London.) (I) Hyperglycemia. (i) Conventional CT and (ii) narrow window CT show faint hyperintensity in the left striatum, which is not seen well on FLAIR (iii), but clearly seen on T_1 MRI (iv). Figure (iv) is taken with motion artifact from the movement disorder.

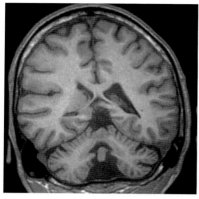

Figure 17.17 Isolated cerebellar atrophy.

gene; most notable are ataxia and myoclonus, but also dystonia and parkinsonism. Cerebellar nuclei, cerebellar cortex, and cerebellar–thalamic connections, and thalamic nuclei can be abnormal on T_2 MRI, with progression of the T_2 hyperintensity over time (Figure 17.21) [23]. This mitochondrial disorder shows lesions more specific to movement disorders, unlike other mitochondrial disorders which can have no or a non-specific MRI abnormality (e.g. myoclonic epilepsy with ragged red fibers [MERRF]) or mitochondrial encephalopathy with lactic acidosis and stroke-like episodes (MELAS).

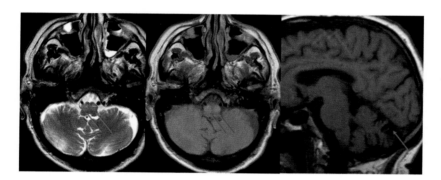

Figure 17.18 The syndrome of progressive ataxia with palatal tremor (PAPT) shows cerebellar atrophy combined with hyperintensity in the inferior olivary nuclei on T_2 or proton density MRI.

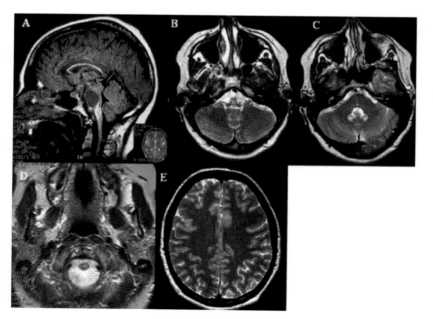

Figure 17.19 Adult onset Alexander disease. Brainstem atrophy and high signal on: (A) axial FLAIR, (B) axial T_2, (C) dentate high signal on T_2, (D) marked spinal cord atrophy, and (E) no cerebral pathology. (With permission from Sreedharan et al. [21].)

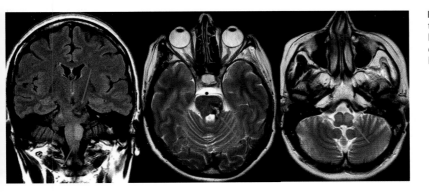

Figure 17.20 Symptomatic palatal tremor from upper brainstem hemorrhage involving the left superior cerebellar peduncle, leading to ipsilateral left inferior olivary hypertrophy.

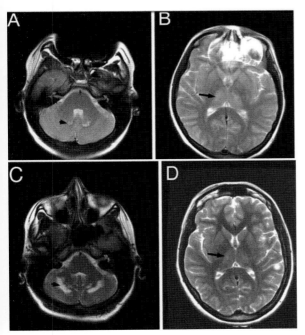

Figure 17.21 POLG mutation. (A and B) Aged 15 years. Axial brain MRI revealing bilateral T$_2$ hyperintense signal in dentate nuclei (arrowheads) and thalami (arrows). (C and D) More extensive signal change in the cerebellar hemispheres at age 20 years. (With permission from Hinnell et al. [23].)

Acquired

MRI cannot distinguish the etiology of global cerebellar atrophy from hypoxia, drug intoxication, or excessive alcohol ingestion. Demyelinating lesions from acute disseminated encephalomyelitis (ADEM) or multiple sclerosis can be readily identified in the cerebellum or its connections (Figure 17.22). Tremor and ataxia are the most common movement disorder presentations in these disorders.

An autoimmune disorder of mixed movement disorders, but typically cranial dystonia and myoclonus in the setting of encephalopathy and seizures in middle-aged adults, is associated with anti-N-methyl-D-aspartate (NMDA) receptor antibodies [24], and is usually associated with covert tumors, most notably ovarian in females. MRI can be non-specifically abnormal as in other encephalopathies (Figure 17.23). Non-specific high FLAIR signal was reported in three of four cases and in two, frontotemporal atrophy was seen within 11 months [24] but the absence of these signs should not steer away from searching extensively for this condition in an appropriate clinical setting. The basal ganglia may appear normal. The atrophy may resolve at 5–7 years [25].

Prion disease typically has movement disorders in the course of the illness, although not always at presentation. The most common disorder is sporadic Creutzfeld–Jakob disease. In this, the most common movement disorder is ataxia/myoclonus. MRI shows hyperintensity subcortically in the caudate, putamen, and thalami, with a gradient of intensity (brighter–darker) from anterior to posterior (Figures 17.24A and B) [26]. Cortical and insular hyperintensity is best seen on DWI rather than T$_2$ sequences (Figures 17.24B, C, and D). These radiological signal changes can predate the onset of the movement disorder, and can steer the diagnosis to prion disease in a patient presenting with rapid-onset dementia. With the possible exception of variant Creutzfeld–Jakob disease (Figure 17.25), MRI is not able to distinguish reliably the other forms of prion diseases.

259

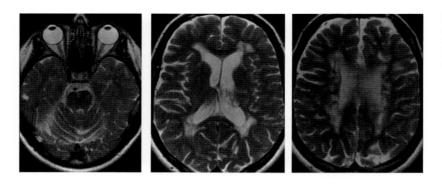

Figure 17.22 Multiple sclerosis with multiple infero- and supratentorial demyelinating plaques affecting brainstem, putamen, thalamus, and periventricular white matter.

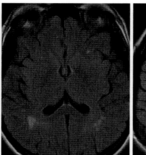 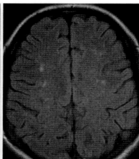

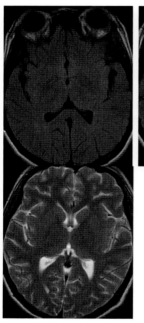

Figure 17.23 Anti-NMDA receptor antibody encephalopathy (see text). (Courtesy of Dr. N. Moran, King's College Hospital.)

Infective/Post-infective

Cavitating lesions can be seen in the basal ganglia and surprisingly may not lead to movement disorders. Nonetheless, appearances can help to direct investigations. A list of bacterial, fungal, and parasitic infections is outside the scope of this chapter. Gadolinium-enhanced T_1 MRI can show the structure of the wall of the cysts and T_2 or FLAIR show the effect of edema on the surrounding tissue. DWI can be abnormal but does not add to the specificity of diagnosis. Toxoplasmosis is the most common, usually presenting as a single lesion (Figure 17.26A).

The differential diagnosis is a cavitating neoplasm or bacterial abscess. Basal ganglia clumped lesions, as in Figure 17.26B, can be seen in cryptococcal infections [27]. Both are mostly seen in immunocompromised individuals. Discrete but multiple cavitating lesions suggest other bacterial infections, tuberculosis or multiple cavitating lesions from vasculitis.

In both adults and children, herpetic viral infections do not often lead to movement disorders. The cerebral structures typically affected on MRI in encephalopathic presentations (white and gray

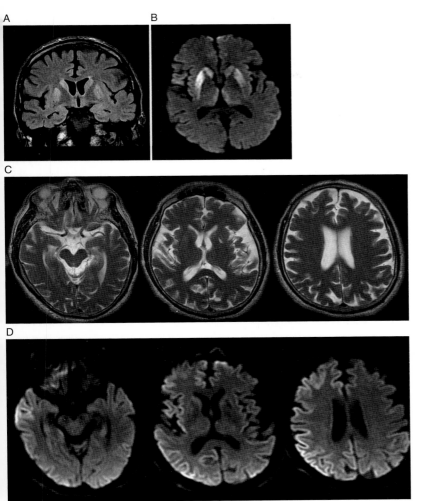

Figure 17.24. Sporadic Creutzfeld–Jakob disease. (A) Coronal FLAIR MRI shows hyperintensity in the caudate nucleus, putamen, and cingulate gyri bilaterally. (B) DWI shows corresponding restricted diffusion in the caudate and putamen as well as the medial thalami bilaterally. (With permission from Hinnell *et al.* [26].) (C) T_2 MRI normal cortex. (D) DWI MRI hyperintense cortex.

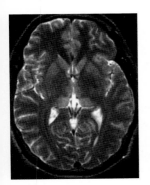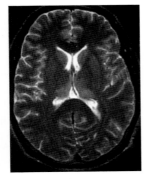

Figure 17.25 Variant Creutzfeld–Jakob disease. The posterior thalami are hyperintense on T_2.

matter of the temporal and frontal lobes) are distinct from those affecting movement disorders. A cerebellar presentation can occur, more often in childhood, but usually the cerebellum appears normal on MRI [28]. Post-infective disorders, for example Sydenham's chorea, other post-streptococcal neuropsychiatric disorders, and encephalitis lethargica, usually have normal imaging, although there are very rare reports of symmetrical, transient, T_2 hyperintensity in the basal ganglia [18]. Normality of the MRI should not deter further investigations to confirm these diagnoses.

A

B

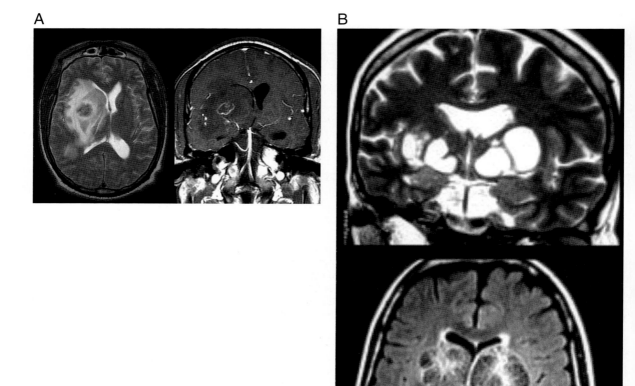

Figure 17.26 (A) Single basal ganglia toxoplasmosis lesion. T_2 and gadolinium- enhanced T_1 show a walled cyst, with mass effect and surrounding vasogenic oedema. (B) Multiple basal ganglia lesions of cryptococcal abscesses on T_2 and FLAIR MRI. With permission from Camargos *et al.* [27].

References

1. Aoki S, Okada Y, Nishimura K, *et al.* Normal deposition of brain iron in childhood and adolescence: MR imaging at 1.5 T. *Radiology.* 1989;**172**(2):381–5.

2. O'Gorman RL, Shmueli K, Ashkan K, *et al.* Optimal MRI methods for direct stereotactic targeting of the subthalamic nucleus and globus pallidus. *Eur Radiol.* 2011;**21**(1):130–6. Epub 2010/07/21.

3. Schneider SA, Bhatia KP. Syndromes of neurodegeneration with brain iron accumulation. *Semin Pediatr Neurol.* 2012;**19**(2):57–66.

4. McNeill A, Birchall D, Hayflick SJ, *et al.* T2* and FSE MRI distinguishes four subtypes of neurodegeneration with brain iron accumulation. *Neurology.* 2008;**70**:1614–19.

5. Shivakumar R, Thomas SV. Teaching Neuro*Images*: face of the giant panda and her cub. MRI correlates of Wilson disease. *Neurology.* 2009;**72**(11):e50.

6. da Costa Mdo D, Spitz M, Bacheschi LA, et al. Wilson's disease: two treatment modalities. Correlations to pretreatment and posttreatment brain MRI. Neuroradiology. 2009;51:627–633.

7. Saporta MA, André C, Bahia PR, et al. Acquired hepatocerebral degeneration without overt liver disease. Neurology. 2004;63: 1981–1982.

8. Ferrara J, Jankovic J. Acquired hepatocerebral degeneration. J Neurol. 2009;256:320–32.

9. Stamelou M, Bhatia KP. A new treatable genetic disorder of manganese metabolism causing dystonia-parkinsonism and cirrhosis: The "new" Wilson's disease? Mov Disord. 2012;27(8): 962. doi: 10.1002/mds.25031.

10. Hughes EF, Fairbanks L, Simmonds HA, Robinson RO. Molybdenum cofactor deficiency-phenotypic variability in a family with late-onset variant. Dev Med Child Neurol. 1998;40:57–61.

11. Alkufri F, Harrower T, Rahman Y, et al. Molybdenum Cofactor Deficiency Presenting With a Parkinsonism-Dystonia Syndrome. Mov Disord. 2013; 28(3):399–401.

12. Vijayakumar K, Gunny R, Grunewald S, et al. Clinical neuroimaging features and outcome in molybdenum cofactor deficiency. Pediatr Neurol. 2011;45:246–52.

13. Massey LA, Micallef C, Paviour DC, et al. Conventional magnetic resonance imaging in confirmed progressive supranuclear palsy and multiple system atrophy. Mov Disord. 2012;27(14):1754–62. doi: 10.1002/mds.24968.

14. Kato N, Arai K, Hattori T. Study of the rostral midbrain atrophy in progressive supranuclear palsy. J Neurol Sci. 2003;210(1–2):57–60.

15. Schrag A, Good CD, Miszkiel K, et al. Differentiation of atypical parkinsonian syndromes with routine MRI. Neurology. 2000;54(3):697–702.

16. Lee YC, Liu CS, Wu HM, et al. The 'hot cross bun' sign in the patients with spinocerebellar ataxia. Eur J Neurol. 2009; (4):513–16.

17. Brunberg JA, Jacquemont S, Hagerman RJ, et al. Fragile X premutation carriers: characteristic MR imaging findings of adult male patients with progressive cerebellar and cognitive dysfunction. AJNR Am J Neuroradiol. 2002;23(10): 1757–66.

18. Martino D, Church A, Giovannoni G. Are antibasal ganglia antibodies important and clinically useful? Prat Neurol. 2007;7(1):32–41.

19. Postuma RB, Lang AE. Hemiballism: revisiting a classic disorder. Lancet Neurol. 2003;2(11):661–8.

20. Samuel M, Torun N, Tuite PJ, Sharpe JA, Lang AE. Progressive ataxia and palatal tremor (PAPT): clinical and MRI assessment with review of palatal tremors. Brain. 2004;127:1252–68.

21. Sreedharan J, Shaw CE, Jarosz J, Samuel M. Alexander disease with hypothermia, microcoria, and psychiatric and endocrine disturbances. Neurology. 2007;68(16):1322–3.

22. Li R, Johnson AB, Salomons G, et al. Glial fibrillary acidic protein mutations in infantile, juvenile, and adult forms of Alexander disease. Ann Neurol. 2005;57 (3):310–26.

23. Hinnell C, Haider S, Delamont S, et al. Dystonia in mitochondrial spinocerebellar ataxia and epilepsy syndrome associated with novel recessive POLG mutations. Mov Disord. 2012;27(1):162–3. doi: 10.1002/mds.23960. Epub 2011/11/28. No abstract available.

24. Iizuka T, Sakai F, Ide T, et al. Anti-NMDA receptor encephalitis in Japan: long-term outcome without tumor removal. Neurology. 2008;70:504–11.

25. Iizuka T, Yoshii S, Kan S, et al. Reversible brain atrophy in anti-NMDA receptor encephalitis: a long-term observational study. J Neurol. 2010;257(10):1686–91.

26. Hinnell C, Buxton-Thomas M, Sibtain N, Samuel M. Striatal 123I-Ioflupane SPECT abnormality in sporadic Creutzfeldt–Jakob disease. J Neurol. 2011;258:948–50.

27. Camargos ST, Teixeira AL, Jr., Cardoso F. Parkinsonism associated with basal ganglia cryptococcal abscesses in an immunocompetent patient. Mov Disord. 2006;21(5):714–15.

28. Tlili-Graiess K, Mhiri Souei M, Mlaiki B, et al. [Imaging of acute cerebellitis in children. Report of 4 cases]. J Neuroradiol. 2006;33(1):38–44. [Article in French]

263

MRI in clinical trials

Norbert Schuff

Introduction

As efforts are growing to develop disease-modifying treatments for Parkinson's disease (PD), such as neuroprotective or cellular restorative therapies, there is a huge need for objective and sensitive markers to assess the efficacy of these therapeutic interventions. Although clinical ratings, such as the Unified Parkinson's Disease Rating Scale (UPDRS) [1], are well established in clinical trials, they may not be sufficiently sensitive to detect subtle slowing in disease progression, which one expects from a successful therapy. Moreover, clinical ratings may change very slowly, potentially leading to premature dismissals of disease-modifying treatments. Conversely, long-term symptomatic effects that persist for some time after medication washout may bias clinical ratings [2]. Radiotracer position emission tomography (PET) and single-photon emission computed tomography (SPECT) imaging of striatal dopamine depletion, a hallmark of PD, have traditionally been the imaging choices for studies of PD progression [3] and disease-modifying interventions [2, 4]. There is, however, controversy about the accuracy of these techniques to reflect dopaminergic neuron loss. In addition, the quantification of these radiotracers, relying on simplifying assumptions, is not without problems. Moreover, these tracer studies depend on the notion that the pathology in PD is confined to the nigrostriatal neurons, which may be overly restrictive given that other neural pathways are likely involved in PD progression, even at an early stage of the illness. Complementary information to radiotracer imaging is therefore desirable.

Magnetic resonance imaging (MRI) has attracted considerable interest as a complementary imaging tool to study PD progression and to assess therapeutic interventions, in part because MRI offers a broad scope of brain assessments that range from structural changes at the macro- and microscopic level to functional changes as well as changes in brain metabolites. The growing attention on MRI has also been fueled by new possibilities to quantify alterations of brain networks in PD using advanced MRI methods, such as MRI tractography for studies of structural connectivity [5] and resting-state functional MRI (fMRI) for studies of functional connectivity [6]. A boost for MRI has also come from ongoing international large-scale multicenter biomarker studies of disease progression, such as the Alzheimer's Disease Neuroimaging Initiative (ADNI) [7], the Parkinson's Disease Progression Marker Initiative (PPMI) [8], and the Dementia and Parkinson's Disease (DEMPARK) project in Europe [9]. These initiatives aim – among other goals – to establish standardized protocols for acquisition, transfer, and analysis of MRI data and to share extensive reference databases of clinical, bio-specimen, and imaging data with the research community.

In this chapter emerging MRI strategies for assessing therapeutic interventions in PD and related conditions will be reviewed. The challenges for MRI in this field as well as the prospect of new developments will also be discussed.

Characteristic of an ideal outcome measure for clinical trials

First, the general role of imaging in clinical trials will be described and the characteristic of an ideal outcome measure defined. As for radiotracer imaging, an extensive review of the role of radiotracers in clinical trials in PD has been published elsewhere [10] and the latest advancements in dopamine imaging have been discussed more recently in other publications [11, 12]. The best method to establish the efficacy of a neuro-protective or restorative therapy would be to compare directly the number and functional viability of neurons before and after a therapeutic intervention. However, this is currently impossible in patients. Instead surrogate outcome markers, which are believed to reflect viable neurons in a clinically meaningful way, have to be used. Most clinical trials use a change in clinical measures of disease severity for this purpose, such as a change in UPDRS. Although clinical measures undoubtedly reflect an important aspect of disease progression and remain the primary clinical endpoint for the assessment of drug efficiency, they also have several serious limitations. Two fundamental ones are first the difficulty in differentiating between disease-modifying and purely symptomatic effects from an intervention and second the inability to detect changes at a preclinical stage of the illness when an intervention might be most effective [13]. As a consequence of these shortcomings, there is great need for more objective and sensitive outcome markers. The ideal outcome marker should fulfill the following criteria: First, the relationship between the outcome marker and the desired clinical effect, for example the prevention of motor deficits in PD, should have been clearly established. Second, the outcome marker should be objective and reproducible, allowing assessments of treatment efficacy with high statistical confidence. Third, the outcome marker should be specific to the expected treatment action. Fourth, the assessment should be non-invasive and well tolerated. Last, the assessment should be inexpensive and widely available. Since MRI meets some of these criteria, in particular objectivity and non-invasiveness, the ability of MRI to benefit assessments of clinical trials is increasingly being investigated. In the next sections, the usefulness of various MRI methods for clinical trials with focus on PD will be discussed.

Potential MRI measures for clinical trials
Structural MRI

Serial structural MRI scans can be used to measure macroscopic changes in brain structure, such as the rate of regional brain volume loss and cortical thinning. Pathologically, brain atrophy in most neurodegenerative diseases, such as PD, results from degeneration and death of neuronal cell bodies and the related loss of axons and potentially secondary loss of glia. Notably in Alzheimer's disease, it has been shown that structural MRI in conjunction with automated brain volume measurements can detect significant slowing of atrophy rates within less than a year of treatment interventions [14, 15]. Several movement disorders, including multiple system atrophy (MSA) [16], progressive supranuclear palsy (PSP) [17], and Huntington disease (HD) [18], are also associated with significant brain atrophy rates, implying structural MRI could potentially be useful as an outcome measure in clinical trials of these conditions. In PD, by contrast, atrophy seems to be much more subtle and barely differs from the atrophy rates that are seen in normal elderly subjects [16], unless PD patients show also signs of cognitive decline [19]. Given the absence of significant brain atrophy in PD based on current MRI methodology, it might appear unlikely that structural MRI will become a prominent outcome measure in clinical trials of PD. However, the method may still play an important role for assessing the safety of pharmacological interventions. For example, a human therapeutic PD trial using infusion of glial cell-derived neurotrophic factors (GDNF) into the putamen was abruptly terminated after findings of cerebellar lesions in monkeys given high-dose GDNF raised safety concerns [20]. However, structural MRI on most PD patients in the GDNF trial found no evidence for volume or other morphological brain changes between pre- and post-treatment scans over a 1-year period, suggesting that a GDNF infusion at a typical therapeutic dose levels for humans has no detectable adverse effect on the brain.

Diffusion MRI

Although white matter does not play a prominent role in the classical picture of PD pathology, the interest in studying white matter in PD has been growing recently. This trend is being fueled by findings of white matter alterations in PD adjacent to motor control regions [21–24] and in the olfactory system [25–27] using diffusion tensor imaging (DTI). DTI is an MRI variant that captures uniquely the microstructural architecture of tissue by measuring the systematic directionality of water diffusion. The degree of diffusion directionality is usually expressed as fractional anisotropy (FA), with values increasing from zero to one for more directional diffusion [28].

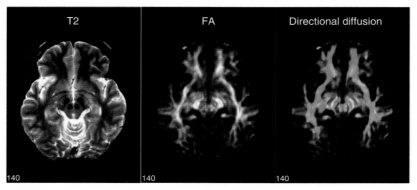

Figure 18.1 Representative maps of fractional anisotropy (FA) and directional diffusivity at the level of the substantia, illustrating the richness of information from diffusion tensor imaging. Color coding in the directional map: red = left/right, blue = head/foot, green = anterior/posterior. The corresponding T_2-weighted MR image is also shown for comparison. The DTI maps are corrected for geometrical distortion, co-registered to the structural T_2-weighted images, and interpolated to the high resolution (1 mm^3) of structural MRI, following the standardized procedures for DTI processing of the Parkinson's Marker Progression Initiative (PPMI). Details for the processing protocol are available at http://www.ppmi-info.org/wp-content/uploads/2011/12/DTI-processing-Pipeline3.pdf.

Although the biological underpinning of DTI alterations is a matter of debate, DTI-derived measures correlated strongly with the loss of dopaminergic neurons in a toxin-induced mouse model of PD [29]. Information from DTI can also be used for mapping fiber tracts and for studies of structural connectivity and brain plasticity using the concept of tractography [30]. The unique information from DTI is illustrated in Figure 18.1, showing parametric maps of FA and the corresponding directional information of water diffusivity at the level of the substantia nigra. A conventional T_2-weighted structural MR image is shown for comparison.

Little is known so far about rates of DTI changes in PD that would establish a strong indication for the use of DTI in clinical trials. However, in a small treatment study of dystonia patients using intramuscular botulinum neurotoxin injections, the treatment of choice for this condition, initial FA abnormalities in white matter regions close to the basal ganglia and thalamus disappeared rapidly following treatment [31]. The findings raise the possibility that activity-dependent white matter plasticity can be observed with DTI. The findings further demonstrate that white matter alterations can change rapidly under certain pathological conditions. Additional support for the potential use of DTI as an outcome marker in neuroprotective therapies comes from various neurological conditions, such as multiple sclerosis, which also showed relatively fast white matter DTI changes within a year of treatment [32]. Whether DTI also has value for clinical trials of PD needs to be

determined. DTI may also be useful for assessing the safety of pharmacological interventions, similar to structural MRI. Potentially, DTI may be even more sensitive than structural MRI in detecting adverse brain reactions given the high sensitivity of various diffusion measures to cerebral edema and inflammation.

Functional MRI

fMRI is increasingly being used to study neurodegenerative disorders, such as PD, because – unlike functional PET – the method does not involve radiation that restricts how often subjects can be scanned. Furthermore, fMRI offers sufficient temporal resolution to monitor dynamic changes. On the other hand, the blood oxygen level-dependent (BOLD) signal of fMRI is only an indirect marker of neuronal activity and does not correspond to a simple quantity, complicating comparisons across individuals and even within subjects between studies. Current fMRI methodology comes in two flavors: In the traditional form of fMRI, subjects are required to participate in a behavioral paradigm while the modulation of the BOLD signal is studied. In the other form, also known as resting-state fMRI, the subject is refraining from any explicit task while modulations of the BOLD signal are analyzed for regional correlations that are thought to reflect functional brain networks.

Both forms of fMRI have been used to study the multiple roles of dopamine and dopaminergic medication in the brain, including not only motor

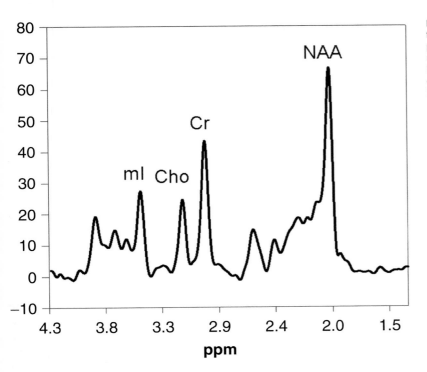

Figure 18.2 Typical ^{1}H MR spectrum from a section of the brain, here the posterior cingulate cortex. The prominent resonance peaks correspond to the main brain metabolites N-acetylaspartate (NAA), choline (Cho), creatine (Cr) and myo-inositol (ml).

functions but also behavioral alterations [33–35], cognitive changes [36], and altered functional brain connectivity [37, 38]. In particular, functional brain connectivity studies using resting-state fMRI have emerged as an area of great interest to assess the modulation of brain networks in PD patients on and off medication. In general, PD patients off medication exhibit reduced connectivity between the putamen and the supplementary motor areas, prefrontal cortex, and inferior parietal cortex compared to controls [6, 39, 40]. These findings are at least partially reversed by medication. Furthermore, a direct positive relation was observed between reduced striatal dopamine transporter (DAT) measures, a putative index of dopaminergic neuron loss, and lower regional BOLD magnitudes [41]. Nonetheless, the value of fMRI as an outcome marker of clinical trials, including restorative therapies, remains undetermined and more studies in this field are required.

Proton magnetic resonance spectroscopy

Proton magnetic resonance spectroscopy (^{1}H MRS) is a useful non-invasive method to study certain brain metabolites, such as N-acetylaspartate (NAA, an amino acid contained almost exclusively within neurons and therefore considered a putative neuronal marker) and *myo*-inositol (*myo*-Ins, a compound contained within glial cells). In addition, other prominent ^{1}H MRS signals correspond to choline (Cho) and creatine (Cr) compounds which are involved respectively in phospholipid membrane synthesis and cellular energy buffering systems. A typical ^{1}H MR spectrum from a section of the brain – here the posterior cingulate cortex – is shown in Figure 18.2. Although ^{1}H MRS of the basal ganglia has yielded variable results in PD, the method has shown promise for differentiating idiopathic PD from atypical parkinsonian syndromes, such as MSA and PSP (for a review see Firbank *et al.* [42]).

A few ^{1}H MRS studies investigated brain metabolite alterations in PD in response to therapy. One study found that 6-month therapy of de novo PD patients with a dopamine agonist (pergolide) was associated with the normalization of initially reduced Cho/Cr ratios in the motor cortex, whereas NAA and *myo*-Ins did not change significantly relative to Cr before and after therapy [43]. The investigators suggested that the normalization of the Cho/Cr ratio was driven by an increase in Cho, potentially reflecting the restoration of cell membranes.

In another ^{1}H MRS study of therapeutic interventions in PD that involved autologous implantation of bone marrow-derived stem cells, an increase of the NAA/Cr ratio was observed in the basal ganglia [44], suggesting neuronal restoration. It is important to note, however, that most patients in this study were also taking other medication for symptom control that may have interfered with the NAA findings, although one PD patient, who had never taken medication, also showed increased NAA/Cr as well as clinical improvements after treatment. A low magnetic field (1.0 Tesla) ^{1}H MRS study on PD patients who underwent bilateral surgery for deep brain stimulation (DBS) in the subthalamic nucleus reported substantial increases of NAA/Cr and Cho/Cr in the fronto-basal cortex post-surgery [45]. The underlying mechanism of these metabolite changes following DBS needs to be elucidated. One explanation for the changes is that DBS might increase neuronal metabolism.

Other MRI uses

Aside from the potential use of MRI as an outcome measure in clinical trials, intraoperative MRI methods can be helpful in monitoring targeted cell and gene infusions. In particular, the unique sensitivity of the MRI signal relaxation to changes in cellular morphology can be utilized to visualize and quantify the volume and distribution of infusions. Toward this goal, T_2-weighted MRI has recently been used to monitor the convection-enhanced delivery of a gene vector to the putamen for the treatment of PD [46]. Changes in T_2 were seen in patients within about 4 hours of the infusion and the region altered overlapped areas with increased PET uptake. This suggests that T_2-weighted MRI allows visualization of a substantial part of the therapeutic gene distribution. Since the controlled distribution of therapeutic agents within targeted brain structures is essential for optimizing treatment efficacy, MRI could become an important tool in PD trials involving cellular infusion.

Discussion

The use of MRI as an outcome measure in clinical trials of PD is still in its infancy, but further progress can be expected from new technical developments. For example, methodological advancements in measuring changes in brain shape, which is expected to improve the detection of brain atrophy, might benefit PD treatment studies that target neuron loss [47]. Additional benefits can be expected from new strategies evaluating structural and diffusion MRI data together. Complementary information from structural and diffusion MRI can be used for instance to improve visualization and delineation of complex brain structures, such as the nuclei of the thalamus [48] and the brainstem [49], including the pedunculopontine nucleus, which is considered an early target of PD pathology. Furthermore, other advanced MRI methods, such as arterial spin labeling (ASL) MRI [50], which measures regional cerebral blood non-invasively and $T_{1\rho}$ and $T_{2\rho}$ MRI [51], which are sensitive to cellular changes and presence of iron, offer new opportunities to study treatment effects. Recent methodological advancements in evaluating functional connectivity between brain regions using resting-state fMRI as well as structural connectivity using MRI tractography allow probing brain responses to therapy in new ways [52]. In particular, studies fusing analyses of functional and structural connectivity could be highly informative in providing new insight into large-scale alterations in neuronal communication as a result of restorative therapies. Another potential benefit for future MRI trials of PD not to be overlooked is the growing availability of rich databases including MR images (raw and processed), biomarkers, and clinical data of natural progression that are collected in a standardized format as part of ongoing large multicenter imaging studies, such as the PPMI [8] and ADNI [7]. Since these databases are open to the research community, they can serve a wide range of useful functions, particularly for MRI, such as providing reference values, test sets for cross-validation and data enrichment for greater statistical power.

In summary, structural, diffusion, functional, and spectroscopic MRI each provide meaningful information about brain changes that accompany PD progression. These MRI methods hold promise to elucidate the benefits and complications of neuroprotective and restorative therapeutic intervention for PD.

Acknowledgements

The work was supported in part by funds from the National Center for Research Resources (P41 RR 023953) and by grants from the Department of Defense (W81XWH-10–2–0078), and by the Michael J. Fox Foundation for Parkinson's Research.

References

1. Goetz CG, Tilley BC, Shaftman SR, et al. Movement Disorder Society-sponsored revision of the Unified Parkinson's Disease Rating Scale (MDS-UPDRS): scale presentation and clinimetric testing results. Mov Disord. 2008;23(15):2129–70.

2. Fahn S, Sulzer D. Neurodegeneration and neuroprotection in Parkinson disease. NeuroRx. 2004;1(1):139–54.

3. Marek K, Jennings D, Seibyl J. Imaging the dopamine system to assess disease-modifying drugs: studies comparing dopamine agonists and levodopa. Neurology. 2003;61(6 Suppl 3):S43–8.

4. Parkinson Study Group. Dopamine transporter brain imaging to assess the effects of pramipexole vs levodopa on Parkinson disease progression. JAMA. 2002;287(13):1653–61.

5. Hagmann P, Kurant M, Gigandet X, et al. Mapping human whole-brain structural networks with diffusion MRI. PLoS One. 2007;2(7):e597.

6. Helmich RC, Derikx LC, Bakker M, et al. Spatial remapping of cortico-striatal connectivity in Parkinson's disease. Cereb Cortex. 2010;20(5):1175–86.

7. Weiner MW, Veitch DP, Aisen PS, et al. The Alzheimer's Disease Neuroimaging Initiative: a review of papers published since its inception. Alzheimers Dement. 2012;8(1 Suppl):S1–68.

8. Parkinson Progressive Marker Initiative. The Parkinson Progression Marker Initiative (PPMI). Prog Neurobiol. 2011;95(4):629–35.

9. Balzer-Geldsetzer M, Costa AS, Kronenburger M, et al. Parkinson's disease and dementia: a longitudinal study (DEMPARK). Neuroepidemiology. 2011;37(3–4):168–76.

10. Ravina B, Eidelberg D, Ahlskog JE, et al. The role of radiotracer imaging in Parkinson disease. Neurology. 2005;64(2):208–15.

11. Shen LH, Liao MH, Tseng YC. Recent advances in imaging of dopaminergic neurons for evaluation of neuropsychiatric disorders. J Biomed Biotechnol. 2012;2012:259349.

12. Varrone A, Halldin C. New developments of dopaminergic imaging in Parkinson's disease. Q J Nucl Med Mol Imaging. 2012;56(1):68–82.

13. Picconi B, Piccoli G, Calabresi P. Synaptic dysfunction in Parkinson's disease. Adv Exp Med Biol. 2012;970:553–72.

14. Schuff N, Suhy J, Goldman R, et al. An MRI substudy of a donepezil clinical trial in mild cognitive impairment. Neurobiol Aging. 2011;32(12):2318.e31–41.

15. Weiner MW, Sadowsky C, Saxton J, et al. Magnetic resonance imaging and neuropsychological results from a trial of memantine in Alzheimer's disease. Alzheimers Dement. 2011;7(4):425–35.

16. Paviour DC, Price SL, Jahanshahi M, Lees AJ, Fox NC. Longitudinal MRI in progressive supranuclear palsy and multiple system atrophy: rates and regions of atrophy. Brain. 2006;129(Pt 4):1040–9.

17. Josephs KA, Whitwell JL, Boeve BF, et al. Rates of cerebral atrophy in autopsy-confirmed progressive supranuclear palsy. Ann Neurol. 2006;59(1):200–3.

18. Aylward EH, Rosenblatt A, Field K, et al. Caudate volume as an outcome measure in clinical trials for Huntington's disease: a pilot study. Brain Res Bull. 2003;62(2):137–41.

19. Hu MT, White SJ, Chaudhuri KR, et al. Correlating rates of cerebral atrophy in Parkinson's disease with measures of cognitive decline. J Neural Transm. 2001;108(5):571–80.

20. Chebrolu H, Slevin JT, Gash DA, et al. MRI volumetric and intensity analysis of the cerebellum in Parkinson's disease patients infused with glial-derived neurotrophic factor (GDNF). Exp Neurol. 2006;198(2):450–6.

21. Vaillancourt DE, Spraker MB, Prodoehl J, et al. High-resolution diffusion tensor imaging in the substantia nigra of de novo Parkinson disease. Neurology. 2009;72(16):1378–84.

22. Gattellaro G, Minati L, Grisoli M, et al. White matter involvement in idiopathic Parkinson disease: a diffusion tensor imaging study. AJNR Am J Neuroradiol. 2009;30(6):1222–6.

23. Zhang K, Yu C, Zhang Y, et al. Voxel-based analysis of diffusion tensor indices in the brain in patients with Parkinson's disease. Eur J Radiol. 2011;77(2):269–73.

24. Zhan W, Kang GA, Glass GA, et al. Regional alterations of brain microstructure in Parkinson's disease using diffusion tensor imaging. Mov Disord. 2012;27(1):90–7.

25. Scherfler C, Schocke MF, Seppi K, et al. Voxel-wise analysis of diffusion weighted imaging reveals disruption of the olfactory tract in Parkinson's disease. Brain. 2006;129(Pt 2):538–42.

26. Ibarretxe-Bilbao N, Junque C, Marti MJ, et al. Olfactory impairment in Parkinson's disease and white matter abnormalities in central olfactory areas: a voxel-based diffusion tensor imaging study. Mov Disord. 2010;25(12):1888–94.

27. Rolheiser TM, Fulton HG, Good KP, et al. Diffusion tensor imaging and olfactory identification testing in early-stage Parkinson's disease. J Neurol. 2011;258(7):1254–60.

28. Pierpaoli C, Basser PJ. Toward a quantitative assessment of diffusion anisotropy. Magn Reson Med. 1996;36(6):893–906.

29. Boska MD, Hasan KM, Kibuule D, *et al.* Quantitative diffusion tensor imaging detects dopaminergic neuronal degeneration in a murine model of Parkinson's disease. *Neurobiol Dis.* 2007;**26**(3):590–6.

30. Basser PJ, Pajevic S, Pierpaoli C, Duda J, Aldroubi A. In vivo fiber tractography using DT-MRI data. *Magn Reson Med.* 2000;**44**(4):625–32.

31. Blood AJ, Tuch DS, Makris N, *et al.* White matter abnormalities in dystonia normalize after botulinum toxin treatment. *Neuroreport.* 2006;**17**(12):1251–5.

32. Fox RJ, Cronin T, Lin J, *et al.* Measuring myelin repair and axonal loss with diffusion tensor imaging. *AJNR Am J Neuroradiol.* 2011;**32**(1):85–91.

33. van Eimeren T, Ballanger B, Pellecchia G, *et al.* Dopamine agonists diminish value sensitivity of the orbitofrontal cortex: a trigger for pathological gambling in Parkinson's disease? *Neuropsychopharmacology.* 2009;**34**(13):2758–66.

34. Harrington DL, Castillo GN, Greenberg PA, *et al.* Neurobehavioral mechanisms of temporal processing deficits in Parkinson's disease. *PLoS One.* 2011;**6**(2):e17461.

35. Voon V, Gao J, Brezing C, *et al.* Dopamine agonists and risk: impulse control disorders in Parkinson's disease. *Brain.* 2011;**134**(Pt 5):1438–46.

36. MacDonald PA, MacDonald AA, Seergobin KN, *et al.* The effect of dopamine therapy on ventral and dorsal striatum-mediated cognition in Parkinson's disease: support from functional MRI. *Brain.* 2011;**134**(Pt 5):1447–63.

37. Honey GD, Suckling J, Zelaya F, *et al.* Dopaminergic drug effects on physiological connectivity in a human cortico-striato-thalamic system. *Brain.* 2003; **126**(Pt 8):1767–81.

38. Delaveau P, Salgado-Pineda P, Fossati P, *et al.* Dopaminergic modulation of the default mode network in Parkinson's disease. *Eur Neuropsychopharmacol.* 2010;**20**(11):784–92.

39. Wu T, Long X, Wang L, *et al.* Functional connectivity of cortical motor areas in the resting state in Parkinson's disease. *Hum Brain Mapp.* 2011;**32**(9):1443–57.

40. Wu T, Wang L, Chen Y, *et al.* Changes of functional connectivity of the motor network in the resting state in Parkinson's disease. *Neurosci Lett.* 2009; **460**(1):6–10.

41. Lotze M, Reimold M, Heymans U, *et al.* Reduced ventrolateral fMRI response during observation of emotional gestures related to the degree of dopaminergic impairment in Parkinson disease. *J Cogn Neurosci.* 2009;**21**(7): 1321–31.

42. Firbank MJ, Harrison RM, O'Brien JT. A comprehensive review of proton magnetic resonance spectroscopy studies in dementia and Parkinson's disease. *Dement Geriatr Cogn Disord.* 2002;**14**(2):64–76.

43. Lucetti C, Del Dotto P, Gambaccini G, *et al.* Influences of dopaminergic treatment on motor cortex in Parkinson disease: a MRI/MRS study. *Mov Disord.* 2007;**22**(15):2170–5.

44. Brazzini A, Cantella R, De la Cruz A, *et al.* Intraarterial autologous implantation of adult stem cells for patients with Parkinson disease. *J Vasc Interv Radiol.* 2010;**21**(4):443–51.

45. Llumiguano C, Kovacs N, Usprung Z, *et al.* 1H-MRS experiences after bilateral DBS of the STN in Parkinson's disease. *Parkinsonism Relat Disord.* 2008;**14**(3):229–32.

46. Valles F, Fiandaca MS, Eberling JL, *et al.* Qualitative imaging of adeno-associated virus serotype 2-human aromatic L-amino acid decarboxylase gene therapy in a phase I study for the treatment of Parkinson disease. *Neurosurgery.* 2010;**67**(5):1377–85.

47. Singh N, Fletcher PT, Preston JS, *et al.* Multivariate statistical analysis of deformation momenta relating anatomical shape to neuropsychological measures. *Med Image Comput Comput Assist Interv.* 2010;**13**(Pt 3):529–37.

48. Johansen-Berg H, Behrens TE, Sillery E, *et al.* Functional-anatomical validation and individual variation of diffusion tractography-based segmentation of the human thalamus. *Cereb Cortex.* 2005;**15**(1):31–9.

49. Yeo SS, Kim SH, Ahn YH, Son SM, Jang SH. Anatomical location of the pedunculopontine nucleus in the human brain: diffusion tensor imaging study. *Stereotact Funct Neurosurg.* 2011;**89**(3):152–6.

50. Kamagata K, Motoi Y, Hori M, *et al.* Posterior hypoperfusion in Parkinson's disease with and without dementia measured with arterial spin labeling MRI. *J Magn Reson Imaging.* 2011;**33**(4):803–7.

51. Michaeli S, Oz G, Sorce DJ, *et al.* Assessment of brain iron and neuronal integrity in patients with Parkinson's disease using novel MRI contrasts. *Mov Disord.* 2007;**22**(3):334–40.

52. Hagmann P, Cammoun L, Gigandet X, *et al.* Mapping the structural core of human cerebral cortex. *PLoS Biol.* 2008;**6**(7):e159.

Index

271